Essentials of
Nursing Leadership
and Management

fifth edition

Essentials of
Nursing Leadership
and Management

fifth edition

Diane K. Whitehead, EdD, RN, ANEF
Associate Dean, Nursing
Nova Southeastern University
Fort Lauderdale, Florida

Sally A. Weiss, EdD, RN, CNE
Associate Chair, Nursing
Nova Southeastern University
Fort Lauderdale, Florida

Ruth M. Tappen, EdD, RN, FAAN
Christine E. Lynn Eminent Scholar and Professor
Florida Atlantic University College of Nursing
Boca Raton, Florida

F.A. Davis Company • Philadelphia

F. A. Davis Company
1915 Arch Street
Philadelphia, PA 19103
www.fadavis.com

Printed in United States of America

Last digit indicates print number: 10 9 8 7 6 5 4 3 2 1

Acquisition Editor: Joanne Patzek DaCunha, RN, MSN
Project Editors: Kim DePaul, Tyler Baber
Manager of Art & Design: Carolyn O'Brien

As new scientific information becomes available through basic and clinical research, recommended treatments and drug therapies undergo changes. The author(s) and publisher have done everything possible to make this book accurate, up to date, and in accord with accepted standards at the time of publication. The author(s), editors, and publisher are not responsible for errors or omissions or for consequences from application of the book, and make no warranty, expressed or implied, in regard to the contents of the book. Any practice described in this book should be applied by the reader in accordance with professional standards of care used in regard to the unique circumstances that may apply in each situation. The reader is advised always to check product information (package inserts) for changes and new information regarding dose and contraindications before administering any drug. Caution is especially urged when using new or infrequently ordered drugs.

Library of Congress Cataloging-in-Publication Data

Whitehead, Diane K., 1945-
Essentials of nursing leadership and management / Diane K. Whitehead, Sally A. Weiss, Ruth M. Tappen. -- 5th ed.
    p. ; cm.
Includes bibliographical references and index.
ISBN 978-0-8036-2208-1 (pbk. : alk. paper)
1. Nursing services--Administration. 2. Leadership. I. Weiss, Sally A., 1950- II. Tappen, Ruth M. III. Title.
[DNLM: 1. Nursing--United States. 2. Leadership--United States. 3. Nursing--organization & administration--United States. 4. Nursing Services--organization & administration--United States. WY 16 W592e 2010]
RT89.T357 2010
362.1'73068--dc22   2009017339

Dedication

To my sister Michele:
Your bravery and spirit inspire me every day.
Diane K. Whitehead

To my granddaughter Sydni,
Whose curiosity and wonder continuously remind me
of the reasons I became a nurse educator.
Sally A. Weiss

To students, colleagues, family and friends,
Who have taught me just about everything I know.
Ruth M. Tappen

Preface

We are delighted to bring our readers this Fifth Edition of *Essentials of Nursing Leadership and Management*. This new edition has been updated to reflect the current health-care environment. As in our previous editions, the content, examples, and diagrams were designed with the goal of assisting the new graduate to make the transition to professional nursing practice.

The Fifth Edition of *Essentials of Nursing Leadership and Management* focuses on the necessary knowledge and skills needed by the staff nurse as a vital member of the health-care team and manager of patient care. Issues related to setting priorities, delegation, quality improvement, legal parameters of nursing practice, and ethical issues were updated for this edition.

We are especially excited to introduce a new chapter, Quality and Safety. This chapter focuses on the current quality and safety issues and initiatives that affect the current health-care environment. In addition, the updated finance chapter and a new chapter on health-care policy will be available on the F.A. Davis Web site, *DavisPlus*.

We continue to bring you comprehensive, practical information on developing a nursing career. Updated information on leading, managing, followership, and workplace issues continues to be included.

Essentials of Nursing Leadership and Management continues to provide a strong foundation for the beginning nurse leader. We want to thank the people at F.A. Davis for their assistance as well as our contributors, reviewers, and students for their guidance and support.

Diane K. Whitehead
Sally A. Weiss
Ruth M. Tappen

Contributors

Patricia Bradley, *MEd, PhD, RN*
Coordinator, Internationally Educated Nurses
    Program
Faculty, Nursing Department
York University
Toronto, Ontario, Canada

Kristie Campoe, *MSN, RN*
Adjunct Faculty
Nursing Department
Nova Southeastern University
Fort Lauderdale, Florida

Patricia Welch Dittman, *PhD, RN, CDE*
Graduate Program Director/Assistant Professor
Nursing Department
Nova Southeastern University
Fort Lauderdale, Florida

Denise Howard, *BSN, RN*
Adjunct Faculty
Nursing Department
Nova Southeastern University
Fort Lauderdale, Florida

Marcie Rutherford, *PhD, MBA, MSN, RN*
Assistant Professor
Nursing Department
Nova Southeastern University
Fort Lauderdale, Florida

Wendy Thomson, *EdD(c), MSN, BSBA, RN, CNE, IBCLC*
Assistant Director of Technology and
    Simulation/Assistant Professor
Nursing Department
Nova Southeastern University
Fort Lauderdale, Florida

Table of Contents

Appendices

Bonus Chapters on DavisPlus

Finance

Triaxial of Action: Policy, Politics, and Nursing

Canadian Nursing Practice and the Law

Professional Considerations

chapter 1

Leadership and Followership

⦿ ○ ○ ○ ○ ○ ○ ○ ○ ○ ○

OBJECTIVES

After reading this chapter, the student should be able to:

- Define the terms leadership and followership.
- Discuss the importance of effective leadership and followership for the new nurse.
- Discuss the qualities and behaviors that contribute to effective followership.
- Discuss the qualities and behaviors that contribute to effective leadership.

OUTLINE

Nurses work with an extraordinary variety of people: physicians, respiratory therapists, physical therapists, social workers, psychologists, technicians, aides, unit managers, housekeepers, clients, and clients' families.

The reason why nurses study leadership is to learn how to work well, or *effectively*, with other people. In this chapter, *leadership* and *followership* and the relationships between them are defined. The characteristics and behaviors that can make you, a new nurse, an effective leader and follower are discussed.

Leadership

Are You Ready to Be a Leader?

You may be thinking, "I'm just beginning my career in nursing. How can I be expected to be a leader now?" This is an important question. You will need time to refine your clinical skills and learn how to function in a new environment. But you can begin to assume some leadership right away within your new nursing roles. Consider the following example:

Billie Blair Thomas was a new staff nurse at Green Valley Nursing Care Center. After orientation, she was assigned to a rehabilitation unit with high admission and discharge rates. Billie noticed that admissions and discharges were assigned rather haphazardly. Anyone who was "free" at the moment was directed to handle them. Sometimes, unlicensed assistant personnel were directed to admit or discharge residents. Billie believed that using them was inappropriate because their assessment skills were limited and they had no training in discharge planning.

Billie thought there was a better way to do this but was not sure that she should say so because she was so new. "Maybe they've already thought of this," she said to a former classmate. "It's such an obvious solution." They began to talk about what they had learned in their leadership course before graduation. "I just keep hearing our instructor saying, 'There's only one manager, but anyone can be a leader of our group.'"

"If you want to be a leader, you have to act on your idea," her friend said.

"Maybe I will," Billie replied.

Billie decided to speak with her nurse manager, an experienced rehabilitation nurse who seemed not only approachable but also open to new ideas. "I have been so busy getting our new record system on line before the surveyors come that I wasn't

paying attention to that," the nurse manager told her. "I'm so glad you brought it to my attention."

Billie's nurse manager raised the issue at the next executive meeting, giving credit to Billie for having brought it to her attention. The other nurse managers had the same response. "We were so focused on the new record system that we overlooked that. We need to take care of this situation as soon as possible. Billie Blair Thomas has leadership potential."

Leadership Defined

Leadership is a much broader concept than is management. Although managers should also be leaders, management is focused on the achievement of organizational goals. Leadership, on the other hand:

...occurs whenever one person attempts to influence the behavior of an individual or group—up, down, or sideways in the organization—regardless of the reason. It may be for personal goals or for the goals of others, and these goals may or may not be congruent with organizational goals. Leadership is influence (Hersey & Campbell, 2004, p. 12)

In order to lead, one must develop three important competencies: (1) ability to diagnose or understand the situation you want to influence, (2) adaptation in order to allow your behaviors and other resources to close the gap between the current situation and what you are hoping to achieve, and (3) communication. No matter how much you diagnose or adapt, if you cannot communicate effectively, you will probably not meet your goal (Hersey & Campbell, 2004).

Effective nurse leaders are those who engage others to work together effectively in pursuit of a shared goal. Examples of shared goals are providing excellent client care, designing a cost-saving procedure, and challenging the ethics of a new policy.

Followership

Followership and leadership are separate but reciprocal roles. Without followers, one cannot be a leader; conversely, one cannot be a follower without a leader (Lyons, 2002).

Being an effective follower is as important to the new nurse as is being an effective leader. In fact, most of the time most of us are followers: members of a team, attendees at a meeting, staff of a nursing care unit, and so forth.

Followership Defined

Followership is not a passive role. On the contrary, the most valuable follower is a skilled, self-directed employee, one who participates actively in setting the group's direction, invests his or her time and energy in the work of the group, thinks critically, and advocates for new ideas (Grossman & Valiga, 2000). Imagine working on a client care unit where all staff members, from the unit secretary to the assistant nurse manager, willingly take on extra tasks without being asked (Spreitzer & Quinn, 2001), come back early from coffee breaks, complete their charting on time, suggest ways to improve client care, and are proud of the high quality care they provide. Wouldn't it be wonderful to be a part of that team?

Becoming a Better Follower

There are a number of things you can do to become a better follower:

- If you discover a problem, inform your team leader or manager right away.
- Even better, include a suggestion in your report for solving the problem.
- Freely invest your interest and energy in your work.
- Be supportive of new ideas and new directions suggested by others.
- When you disagree, explain why you do not support an idea or suggestion.
- Listen carefully, and reflect on what your leader or manager says.
- Continue to learn as much as you can about your specialty area.
- Share what you learn.

Being an effective follower will not only make you a more valuable employee but will also increase the meaning and satisfaction that you can get from your work.

Most team leaders and nurse managers will respond very positively to having staff who are good followers. Occasionally you will encounter a poor leader or manager who can confuse, frustrate, and even distress you. Here are a few suggestions for handling this:

- Avoid adopting the ineffective behaviors of this individual.
- Continue to do your best work and to provide leadership for the rest of the group.

- If the situation worsens, enlist the support of others on your team to seek a remedy; do not try to do this alone as a new graduate.
- If the situation becomes intolerable, consider the option of transferring to another unit or seeking another position (Deutschman, 2005; Korn, 2004).

What Makes a Person a Leader?

Leadership Theories

There are many different ideas about how a person becomes a good leader. Despite years of research on this subject, no one idea has emerged as the clear winner. The reason for this may be that different qualities and behaviors are most important in different situations. In nursing, for example, some situations require quick thinking and fast action. Others require time to figure out the best solution to a complicated problem. Different leadership qualities and behaviors are needed in these two instances. The result is that there is not yet a single best answer to the question, "What makes a person a leader?"

Consider some of the best-known leadership theories and the many qualities and behaviors that have been identified as those of the effective nurse leader (Pavitt, 1999; Tappen, 2001).

Trait Theories

At one time or another, you have probably heard someone say, "Leaders are born, not made." In other words, some people are natural leaders, and others are not. In reality, leadership may come more easily to some than to others, but everyone can be a leader, given the necessary knowledge and skill. Research into the traits of leaders is a continuing process. A 5-year study of 90 outstanding leaders by Warren Bennis (1984) identified four common traits shared by all of these leaders. These traits continue to hold true:

1. Management of attention. These leaders were able to communicate a sense of goal or direction to attract followers.
2. Management of meaning. These leaders created and communicated meaning with clarity and purpose.
3. Management of trust. These leaders demonstrated reliability and consistency.
4. Management of self. These leaders were able to know self and work within their strengths and weaknesses (Bennis, 1984).

Behavioral Theories

The behavioral theories are concerned with what the leader does. One of the most influential theories is concerned with leadership style (White & Lippitt, 1960) (Table 1-1).

The three styles are:

- **Autocratic leadership** (also called *directive, controlling,* or *authoritarian*). The autocratic leader gives orders and makes decisions for the group. For example, when a decision needs to be made, an autocratic leader says, "I've decided that this is the way we're going to solve our problem." Although this is an efficient way to run things, it usually dampens creativity and may inhibit motivation.
- **Democratic leadership** (also called *participative*). Democratic leaders share leadership. Important plans and decisions are made with the team (Chrispeels, 2004). Although this is often a less efficient way to run things, it is more flexible and usually increases motivation and creativity. Democratic leadership is characterized by guidance from rather than control by the leader.
- **Laissez-faire leadership** (also called *permissive* or *nondirective*). The laissez-faire ("let someone do") leader does very little planning or decision making and fails to encourage others to do so. It is really a lack of leadership. For example, when a decision needs to be made, a laissez-faire leader may postpone making the decision or never make the decision. In most instances, the laissez-faire leader leaves people feeling confused and frustrated because there is no goal, no guidance, and no direction. Some very mature individuals thrive under laissez-faire leadership

because they need little guidance. Most people, however, flounder under this kind of leadership.

Pavitt summed up the difference among these three styles: a democratic leader tries to move the group toward its goals; an autocratic leader tries to move the group toward the leader's goals; and a laissez-faire leader makes no attempt to move the group (1999, pp. 330ff).

Task Versus Relationship

Another important distinction in leadership style is between a task focus and a relationship focus (Blake, Mouton, & Tapper, 1981). Some nurses emphasize the tasks (e.g., reducing medication errors, completing patient records) and fail to realize that interpersonal relationships (e.g., attitude of physicians toward nursing staff, treatment of housekeeping staff by nurses) affect the morale and productivity of employees. Other nurses focus on the interpersonal aspects and ignore the quality of the job being done as long as people get along with each other. The most effective leader is able to balance the two, attending to both the task and the relationship aspects of working together.

Motivating Theories

The concept of motivation seems fairly simple. We do things to get what we want and avoid things that we don't want. However, motivation is still surrounded in mystery. The study of motivation as a focus of leadership began in the 1920s with the historic Hawthorne study. Several experiments were conducted to see if increasing light and, later, improved working conditions would improve productivity of workers in the Hawthorne, Illinois,

---

table 1-1			

Comparison of Autocratic, Democratic, and Laissez-Faire Leadership Styles

	Autocratic	**Democratic**	**Laissez-Faire**
Amount of freedom	Little freedom	Moderate freedom	Much freedom
Amount of control	High control	Moderate control	Little control
Decision making	By the leader	Leader and group together	By the group or by no one
Leader activity level	High	High	Minimal
Assumption of responsibility	Leader	Shared	Abdicated
Output of the group	High quantity, good quality	Creative, high quality	Variable, may be poor quality
Efficiency	Very efficient	Less efficient than autocratic style	Inefficient

Adapted from White, R.K., & Lippitt, R. (1960). Autocracy and Democracy: An Experimental Inquiry. New York: Harper & Row.

electrical plant. Those workers who had the improved working conditions taken away continued to show improved productivity. Therefore, the answers were found not in the *conditions* of the experiments but in the *attention* given to the workers by the experimenters. Similar to the 1954 Maslow Hierarchy of Needs theory, the 1959 Motivation-Hygiene theory developed by Frederick Herzberg looked at factors that motivated workers in the workplace. Following closely after Herzberg was David McClelland and his 1961 Theory of Needs. Clayton Alderfer responded to Maslow's theory with his own Existence, Relatedness, and Growth (ERG) theory. Table 1-2 summarizes these four historical motivation theories.

Emotional Intelligence

The relationship aspects of leadership are a focus of the work on emotional intelligence (Goleman, Boyatzes, & McKee, 2002). Part of what distinguishes ordinary leaders from leadership "stars" is consciously addressing the effect of people's feelings on the team's emotional reality. How is this done?

First, learn how to recognize and understand your own emotions, and learn how to manage them, channel them, stay calm and clear-headed, and suspend judgment until all the facts are in when a crisis occurs (Baggett & Baggett, 2005). The emotionally intelligent leader welcomes constructive criticism, asks for help when needed, can juggle multiple demands without losing focus, and can turn problems into opportunities.

Second, the emotionally intelligent leader listens attentively to others, perceives unspoken concerns, acknowledges others' perspectives, and brings people together in an atmosphere of respect, cooperation, collegiality, and helpfulness so they can direct their energies toward achieving the team's goals. "The enthusiastic, caring, and supportive leader generates those same feelings throughout the team," wrote Porter-O'Grady of the emotionally intelligent leader (2003, p. 109).

Situational Theories

People and leadership situations are far more complex than the early theories recognized. In addition, situations can change rapidly, requiring more complex

table 1-2

Leading Motivation Theories

Theory	Summary of Motivation Requirements
Maslow, 1954	Categories of Need: Lower needs (below, listed first) must be fulfilled before others are activated. *Physiological* *Safety* *Belongingness* *Esteem* *Self-actualization*
Alderfer, 1972	Three categories of needs, also ordered into a hierarchy: **1.** *Existence:* Physical well-being **2.** *Relatedness:* Satisfactory relations with others **3.** *Growth:* Development of competence and realization of potential
Herzberg, 1959	Two factors that influence motivation. The absence of hygiene factors can create job dissatisfaction, but their presence does not motivate or increase satisfaction. **1.** *Hygiene factors:* Company policy, supervision, interpersonal relations, working conditions, salary **2.** *Motivators:* Achievement, recognition, the work itself, responsibility, advancement
McClelland, 1961	Motivation results from three dominant needs. Usually all three needs are present in each individual but vary in importance depending on the position a person has in the workplace. Needs are also shaped over time by culture and experience. **1.** *Need for achievement:* Performing tasks on a challenging and high level **2.** *Need for affiliation:* Good relationships with others **3.** *Need for power:* Being in charge

Adapted from Hersey, P. & Campbell, R. (2004). Leadership: A Behavioral Science Approach. Calif.: Leadership Studies Publishing.

theories to explain leadership (Bennis, Spreitzer, & Cummings, 2001).

Adaptability is the key to the situational approach (McNichol, 2000). Instead of assuming that one particular approach works in all situations, situational theories recognize the complexity of work situations and encourage the leader to consider many factors when deciding what action to take.

Situational theories emphasize the importance of understanding all the factors that affect a particular group of people in a particular environment. The most well-known and still practiced theory is the Situational Leadership Model by Dr. Paul Hersey. The appeal of this model is that it focuses on the task and the follower. The key is to marry the readiness of the follower with the task behavior at hand. "Readiness is defined as the extent to which a follower demonstrates the ability and willingness to accomplish a specific task" (Hersey & Campbell, 2004, p. 114). The task behavior is defined as "the extent to which the leader engages in spelling out the duties and responsibilities of an individual and a group" (Hersey & Campbell, 2004, p. 114).

Followers' readiness levels can range from unable and unwilling (or insecure) to able, willing, and confident. The leader's behavior will focus on appropriately fulfilling the follower's needs, which are identified by their readiness level and the task. Leader behaviors will range from telling, guiding, and directing to delegating, observing, and monitoring.

Where did you fall in this model during your first clinical rotation compared with where you are now? In the beginning, the clinical instructor was giving you clear instructions and guiding and directing you. Now, she or he is most likely delegating, observing, and monitoring. However, as you move into your first nursing position, you may return to the guiding and directing stage. On the other hand, you may have become a leader/instructor for new students, and you may be guiding and directing them.

Transformational Leadership

Although the situational theories were an improvement over earlier theories, there was still something missing. Meaning, inspiration, and vision were not given enough attention (Tappen, 2001). These are the distinguishing features of transformational leadership.

The transformational theory of leadership emphasizes that people need a sense of mission that goes beyond good interpersonal relationships or the appropriate reward for a job well done (Bass & Avolio, 1993). This is especially true in nursing. Caring for people, sick or well, is the goal of the profession. Most people chose nursing in order to do something for the good of humankind: this is their vision. One responsibility of leadership is to help nurses achieve their vision.

Transformational leaders can communicate their vision in a manner that is so meaningful and exciting that it reduces negativity (Leach, 2005) and inspires commitment in the people with whom they work (Trofino, 1995). If successful, the goals of the leader and staff will "become fused, creating unity, wholeness, and a collective purpose" (Barker, 1992, p. 42).

Moral Leadership

The corporate scandals of recent years have redirected attention to the values and ethics that underlie the practice of leadership as well as that of client care (Dantley, 2005). Caring about the people who work for you as people as well as employees (Spears & Lawrence, 2004) is part of moral leadership. This can be a great challenge in times of limited financial resources.

Molly Benedict was a team leader on the acute geriatric unit (AGU) when a question of moral leadership arose. Faced with large budget cuts in the middle of the year and feeling a little desperate to figure out how to run the AGU with fewer staff, her nurse manager suggested that reducing the time that unlicensed assistive personnel (UAP) spent ambulating the clients would enable him to increase UAP workload from 10 to 15 clients. "George," responded Molly, "you know that inactivity has many harmful effects, from emboli to disorientation in our very elderly population. Instead, let's try to figure out how to encourage more self-care or even family involvement in care so the UAP can still walk clients and prevent their becoming nonambulatory." Molly based her response on important values, particularly those of prevention.

Qualities of an Effective Leader

If leadership is seen as the ability to influence, what qualities must the leader possess in order to be able to do that? Integrity, courage, attitude, initiative, energy, optimism, perseverance, balance, ability to handle stress, and self-awareness are some of the qualities of effective leaders in nursing (Fig. 1.1):

- **Integrity.** Integrity is expected of health-care professionals. Clients, colleagues, and employers all expect nurses to be honest, law-abiding, and trustworthy. Adherence to both a code of personal ethics and a code of professional ethics (Appendix 1, American Nurses Association Code for Nurses) is expected of every nurse. Would-be leaders who do not exhibit these characteristics cannot expect them of their followers. This is an essential component of moral leadership.
- **Courage.** Sometimes, being a leader means taking some risks. In the story of Billie Blair Thomas, for example, Billie needed some courage to speak to her nurse manager about a problem she had observed.
- **Attitude.** A good attitude goes a long way in making a good leader. In fact, many outstanding leaders cite attitude as the single greatest reason for not hiring someone (Maxwell, 1993, p. 98). A leader's attitude is noticed by the followers more quickly than are the actions.
- **Initiative.** Good ideas are not enough. To be a leader, you must act on those good ideas. This requires initiative on your part.
- **Energy.** Leadership requires energy. Both leadership and followership are hard but satisfying endeavors that require effort. It is also important that the energy be used wisely.
- **Optimism.** When the work is difficult and one crisis seems to follow another in rapid succession, it is easy to become discouraged. It is important not to let discouragement keep you and your coworkers from seeking ways to resolve the problems. In fact, the ability to see a problem as an opportunity is part of the optimism that makes a person an effective leader. Like energy, optimism is "catching." Holman (1995) called this being a *winner* instead of a *whiner* (Table 1-3).
- **Perseverance.** Effective leaders do not give up easily. Instead, they persist, continuing their efforts when others are tempted to stop trying. This persistence often pays off.
- **Balance.** In the effort to become the best nurses they can be, people may forget that other aspects of life are equally important. As important as clients and colleagues are, family and friends are important, too. Although school and work are meaningful activities, cultural, social, recreational, and spiritual activities also have meaning. People need to find a balance between work and play.
- **Ability to handle stress.** There is some stress in almost every job. Coping with stress in as positive and healthy a manner as possible helps to conserve energy and can be a model for others. Maintaining balance and handling stress are reviewed in Chapter 10.
- **Self-awareness.** How is your emotional intelligence? People who do not understand themselves are limited in their ability to understand the motivations of others. They are far more likely to fool themselves than are self-aware people. For example, it is much easier to be fair with a coworker you like than with one you do not

Qualities

Integrity	Perseverance
Courage	Balance
Initiative	Ability to handle stress
Energy	
Optimism	Self-awareness

Behaviors

Think critically	Set goals, share vision
Solve problems	
Communicate skillfully	Develop self and others

Figure 1.1 Keys to effective leadership.

table 1-3	
Winner or Whiner—Which Are You?	
A winner says:	**A whiner says:**
"We have a real challenge here."	"This is really a problem."
"I'll give it my best."	"Do I have to?"
"That's great!"	"That's nice, I guess."
"We can do it!"	"That will never succeed."
"Yes!"	"Maybe...."

Adapted from Holman, L. (1995). Eleven Lessons in Self-leadership: Insights for Personal and Professional Success. Lexington, Ky.: A Lessons in Leadership Book.

like. Recognizing that you like some people more than others is the first step in avoiding unfair treatment based on personal likes and dislikes.

Behaviors of an Effective Leader

Leadership requires action. The effective leader chooses the action carefully. Important leadership behaviors include setting specific goals, thinking critically, solving problems, respecting people, communicating skillfully, communicating a vision for the future, and developing oneself and others.

- **Setting priorities.** Whether planning care for a group of clients or setting the strategic plan for an organization, priorities continually shift and demand attention. As a leader you will need to remember the three "E's" of prioritization: evaluate, eliminate, and estimate. Continually evaluate what you need to do, eliminate tasks that someone else can do, and estimate how long your top priorities will take you to complete.
- **Thinking critically.** Critical thinking is the careful, deliberate use of reasoned analysis to reach a decision about what to believe or what to do (Feldman, 2002). The essence of critical thinking is a willingness to ask questions and to be open to new ideas, new ways to do things. To avoid falling prey to assumptions and biases of your own and those of others, ask yourself frequently, "Do I have the information I need? Is it accurate? Am I prejudging a situation?" (Jackson, Ignatavicius, & Case, 2004).
- **Solving problems.** Client problems, paperwork problems, staff problems: these and others occur frequently and need to be solved. The effective leader helps people to identify problems and to work through the problem-solving process to find a reasonable solution.
- **Respecting the individual.** Although people have much in common, each individual has different wants and needs and has had different life experiences. For example, some people really value the psychological rewards of helping others; other people are more concerned about earning a decent salary. There is nothing wrong with either of these points of view; they are simply different. The effective leader recognizes these differences in people and helps them find the rewards in their work that mean the most to them.

- **Skillful communication.** This includes listening to others, encouraging exchange of information, and providing feedback:

1. *Listening to others.* Listening is separate from talking with other people: listening emphasizes that communication involves both giving and receiving information. The only way to find out people's individual wants and needs is to watch what they do and to listen to what they say. It is amazing how often leaders fail simply because they did not listen to what other people were trying to tell them.
2. *Encouraging exchange of information.* Many misunderstandings and mistakes occur because people fail to share enough information with each other. The leader's role is to make sure that the channels of communication remain open and that people use them.
3. *Providing feedback.* Everyone needs some information about the effectiveness of his or her performance. Frequent feedback, both positive and negative, is needed so people can continually improve their performance. Some nurse leaders find it difficult to give negative feedback because they fear that they will upset the other person. How else can the person know where improvement is needed? Negative feedback can be given in a manner that is neither hurtful nor resented by the individual receiving it. In fact, it is often appreciated. Other nurse leaders, however, fail to give positive feedback, assuming that coworkers will know when they are doing a good job. This is also a mistake because everyone appreciates positive feedback. In fact, for some people, it is the most important reward they get from their jobs.

- **Communicating a vision for the future.** The effective leader has a vision for the future. Communicating this vision to the group and involving everyone in working toward that vision create the inspiration that keeps people going when things become difficult. Even better, involving people in creating the vision is not only more satisfying for employees but also has the potential for the most creative and innovative outcomes (Kerfott, 2000). It is this vision that helps make work meaningful.
- **Developing oneself and others.** Learning does not end on leaving school. In fact, experienced nurses say that school is just the beginning, that

school only prepares you to continue learning throughout your career. As new and better ways to care for clients are discovered, it is your responsibility as a professional to critically analyze these new approaches and decide whether they would be better for your clients than current approaches to care. Effective leaders not only continue to learn but also encourage others to do the same. Sometimes, leaders function as teachers. At other times, their role is primarily to encourage and guide others to seek more knowledge. Observant, reflective, analytical practitioners know that learning takes place every day if people are open to it (Kagan, 1999).

Conclusion

Leadership ability determines a person's level of effectiveness. To be an effective nurse, you must be an effective leader. Your patients, your peers, and your organization are depending on you to influence others. Leadership develops daily. True leaders never stop learning and growing. John Maxwell (1998), one of America's experts on leadership, states "who we are is who we attract" (p. xi). To attract leaders, people need to start leading and never stop learning to lead.

The key elements of leadership and followership have been discussed in this chapter. Many of the leadership qualities and behaviors mentioned here are discussed in more detail in later chapters.

Study Questions

1. Why is it important for nurses to be good leaders? What qualities have you observed from nurses on the units that exemplify effective leadership in action? How do you think these behaviors might have improved the outcomes of their patients?

2. Why are effective followers as important as effective leaders?

3. Review the various leadership theories discussed in the chapter. Which ones might apply to leading in today's health-care environment? Support your answer with specific examples.

4. Select an individual whose leadership skills you particularly admire. What are some qualities and behaviors that this individual displays? How do these relate to the leadership theories discussed in this chapter? In what ways could you emulate this person?

5. As a new graduate, what leadership and followership skills will you work on developing or enhancing during the first 3 months of your first nursing position? Why?

Case Study to Promote Critical Reasoning

Two new associate-degree graduates were hired for the pediatric unit. Both worked three 12-hour shifts a week, Jan in the day-to-evening shift and Ronnie at night. Whenever their shifts connected, they would compare notes on their experience. Jan felt she was learning rapidly, gaining clinical skills and beginning to feel at ease with her colleagues.

Ronnie, however, still felt unsure of herself and often isolated. "There have been times," she told Jan, "that I am the only registered nurse on the unit all night. The aides and LPNs are really experienced, but that's not enough. I wish I could work with an experienced nurse as you are doing."

"Ronnie, you are not even finished with your 3-month orientation program," said Jan. "You should never be left alone with all these sick children. Neither of us is ready for that kind of responsibility. And how will you get the experience you need with no experienced nurses to help you? You must speak to our nurse manager about this."

"I know I should, but she's so hard to reach. I've called several times, and she's never available. She leaves all the shift assignments to her assistant. I'm not sure she even reviews the schedule before it's posted."

"You will have to try harder to reach her. Maybe you could stay past the end of your shift one morning and meet with her," suggested Jan. "If something happens when you are the only nurse on the unit, you will be held responsible."

1. In your own words, summarize the problem that Jan and Ronnie are discussing. To what extent is this problem due to a failure to lead? Who has failed to act?

2. What style of leadership was displayed by Ronnie and the nurse manager? How effective was their leadership? Did Jan's leadership differ from that of Ronnie and the nurse manager? In what way?

3. In what ways has Ronnie been an effective follower? In what ways has Ronnie not been so effective as a follower?

4. If an emergency occurred and was not handled well while Ronnie was the only nurse on the unit, who would be responsible? Explain why this person or persons would be responsible.

5. If you found yourself in Ronnie's situation, what steps would you take to resolve the problem? Show how the leader characteristics and behaviors found in this chapter support your solution to the problem.

References

Baggett, M.M., & Baggett, F.B. (2005). Move from management to high-level leadership. *Nursing Management, 36*(7), 12.

Barker, A.M. (1992). *Transformational Nursing Leadership: A Vision for the Future.* New York: National League for Nursing Press.

Bass, B.M., & Avolio, B.J. (1993). Transformational leadership: A response to critiques. In Chemers, M.M., & Ayman, R. (eds.). *Leadership Theory and Research: Perspectives and Direction.* San Diego: Academic Press.

Bennis, W. (1984). The four competencies of leadership. *Training and Development Journal,* August, 1984, pp. 15–19.

Bennis, W., Spreitzer, G.M., & Cummings, T.G. (2001). *The Future of Leadership.* San Francisco: Jossey-Bass.

Blake, R.R., Mouton, J.S., & Tapper, M., et al. (1981). *Grid Approaches for Managerial Leadership in Nursing.* St. Louis: C.V. Mosby.

Chrispeels, J.H. (2004). *Learning to Lead Together.* Thousand Oaks, Calif.: Sage Publications.

Dantley, M.E. (2005). Moral leadership: Shifting the management paradigm. In English, F.W. *The Sage Handbook of Educational Leadership* (pp. 34–46). Thousand Oaks, Calif.: Sage Publications.

Deutschman, A. (2005). Is your boss a psychopath? *Making Change.* Fast Company, 96, 43–51.

Feldman, D.A. (2002). *Critical Thinking: Strategies for Decision Making.* Menlo Park, Calif.: Crisp Publications.

Goleman, D., Boyatzes, R., & McKee, A. (2002). *Primal Leadership: Realizing the Power of Emotional Intelligence.* Boston: Harvard Business School Press.

Grossman, S., & Valiga, T.M. (2000). *The New Leadership Challenge: Creating the Future of Nursing.* Philadelphia: FA Davis.

Hersey, P. & Campbell, R. (2004). *Leadership: A Behavioral Science Approach.* Calif.: Leadership Studies Publishing.

Holman, L. (1995). *Eleven Lessons in Self-Leadership: Insights for Personal and Professional Success.* Lexington, Ky.: A Lessons in Leadership Book.

Jackson, M., Ignatavicius, D., & Case, B. (eds.). (2004). *Conversations in Critical Thinking and Clinical Judgement.* Pensacola, Fla.: Pohl.

Kagan, S.S. (1999). *Leadership Games: Experiential Learning for Organizational Development.* Thousand Oaks, Calif.: Sage Publications.

Kerfott, K. (2000). Leadership: Creating a shared destiny. *Dermatological Nursing, 12*(5), 363–364.

Korn, M. (2004). *Toxic Cleanup: How to Deal With a Dangerous Leader.* Fast Company, 88, 17.

Leach, L.S. (2005). Nurse executive transformational leadership and organizational commitment. *Journal of Nursing Administration, 35*(5), 228–237.

Lyons, M.F. (2002). Leadership and followership. *The Physician Executive,* Jan/Feb, 91–93.

Maxwell, J.C. (1993). *Developing the Leader Within You.* Tenn.: Thomas Nelson Inc.

Maxwell, J. C. (1998). *The 21 Inrrefutable Laws of Leadership.* Tenn.: Thomas Nelson Inc.

McNichol, E. (2000). How to be a model leader. *Nursing Standard, 14*(45), 24.

Pavitt, C. (1999). Theorizing about the group communication-leadership relationship. In Frey, L.R. (ed.). *The Handbook of Group Communication Theory and Research.* Thousand Oaks, Calif.: Sage Publications.

Porter-O'Grady, T. (2003). A different age for leadership, Part II. *Journal of Nursing Administration, 33*(2), 105–110.

Spears, L.C., & Lawrence, M. (2004). *Practicing Servant-Leadership.* New York: Jossey-Bass.

Spreitzer, G.M., & Quinn, R.E. (2001). *A Company of Leaders: Five Disciplines for Unleashing the Power in Your Workforce.* San Francisco: Jossey-Bass.

Tappen, R.M. (2001). *Nursing Leadership and Management: Concepts and Practice.* Philadelphia: FA Davis.

Trofino, J. (1995). Transformational leadership in health care. *Nursing Management, 26*(8), 42–47.

White, R.K., & Lippitt, R. (1960). *Autocracy and Democracy: An Experimental Inquiry.* New York: Harper & Row.

Manager

Every nurse should be a good leader and a good follower. Not everyone should be a manager, however. In fact, new graduates simply are not ready to take on management responsibilities. Once you have had time to develop your clinical and leadership skills, you can begin to think about taking on management responsibilities (Table 2-1).

MANAGEMENT

Are You Ready to Be a Manager?

For most new nurses, the answer is *no,* you should not accept managerial responsibility. The breadth and depth of your experience are still undeveloped. You need to direct your energies to building your own skills before you begin supervising other people.

What Is Management?

The essence of management is getting work done through others. The classic definition of management is Henri Fayol's 1916 list of managerial tasks: planning, organizing, commanding, coordinating, and controlling the work of a group of employees (Wren, 1972). But Mintzberg (1989) argued that managers really do whatever is needed to make sure that employees do their work and do it well. Lombardi (2001) points out that two-thirds of a manager's time is spent on people problems. The rest is taken up by budget work, going to meetings, preparing reports, and other administrative tasks.

Management Theories

There are two major but opposing schools of thought in management: scientific management and the human relations–based approach. As its name implies, the human-relations approach emphasizes the interpersonal aspects of managing people, whereas scientific management emphasizes the task aspects.

Scientific Management

Almost 100 years ago, Frederick Taylor argued that most jobs could be done more efficiently if they were analyzed thoroughly (Lee, 1980; Locke, 1982). With a well-designed task and enough incentive to get the work done, workers could be more productive. For example, Taylor promoted the concept of paying people by the piece instead of by the hour. In health care, the equivalent would be by the number of patients bathed or visited at home rather than by the number of hours worked. This would create an incentive to get the most work done in the least amount of time. Taylorism stresses that there is a best way to do a job. Usually, this is also the fastest way to do the job (Dantley, 2005).

The work is analyzed to improve efficiency. In health care, for example, there has been much discussion about the time it takes to bring patients to radiology or to physical therapy versus bringing the technician or therapist to the patient. Eliminating excess staff or increasing the productivity of remaining employees is also based on this kind of thinking.

Nurse managers who use the principles of scientific management will pay particular attention to the type of assessments and treatments done on the unit, the equipment needed to do this efficiently, and the strategies that would facilitate efficient accomplishment of these tasks. Typically, these nurse managers keep careful records of the amount of work accomplished and reward those who accomplish the most.

Human Relations–Based Management

McGregor's theories X and Y provide a good example of the difference between scientific management and human relations–based management. Theory X, said McGregor (1960), reflects a common attitude among managers that most people do not want to work very hard and that the manager's job is to make sure that they do work hard. To accomplish this, according to Theory X, a manager needs to employ strict rules, constant supervision, and the threat of punishment (reprimands, withheld raises, and threats of job loss) to create industrious, conscientious workers.

table 2-1	
Differences Between Leadership and Management	
Leadership	**Management**
Based on influence and shared meaning	Based on authority
An informal role	A formally designated role
An achieved position	As assigned position
Part of every nurse's responsibility	Usually responsible for budgets, hiring, and firing people
Requires initiative and independent thinking	Improved by the use of effective leadership skills

Theory Y, which McGregor preferred, is the opposite viewpoint. Theory Y managers believe that the work itself can be motivating and that people will work hard if their managers provide a supportive environment. A Theory Y manager emphasizes guidance rather than control, development rather than close supervision, and reward rather than punishment (Fig. 2.1). A Theory Y nurse manager is concerned with keeping employee morale as high as possible, assuming that satisfied, motivated employees will do the best work. Employees' attitudes, opinions, hopes, and fears are important to this type of nurse manager. Considerable effort is expended to work out conflicts and promote mutual understanding to provide an environment in which people can do their best work.

Servant Leadership

The emphasis on people and interpersonal relationships is taken one step further by Greenleaf (2004), who wrote an essay in 1970 that began the servant leadership movement. Like transformational leadership, servant leadership has a special appeal to nurses and other health-care professionals. Despite its name, servant leadership applies more to people in supervisory or administrative positions than to people in staff positions.

The servant leader–style staff manager believes that people have value as people, not just as workers (Spears & Lawrence, 2004). The manager is committed to improving the way each employee is treated at work. The attitude is "employee first," not "manager first." So the manager sees himself or herself as being there for the employee. Here is an example:

Hope Marshall is a relatively new staff nurse at Jefferson County Hospital. When she was invited to be the staff nurse representative on the search committee for a new vice-president for nursing, she was very excited about being on a committee with so many managerial and administrative people. As the interviews of candidates began, she focused on what they had to say. They had very impressive résumés and spoke confidently about their accomplishments. Hope was impressed but did not yet prefer one over the other. Then the final candidate spoke to the committee. "My primary job," he said, "is to make it possible for each nurse to do the very best job he or she can do. I am here to make their work easier, to remove barriers, and to provide them with whatever they need to provide the best patient care possible." Hope had never heard the term servant leadership, but she knew immediately that this candidate, who articulated the essence of servant leadership, was the one she would support for this important position.

QUALITIES OF AN EFFECTIVE MANAGER

Two-thirds of people who leave their jobs say the main reason was an ineffective or incompetent manager (Hunter, 2004). A survey of 3266 newly licensed nurses found that lack of support from their manager was the primary reason for leaving their position, followed by a stressful work environment as the second reason. Following are some of the indicators of their stressful work environment:

- 25% reported at least one needle stick in their first year.
- 39% reported at least one strain or sprain.
- 62% reported experiencing verbal abuse.
- 25% reported a shortage of supplies needed to do their work.

These results underscore the importance of having effective nurse managers who can create an environment in which new nurses thrive (Kovner, Brewer, Fairchild, et al., 2007)

> ## THEORY X
> **Work is something to be avoided**
> **People want to do as little as possible**
> **Use control-supervision-punishment**

> ## THEORY Y
> **The work itself can be motivating**
> **People really want to do their job well**
> **Use guidance-development-reward**

Figure 2.1 Theory X versus Theory Y.

The effective nurse manager possesses a combination of qualities: leadership, clinical expertise, and business sense. None of these alone is enough; it is the combination that prepares an individual for the complex task of managing a unit or team of healthcare providers. Consider each of these briefly:

- **Leadership.** All of the people skills of the leader are essential to the effective manager. They are skills needed to function *as* a manager.
- **Clinical expertise.** It is very difficult to help others develop their skills and evaluate how well they have done so without possessing clinical expertise oneself. It is probably not necessary (or even possible) to know everything all other professionals on the team know, but it is important to be able to assess the effectiveness of their work in terms of patient outcomes.
- **Business sense.** Nurse managers also need to be concerned with the "bottom line," with the *cost* of providing the care that is given, especially in comparison with the benefit received from that care and the funding available to pay for it, whether from insurance, Medicare, Medicaid, or out of the patient's own pocket. This is a complex task that requires knowledge of budgeting, staffing, and measurement of patient outcomes.

There is some controversy over the amount of clinical expertise versus business sense that is needed to be an effective nurse manager. Some argue that a person can be a "generic" manager, that the job of managing people is the same no matter what tasks he or she performs. Others argue that managers must understand the tasks themselves, better than anyone else in the work group. Our position is that equal amounts of clinical skill and business acumen are needed, along with excellent leadership skills.

BEHAVIORS OF AN EFFECTIVE MANAGER

Mintzberg (1989) divided a manager's activities into three categories: interpersonal, decisional, and informational. We use these categories and have added some activities suggested by other authors (Dunham-Taylor, 1995; Montebello, 1994) and by our own observations of nurse managers (Fig. 2.2).

Figure 2.2 Keys to effective management.

Interpersonal Activities

The interpersonal category is one in which leaders and managers have overlapping concerns. However, the manager has some additional responsibilities that are seldom given to leaders. These include the following:

- **Networking.** Nurse managers are in pivotal positions, especially in inpatient settings where they have contact with virtually every service of the institution as well as with most people above and below them in the organizational hierarchy. This provides them with many opportunities to influence the status and treatment of staff nurses and the quality of the care provided to their patients. It is important that they "maintain the line of sight," or connection, between what they do as managers, patient care, and the mission of the organization (Mackoff & Triolo, 2008, p. 123). In other words, they need to keep in mind how their interactions with both their staff members and with administration affects the care provided to the patients for whom they are responsible.

- **Conflict negotiation and resolution.** Managers often find themselves resolving conflicts among employees, patients, and administration. The ineffective manager either lets people go unmanaged emotionally or mismanages feelings in the workplace (Welch & Welch, 2008).
- **Employee development.** Providing for the continuing learning and upgrading of the skills of employees is a managerial responsibility.
- **Coaching.** It is often said that employees are the organization's most valuable asset (Shirey, 2007). This is one of the ways in which nurse managers can share their experience and expertise with the rest of the staff. The goal is to nurture the growth and development of the employee (the "coachee") to do a better job through learning (McCauley & Van Velson, 2004; Shirey, 2007).

Some managers use a directive approach: "This is how it's done. Watch me." or "Let me show you how to do this." Others prefer a nondirective approach: "Let's try to figure out what's wrong here" (Hart & Waisman, 2005). "How do you think we can improve our outcomes?"

You can probably see the parallel with democratic and autocratic leadership styles described in Chapter 1. The decision whether to be directive (e.g., in an emergency) or nondirective (e.g., when developing a long-term plan to improve infection control) will depend on the situation.

- **Rewards and punishments.** Managers are in a position to provide specific (e.g., salary increases, time off) and general (e.g., praise, recognition) rewards as well as punishments.

Decisional Activities

Nurse managers are responsible for making many decisions:

- **Employee evaluation.** Managers are responsible for conducting formal performance appraisals of their staff members. Effective managers regularly tell their staff how well they are doing and where they need improvement (Welch & Welch, 2008).
- **Resource allocation.** In decentralized organizations, nurse managers are often given a set amount of money to run their units or departments and must allocate these resources wisely. This can be difficult when resources are very limited.

- **Hiring and firing employees.** Nurse managers decide either independently or participate in employment and termination decisions for their units.
- **Planning for the future.** The day-to-day operation of most units is complex and time-consuming, and nurse managers must also look ahead in order to prepare themselves and their units for future changes in budgets, organizational priorities, and patient populations. They need to look beyond the four walls of their own organization to become aware of what is happening to their competition and to the health-care system (Kelly & Nadler, 2007).
- **Job analysis and redesign.** In a time of extreme cost sensitivity, nurse managers are often required to analyze and redesign the work of their units to make them as efficient as possible.

Informational Activities

Nurse managers often find themselves in positions within the organizational hierarchy in which they acquire much information that is not available to their staff. They also have much information about their staff that is not readily available to the administration, placing them in a strategic position within the information web of any organization. The effective manager uses this position for the benefit of both the staff and the organization. The following are some examples:

- **Spokesperson.** Nurse managers often speak for administration when relaying information to their staff members. Likewise, they often speak for staff members when relaying information to administration. You could think of them as clearinghouses, acting as gatherers and disseminators of information to people above and below them in the organizational hierarchy (Shirey, Ebright, & McDaniel, 2008, p. 126).
- **Monitoring.** Nurse managers are also expert "sensors," picking up early signs of problems before they grow too big (Shirey, Ebright, & McDaniel, 2008). They are expected to monitor the many and various activities of their units or departments, including the number of patients seen, average length of stay, infection rates, fall rates, and so forth. They also monitor the staff (e.g., absentee rates, tardiness, unproductive time), the budget (e.g., money spent, money left to spend in comparison with money

table 2-2

Bad Management Styles

These are the types of managers you do not want to be and for whom you do not want to work:

Know-it-all	Self-appointed experts on everything, these managers do not listen to anyone else.
Emotionally remote	Isolated from the staff and the work going on, these managers do not know what is going on in the workplace and cannot inspire others.
Pure mean	Mean, nasty, dictatorial, these managers look for problems and reasons to criticize.
Overnice	Desperate to please everyone, these managers agree to every idea and request, causing confusion and spending too much money on useless projects.
Afraid to decide	In the name of fairness, these managers do not distinguish between competent and incompetent, hard-working and unproductive employees, thus creating an unfair reward system.

Based on Welch, J. & Welch, S. (2007, July 23). Bosses who get it all wrong. BusinessWeek, p. 88.

needed to operate the unit), and the costs of procedures and services provided, especially those that are variable such as medical supplies (Dowless, 2007).

■ **Public Relations.** Nurse managers share information with their patients, staff members, and employers. This information may be related to the results of their monitoring efforts, new developments in health care, policy changes, and so forth. Review Table 2-2, "Bad Management Styles," to compare what you have just read about effective nurse managers with descriptions of some of the most common ineffective approaches to being a manager.

Conclusion

Nurse managers have complex, responsible positions in health-care organizations. Ineffective managers may do harm to their employees, their patients, and to the organization, and effective managers can help their staff members grow and develop as health-care professionals while providing the highest quality care to their patients.

Study Questions

1. Why should new graduates decline nursing management positions? At what point do you think a nurse is ready to assume managerial responsibilities?

2. Which theory, scientific management or human relations, do you believe is most useful to nurse managers? Explain your choice.

3. Compare servant leadership with scientific management. Which approach do you prefer? Why?

4. Describe your ideal nurse manger in terms of the person for whom you would most like to work. Then describe the worst nurse manager you can imagine, and explain why this person would be very difficult.

5. List 10 behaviors of nurse managers, then rank them from least to most important. What rationale(s) did you use in ranking them?

Case Study to Promote Critical Reasoning

Joe Garcia has been an operating room nurse for 5 years. He was often on call on Saturday and Sunday, but he enjoyed his work and knew that he was good at it.

Joe was called to come in on a busy Saturday afternoon just as his 5-year-old daughter's birthday party was about to begin. "Can you find someone else just this once?" he asked the nurse manager who called him. "I should have let you know in advance that we have an important family event today, but I just forgot. If you can't find someone else, call me back, and I'll come right in." Joe's manager was furious. "I don't have time to make a dozen calls. If you knew that you wouldn't want to come in today, you should not have accepted on-call duty. We pay you to be on-call, and I expect you to be here in 30 minutes, not one minute later, or there will be consequences."

Joe decided that he no longer wanted to work in the institution. With his 5 years of operating room experience, he quickly found another position in an organization that was more supportive of its staff.

1. What style of leadership and school of management thought seemed to be preferred by Joe Garcia's manager?

2. What style of leadership and school of management were preferred by Joe?

3. Which of the listed qualities of leaders and managers did the nurse manager display? Which behaviors? Which ones did the nurse manager not display?

4. If you were Joe, what would you have done? If you were the nurse manager, what would you have done? Why?

5. Who do you think was right, Joe or the nurse manager? Why?

References

Dantley, M.F. (2005). Moral leadership: Shifting the management paradigm. In English, F.W. *The Sage Handbook of Educational Leadership* (pp. 34–46). Thousand Oaks, Calif.: Sage Publications.

Dowless, R.M. (2007). Your guide to costing methods and terminology. *Nursing Management, 38*(4), 52–57.

Dunham-Taylor, J. (1995). Identifying the best in nurse executive leadership. *Journal of Nursing Administration, 25*(7/8), 24–31.

Greenleaf, R.K. (2004). Who is the servant-leader? In Spears, L.C., & Lawrence, M. *Practicing Servant-Leadership.* New York: Jossey-Bass.

Hart, L.B., & Waisman, C.S. (2005). *The Leadership Training Activity Book.* New York: AMACOM.

Hunter, J.C. (2004). *The World's Most Powerful Leadership Principle.* New York: Crown Business.

Kelly, J., & Nadler, S. (2007, March 3–4). Leading from below. *Wall Street Journal,* p. R4.

Kovner, C.T., Brewer, C.S., Fairchild, S., et al. (2007). Newly licensed RNs' characteristics, work attitudes, and intentions to work. *American Journal of Nursing, 107*(9), 58–70.

Lee, J.A. (1980). *The Gold and the Garbage in Management Theories and Prescriptions.* Athens, Ohio: Ohio University Press.

Locke, E.A. (1982). The ideas of Frederick Taylor: An evaluation. *Academy of Management Review, 7*(1), 14.

Lombardi, D.N. (2001). *Handbook for the New Health Care Manager.* San Francisco: Jossey-Bass/AHA Press.

Mackoff, B.L., & Triolo, P.K. (2008). Why do nurse managers stay? Building a model engagement. Part I: Dimensions of engagement. *Journal of Nursing Administration, 38*(3), 118–124.

McCauley, C.D., & Van Velson, E. (eds.). (2004). *The Center for Creative Leadership Handbook of Leadership Development.* New York: Jossey-Bass.

McGregor, D. (1960). *The Human Side of Enterprise.* New York: McGraw-Hill.

Mintzberg, H. (1989). *Mintzberg on Management: Inside Our Strange World of Organizations.* New York: Free Press.

Montebello, A. (1994). *Work Teams That Work.* Minneapolis: Best Sellers Publishing.

Shirey, M.R. (2007). Competencies and tips for effective leadership. *Journal of Nursing Administration, 37*(4), 167–170.

Shirey, M.R., Ebright, P.R., & McDaniel, A.M. (2008). Sleepless in America: Nurse managers cope with stress and complexity. *Journal of Nursing Administration, 38*(3), 125–131.

Spears, L.C., & Lawrence, M. (2004). *Practicing Servant-Leadership.* New York: Jossey-Bass.

Welch, J., & Welch, S. (2007, July 23). Bosses who get it all wrong. *BusinessWeek,* p. 88.

Welch, J., & Welch, S. (2008, July 28). Emotional mismanagement. *BusinessWeek,* p. 84.

Wren, D.A. (1972). *The Evolution of Management Thought.* New York: Ronald Press.

chapter 3

Nursing Practice and the Law

OBJECTIVES

After reading this chapter, the student should be able to:

- Identify three major sources of laws.
- Explain the differences between various types of laws.
- Differentiate between negligence and malpractice.
- Explain the difference between an intentional and an unintentional tort.
- Explain how standards of care are used in determining negligence and malpractice.
- Describe how nurse practice acts guide nursing practice.
- Explain the purpose of licensure.
- Discuss issues of licensure.
- Explain the difference between internal standards and external standards.
- Discuss advance directives and how they pertain to clients' rights.
- Discuss the legal implications of the Health Insurance Portability and Accountability Act (HIPAA)

OUTLINE

The courtroom seemed cold and sterile. Scanning her surroundings with nervous eyes, Germaine decided she knew how Alice must have felt when the Queen of Hearts screamed for her head. The image of the White Rabbit running through the woods, looking at his watch, yelling, "I'm late! I'm late!" flashed before her eyes. For a few moments, she indulged herself in thoughts of being able to turn back the clock and rewrite the past. The future certainly looked grim at that moment. The calling of her name broke her reverie. Mr. Ellison, the attorney for the plaintiff, wanted her undivided attention regarding the fateful day when she committed a fatal medication error. That day, the client died following a cardiac arrest because Germaine failed to check the appropriate dosage and route for the medication. She had administered 40 mEq of potassium chloride by intravenous push. Her 15 years of nursing experience meant little to the court. Because she had not followed hospital protocol and had violated an important standard of practice, Germaine stood alone. She was being sued for malpractice.

As client advocates, nurses have a responsibility to deliver safe care to their clients. This expectation requires that nurses have professional knowledge at their expected level of practice and be proficient in technological skills. A working knowledge of the legal system, client rights, and behaviors that may result in lawsuits helps nurses to act as client advocates. As long as nurses practice according to established standards of care, they will be able to avoid the kind of day in court that Germaine experienced.

General Principles

Meaning of Law

The word *law* has several meanings. For the purposes of this chapter, *law* means those rules that prescribe and control social conduct in a formal and legally binding manner (Bernzweig, 1996). Laws are created in one of three ways:

1. *Statutory laws* are created by various legislative bodies, such as state legislatures or Congress. Some examples of federal statutes include the Patient Self-Determination Act of 1990 and the Americans With Disabilities Act. State statutes include the state nurse practice acts, the state boards of nursing, and the Good Samaritan Act. Laws that govern nursing practice are statutory laws.

2. *Common law* develops within the court system as judicial decisions are made in various cases and precedents for future cases are set. In this way, a decision made in one case can affect decisions made in later cases of a similar nature. This feature of American law is based on the English tradition of case law: "judge-made law" (Black, 2004). Many times a judge in a subsequent case will follow the reasoning of a judge in a previous case. Therefore, one case sets a precedent for another.

3. *Administrative law* is established through the authority given to government agencies, such as state boards of nursing, by a legislative body. These governing boards have the duty to meet the intent of laws or statutes.

Sources of Law

The Constitution

The U.S. Constitution is the foundation of American law. The Bill of Rights, comprising the first 10 amendments to the Constitution, is the basis for protection of individual rights. These laws define and limit the power of the government and protect citizens' freedom of speech, assembly, religion, and the press and freedom from unwarranted intrusion by government into personal choices. State constitutions can expand individual rights but cannot deprive people of rights guaranteed by the U.S. Constitution.

Constitutional law evolves. As individuals or groups bring suit to challenge interpretations of the Constitution, decisions are made concerning application of the law to that particular event. An example is the protection of freedom of speech. Are obscenities protected? Can one person threaten or criticize another person? The freedom to criticize is protected; threats are not protected. The definition of what constitutes obscenity is often debated and has not been fully clarified by the courts.

Statutes

Localities, state legislatures, and the U.S. Congress create statutes. These can be found in multivolume sets of books and databases.

At the federal level, conference committees comprising representatives of both houses of Congress negotiate the resolution of any differences on wording of a bill before it becomes law. If the bill does not meet with the approval of the executive branch of government, the president can veto it. If that occurs, the legislative branch must have enough votes to override the veto or the bill will not become law.

Nurses have an opportunity to influence the development of statutory law both as citizens and as health-care providers. Writing to or meeting with state legislators or members of Congress is a way to demonstrate interest in such issues and their outcomes in terms of the laws passed. Passage of a new law is often a long process that includes some compromise of all interested individuals.

Administrative Law

The Department of Health and Human Services, the Department of Labor, and the Department of Education are the federal agencies that administer health-care–related laws. At the state level are departments of health and mental health and licensing boards.

Administrative agencies are staffed with professionals who develop the specific rules and regulations that direct the implementation of statutory law. These rules must be reasonable and consistent with existing statutory law and the intent of the legislature. Usually, the rules go into effect only after review and comment by affected persons or groups. For example, specific statutory laws give state nursing boards the authority to issue and revoke licenses, which means that each board of nursing has the responsibility to oversee the professional nurse's competence.

Types of Laws

Another way to look at the legal system is to divide it into two categories: criminal law and civil law.

Criminal Law

Criminal laws were developed to protect society from actions that threaten its existence. Criminal acts, although directed toward individuals, are considered offenses against the state. The perpetrator of the act is punished, and the victim receives no compensation for injury or damages. There are three categories of criminal law:

1. *Felony:* the most serious category, including such acts as homicide, grand larceny, and nurse practice act violation
2. *Misdemeanor:* includes lesser offenses such as traffic violations or shoplifting of a small dollar amount

3. *Juvenile:* crimes carried out by individuals younger than 18 years; specific age varies by state and crime

There are occasions when a nurse breaks a law and is tried in criminal court. A nurse who distributes controlled substances illegally, either for personal use or for the use of others, is violating the law. Falsification of records of controlled substances is a criminal action. In some states, altering a patient record may be a misdemeanor (Northrop & Kelly, 1987). For example:

Nurse V needed to administer a blood transfusion. Because she was in a hurry, she did not check the paperwork properly and therefore did not follow the standard of practice established for blood administration. The client was transfused with incompatible blood, suffered from a transfusion reaction, and died. Nurse V attempted to conceal her conduct and falsified the records. She was found guilty of manslaughter (Northrop & Kelly, 1987).

Civil Law

Civil laws usually involve the violation of one person's rights by another person. Areas of civil law that particularly affect nurses are tort law, contract law, antitrust law, employment discrimination, and labor laws.

Tort

The remainder of this chapter focuses primarily on tort law. A tort is a legal or civil wrong carried out by one person against the person or property of another (Black, 2004). Tort law recognizes that individuals in their relationships with each other have a general duty not to harm each other (Cushing, 1999). For example, as drivers of automobiles, everyone has a duty to drive safely so that others will not be harmed. A roofer has a duty to install a roof properly so that it will not collapse and injure individuals inside the structure. Nurses have a duty to deliver care in such a manner that the consumers of care are not harmed. These legal duties of care may be violated intentionally or unintentionally.

Quasi-Intentional Tort

A quasi-intentional tort has its basis in speech. These are voluntary acts that directly cause injury or anguish without meaning to harm or to cause distress. The elements of cause and desire are present, but the element of intent is missing. Quasi-intentional torts usually involve problems in communication that result in damage to a person's reputation, violation of personal privacy, or infringement of an individual's civil rights. These include defamation of character, invasion of privacy, and breach of confidentiality (Aiken, 2004, p. 139).

Negligence

Negligence is the unintentional tort of acting or failing to act as an ordinary, reasonable, prudent person, resulting in harm to the person to whom the duty of care is owed (Black, 2004). The legal elements of negligence consist of duty, breach of duty, causation, and harm or injury (Cushing, 1999). All four elements must be present in the determination. For example, if a nurse administers the wrong medication to a client, but the client is not injured, then the element of harm has not been met. However, if a nurse administers appropriate pain medication but fails to put up the side rails, and the client falls and breaks a hip, all four elements have been satisfied. The duty of care is the standard of care. The law defines standard of care as that which a reasonable, prudent practitioner with similar education and experience would do or not do in similar circumstances (Prosser & Keeton, 1984).

Malpractice

Malpractice is the term used for professional negligence. When fulfillment of duties requires specialized education, the term malpractice is used. In most malpractice suits, the facilities employing the nurses who cared for a client are named as defendants in the suit. Vicarious liability is the legal principle cited in these cases. *Respondeat superior,* the borrowed servant doctrine, and the captain of the ship doctrine fall under vicarious liability.

An important principle in understanding negligence is *respondeat superior* ("let the master answer") (Aiken, 2004, p. 279). This doctrine holds employers liable for any negligence by their employees when the employees were acting within the realm of employment and when the alleged negligent acts happened during employment (Aiken, 2004).

Consider the following scenario:

A nursing instructor on a clinical unit in a busy metropolitan hospital instructed his students not to administer any medications unless he was present.

Marcos, a second-level student, was unable to find his instructor, so he decided to administer digoxin to his client without supervision. The dose was 0.125 mg. The unit dose came as digoxin 0.5 mg/mL. Marcos administered the entire amount without checking the digoxin dose or the client's blood and potassium levels. The client became toxic, developed a dysrhythmia, and was transferred to the intensive care unit. The family sued the hospital and the nursing school for malpractice. The nursing instructor was also sued under the principle of respondeat superior, even though specific instructions to the contrary had been given to the students.

Other Laws Relevant to Nursing Practice

Good Samaritan Laws

Fear of being sued has often prevented trained professionals from assisting during an emergency. To encourage physicians and nurses to respond to emergencies, many states developed what are now known as the Good Samaritan laws. When administering emergency care, nurses and physicians are protected from civil liability by Good Samaritan laws as long as they behave in the same manner as an ordinary, reasonable, and prudent professional in the same or similar circumstances (Prosser & Keeton, 1984). In other words, when assisting during an emergency, nurses must still observe professional standards of care. However, if a payment is received for the care given, the Good Samaritan laws do not hold.

Confidentiality

It is possible for nurses to be involved in lawsuits other than those involving negligence. For example, clients have the right to confidentiality, and it is the duty of the professional nurse to ensure this right. This assures the client that information obtained by a nurse while providing care will not be communicated to anyone who does not have a need to know. This includes giving information by telephone to individuals claiming to be related to a client, giving information without a client's signed release, or removing documents from a health-care provider with a client's name or other information.

The Health Insurance Portability and Accountability Act (HIPAA) of 1996 was passed as an effort to preserve confidentiality and protect the privacy of health information and improve the portability and continuation of health-care coverage. The HIPAA gave Congress until August 1999 to pass this legislation. Congress failed to act, and the Department of Health and Human Services took over developing the appropriate regulations (Charters, 2003). The latest version of this privacy act was published in the Federal Register in 2002 (Charters, 2003).

The increased use of electronic sources of documentation and transfer of client information presents many confidentiality issues. It is important for nurses to be aware of the guidelines protecting the sharing and transfer of information through electronic sources. Most health-care institutions have internal procedures to protect client confidentiality.

Take the following example:

Bill was admitted for pneumonia. With Bill's permission, an HIV test was performed, and the result was positive. This information was available on the computerized laboratory result printout. A nurse inadvertently left the laboratory results on the computer screen that was partially facing the hallway. One of Bill's coworkers, who had come to visit him, saw the report on the screen. This individual reported the test results to Bill's supervisor. When Bill returned to work, he was fired for "poor job performance," although he had had superior job evaluations. In the process of filing a discrimination suit against his employer, Bill discovered that the information on his health status had come from this source. A lawsuit was filed against the hospital and the nurse involved based on a breach of confidentiality.

Slander and Libel

Slander and libel are categorized as quasi-intentional torts. Nurses rarely think of themselves as being guilty of slander or libel. The term *slander* refers to the spoken word, and *libel* refers to the written word. Making a false statement about a client's condition that may result in an injury to that client is considered slander. Making a written false statement is libel. For example, stating that a client who had blood drawn for drug testing has a substance abuse problem, when in fact the client does not carry that diagnosis, could be considered a slanderous statement.

Slander and libel also refer to statements made about coworkers or other individuals whom you may encounter in both your professional and educational life. Think before you speak and write. Sometimes what may appear to be harmless to you, such as a complaint, may contain statements that damage another person's credibility personally and professionally. Consider this example:

Several nurses on a unit were having difficulty with the nurse manager. Rather than approach the manager or follow the chain of command, they decided to send a written statement to the chief executive officer (CEO) of the hospital. In this letter, they embellished some of the incidents that occurred and took statements out of context that the nurse manager had made, changing the meanings of the remarks. The nurse manager was called to the CEO's office and reprimanded for these events and statements, which in fact had not occurred. The nurse manager sued the nurses for slander and libel based on the premise that her personal and professional reputation had been tainted.

False Imprisonment

False imprisonment is confining an individual against his or her will by either physical (restraining) or verbal (detaining) means. The following are examples:

- Using restraints on individuals without the appropriate written consent
- Restraining mentally handicapped individuals who do not represent a threat to themselves or others
- Detaining unwilling clients in an institution when they desire to leave
- Keeping persons who are medically cleared for discharge for an unreasonable amount of time
- Removing the clothing of clients to prevent them from leaving the institution
- Threatening clients with some form of physical, emotional, or legal action if they insist on leaving

Sometimes clients are a danger to themselves and to others. Nurses need to decide on the appropriateness of restraints as a protective measure. Nurses should try to obtain the cooperation of the client before applying any type of restraints. The first step is to attempt to identify a reason for the risky behavior and resolve the problem. If this fails, document the need for restraints, consult with the physician, and carefully follow the institution's policies and standards of practice. Failure to follow these guidelines may result in greater harm to the client and possibly a lawsuit for the staff. Consider the following:

> *Mr. Harrison, who is 87 years old, was admitted through the emergency department with severe lower abdominal pain of 3 days' duration. Physical assessment revealed severe dehydration and acute distress. A surgeon was called, and an abdominal laparotomy was performed, revealing a ruptured appendix. Surgery was successful, and the client was sent to the intensive care unit for 24 hours. On transfer to the surgical floor the next day, Mr. Harrison was in stable condition. Later that night, he became confused, irritable, and anxious. He attempted to climb out of bed and pulled out his indwelling urinary catheter. The nurse restrained him. The next day, his irritability and confusion continued. Mr. Harrison's nurse placed him in a chair, tying him in and restraining his hands. Three hours later he was found in cardiopulmonary arrest. A lawsuit of wrongful death and false imprisonment was brought against the nurse manager, the nurses caring for Mr. Harrison, and the institution. During discovery, it was determined that the primary cause of Mr. Harrison's behavior was hypoxemia. A violation of law occurred with the failure of the nursing staff to notify the physician of the client's condition and to follow the institution's standard of practice on the use of restraints.*

To protect themselves against charges of negligence or false imprisonment in such cases, nurses should discuss safety needs with clients, their families, or other members of the health-care team. Careful assessment and documentation of client status are also imperative; confusion, irritability, and anxiety often have metabolic causes that need correction, not restraint.

There are statutes and case laws specific to the admission of clients to psychiatric institutions. Most states have guidelines for emergency involuntary hospitalization for a specific period. Involuntary admission is considered necessary when clients are a danger to themselves or others. Specific procedures must be followed. A determination by a judge or administrative agency or certification by a specified number of physicians that a person's mental health justifies the person's detention and treatment may be required. Once admitted, these clients may not be restrained unless the guidelines established by state law and the institution's policies provide. Clients who voluntarily admit themselves to psychiatric institutions are also protected against false imprisonment. Nurses need to find out the policies of their state and employing institution.

Assault and Battery

Assault is threatening to do harm. Battery is touching another person without his or her consent. The significance of an assault is in the threat: "If you don't stop pushing that call bell, I'll give you this injection with the biggest needle I can find" is considered an assaultive statement. Battery would occur if the injection were given when it was refused, even if medical personnel deemed it was for the "client's good." With few exceptions, clients have a right to refuse treatment. Holding down a violent client against his or her will and injecting a sedative is battery. Most medical treatments, particularly surgery, would be battery if it were not for informed consent from the client.

Standards of Practice

Concern for the quality of care is a major part of nursing's responsibility to the public. Therefore, the nursing profession is accountable to the consumer for the quality of its services. One of the defining characteristics of a profession is the ability to set its own standards. Nursing standards were established as guidelines for the profession to ensure acceptable quality of care (Beckman, 1995). Standards of practice are also used as criteria to determine whether appropriate care has been delivered. In practice, they represent the minimum acceptable level of care. Nurses are judged on generally accepted standards of practice for their level of education, experience, position, and specialty area. Standards take many forms. Some are written and appear as criteria of professional organizations, job descriptions, agency policies and procedures, and textbooks. Others, which may be intrinsic to the custom of practice, are not found in writing (Beckman, 1995).

State boards of nursing and professional organizations vary by role and responsibility in relation to standards of development and implementation (ANA, 1998; 2004). Statutes, professional organizations, and health-care institutions establish standards of practice. The nurse practice acts of individual states define the boundaries of nursing practice within the state. In Canada, the provincial and territorial associations define practice.

The courts have upheld the authority of boards of nursing to regulate standards. The boards accomplish this through direct or delegated statutory language (ANA, 1998; 2004). The American Nurses Association (ANA) also has specific standards of practice in general and in several clinical areas (see Appendix 2). In Canada, the colleges of registered nurses and the registered nurses associations of the various provinces and territories have developed published practice standards. These may be found at cna-aiic.ca

Institutions develop internal standards of practice. The standards are usually explained in a specific institutional policy (for example, guidelines for the appropriate administration of a specific chemotherapeutic agent), and the institution includes these standards in policy and procedure manuals. The guidelines are based on current literature and research. It is the nurse's responsibility to meet the institution's standards of practice. It is the institution's responsibility to notify the health-care personnel of any changes and instruct the personnel about the changes. Institutions may accomplish this task through written memos or meetings and in-service education.

With the expansion of advanced nursing practice, it has become particularly important to clarify the legal distinction between nursing and medical practice. It is important to be aware of the boundaries between these professional domains because crossing them can result in legal consequences and disciplinary action. The nurse practice act and related regulations developed by most state legislatures and state boards of nursing help to clarify nursing roles at the various levels of practice.

Use of Standards in Nursing Negligence Malpractice Actions

When omission of prudent care or acts committed by a nurse or those under his or her supervision cause harm to a client, standards of nursing practice are among the elements used to determine whether malpractice or negligence exists. Other criteria may include but are not limited to (ANA, 1998):

- State, local, or national standards
- Institutional policies that alter or adhere to the nursing standards of care
- Expert opinions on the appropriate standard of care at the time
- Available literature and research that substantiates a standard of care or changes in the standard

Patient's Bill of Rights

In 1973 the American Hospital Association approved a statement called the Patient's Bill of Rights. These were revised in October 1992. Patient rights were developed with the belief that hospitals and health-care institutions would support these rights with the goal of delivering effective client care. In 2003 the Patient's Bill of Rights was replaced by the Patient Care Partnership. These standards were derived from the ethical principle of autonomy. This document may be found at aha.org/aha/ptcommunication/partnership/index

Informed Consent

Without consent, many of the procedures performed on clients in a health-care setting may be considered battery or unwarranted touching. When clients consent to treatment, they give health-care personnel the right to deliver care and perform specific treatments without fear of prosecution. Although physicians are responsible for obtaining informed consent, nurses often find themselves involved in the process. It is the physician's responsibility to give information to a client about a specific treatment or medical intervention (*Giese v. Stice*, 1997). The individual institution is not responsible for obtaining the informed consent unless (1) the physician or practitioner is employed by the institution or (2) the institution was aware or should have been aware of the lack of informed consent and did not act on this fact (Guido, 2001). Some institutions require the physician or independent practitioner to obtain his or her own informed consent by obtaining the client's signature at the time the explanation for treatment is given.

The informed consent form should contain all the possible negative outcomes as well as the positive ones. Nurses may be asked to obtain the signatures on this form. The following are some criteria to help ensure that a client has given an informed consent (Guido, 2001; Kozier, Erb, Blais, et al., 1995):

- A mentally competent adult has voluntarily given the consent.
- The client understands exactly to what he or she is consenting.
- The consent includes the risks involved in the procedure, alternative treatments that may be available, and the possible result if the treatment is refused.

■ The consent is written.
■ A minor's parent or guardian usually gives consent for treatment.

Ideally, a nurse should be present when the physician is explaining the treatment to the client. Before obtaining the client's signature, the nurse asks the client to recall exactly what the physician has told him or her about the treatment. If at any point the nurse thinks that the client does not understand the treatment or the expected outcome, the nurse must notify the physician of this fact.

To be able to give informed consent, the client must be fully informed fully. Clients have the right to refuse treatment, and nurses must respect this right. If a client refuses the recommended treatment, a client must be informed of the possible consequences of this decision.

Implied consent occurs when consent is assumed. This may be an issue in an emergency when an individual is unable to give consent, as in the following scenario:

An elderly woman is involved in a car accident on a major highway. The paramedics called to the scene find her unresponsive and in acute respiratory distress; her vital signs are unstable. The paramedics immediately intubate her and begin treating her cardiac dysrhythmias. Because she is unconscious and unable to give verbal consent, there is an implied consent for treatment.

Staying Out of Court

Prevention

Unfortunately, the public's trust in the medical profession has declined over recent years. Consumers are better informed and more assertive in their approach to health care. They demand good and responsible care. If clients and their families believe that behaviors are uncaring or that attitudes are impersonal, they are more likely to sue for what they view as errors in treatment. The same applies to nurses. If nurses demonstrate an interest in and caring behaviors toward clients, a relationship develops. Individuals do not sue those they view as "caring friends." The potential to change the attitudes of health-care consumers is within the power of health-care personnel. Demonstrating care and concern and making clients and families aware of choices and methods can help decrease liability. Nurses who involve clients and their families in decisions about care reduce the likelihood of a lawsuit. Tips to prevent legal problems are listed in Box 3-1.

All health-care personnel are accountable for their own actions and adherence to the accepted standards of health care. Most negligence and malpractice cases arise from a violation of the accepted standards of practice and the policies of the employing institution. Common causes of negligence are listed in Table 3-1. Expert witnesses are called to cite the accepted standards and assist attorneys in formulating the legal strategies pertaining to those standards. For example, most medication errors can be traced to a violation of the accepted standard of medication administration, originally referred to as the Five Rights (Kozier et al., 1995; Taylor, Lillis, & LeMone, 2008), which have been amended to Seven Rights (Balas, Scott, & Rogers, 2004):

1. Right drug
2. Right dose
3. Right route
4. Right time
5. Right client
6. Right reason
7. Right documentation

Appropriate Documentation

The adage "not documented, not done" holds true in nursing. According to the law, if something has not been documented, then the responsible party

---

box 3-1

Tips for Avoiding Legal Problems

- Keep yourself informed regarding new research related to your area of practice.
- Insist that the health-care institution keep personnel apprised of all changes in policies and procedures and in the management of new technological equipment.
- Always follow the standards of care or practice for the institution.
- Delegate tasks and procedures only to appropriate personnel.
- Identify clients at risk for problems, such as falls or the development of decubiti.
- Establish and maintain a safe environment.
- Document precisely and carefully.
- Write detailed incident reports, and file them with the appropriate personnel or department.
- Recognize certain client behaviors that may indicate the possibility of a lawsuit.

table 3-1

Common Causes of Negligence

Problem	Prevention
Client falls	Identify clients at risk.
	Place notices about fall precautions.
	Follow institutional policies on the use of restraints.
	Always be sure beds are in their lowest positions.
	Use side rails appropriately.
Equipment injuries	Check thermostats and temperature in equipment used for heat or cold application.
	Check wiring on all electrical equipment.
Failure to monitor	Observe IV infusion sites as directed by institutional policy.
	Obtain and record vital signs, urinary output, cardiac status, etc., as directed by institutional policy and more often if client condition dictates.
	Check pertinent laboratory values.
Failure to communicate	Report pertinent changes in client status.
	Document changes accurately.
	Document communication with appropriate source.
Medication errors	Follow the Seven Rights.
	Monitor client responses.
	Check client medications for multiple drugs for the same actions.

did not do whatever needed to be done. If a nurse did not "do" something, that leaves the nurse open to negligence or malpractice charges.

Nursing documentation needs to be legally credible. Legally credible documentation is an accurate accounting of the care the client received. It also indicates the competence of the individual who delivered the care.

Charting by exception creates defense difficulties. When this method of documentation is used, investigators need to review the entire patient record in an attempt to reconstruct the care given to the client. Clear, concise, and accurate documentation helps nurses when they are named in lawsuits. Often, this documentation clears the individual of any negligence or malpractice. Documentation is credible when it is:

- **Contemporaneous** (documenting at the time care was provided)
- **Accurate** (documenting exactly what was done)
- **Truthful** (documenting only what was done)
- **Appropriate** (documenting only what could be discussed comfortably in a public setting)

Box 3-2 lists some documentation tips.

Marcos, the nursing student earlier in the chapter, violated the right-dose principle and therefore made a medication error. By signing off on medications for

all clients for a shift before the medications are administered, a nurse is leaving himself or herself open to charges of medication error.

In the case of Mr. Harrison, the institutional personnel were found negligent because of a direct violation of the institution's standards regarding the application of restraints.

Nursing units are busy and often understaffed. These realities exist but should not be allowed to interfere with the safe delivery of health care. Clients have a right to safe and effective health care, and nurses have an obligation to deliver this care.

Common Actions Leading to Malpractice Suits

- Failure to assess a client appropriately
- Failure to report changes in client status to the appropriate personnel
- Failure to document in the patient record
- Altering or falsifying a patient record
- Failure to obtain informed consent
- Failure to report a coworker's negligence or poor practice
- Failure to provide appropriate education to a client and/or family members
- Violation of internal or external standards of practice

box 3-2

Some Documentation Guidelines

Medications:

- Always chart the time, route, dose, and response.
- Always chart PRN medications and the client response.
- Always chart when a medication was not given, the reason (e.g., client in Radiology, Physical Therapy; do not chart that the medication was not on the floor), and the nursing intervention.
- Chart all medication refusals, and report them.

Physician communication:

- Document each time a call is made to a physician, even if he or she is not reached. Include the exact time of the call. If the physician is reached, document the details of the message and the physician's response.
- Read verbal orders back to the physician, and confirm the client's identity as written on the chart. Chart only verbal orders that you have heard from the source, not those told to you by another nurse or unit personnel.

Formal issues in charting:

- Before writing on the chart, check to be sure you have the correct patient record.
- Check to make sure each page has the client's name and the current date stamped in the appropriate area.
- If you forgot to make an entry, chart "late entry," and place the date and time at the entry.
- Correct all charting mistakes according to the policy and procedures of your institution.
- Chart in an organized fashion, following the nursing process.
- Write legibly and concisely, and avoid subjective statements.
- Write specific and accurate descriptions.
- When charting a symptom or situation, chart the interventions taken and the client response.
- Document your own observations, not those that were told to you by another party.
- Chart frequently to demonstrate ongoing care, and chart routine activities.
- Chart client and family teaching and their response.

In the case *Tovar v. Methodist Healthcare* (2005), a 75-year-old female client came to the emergency department complaining of a headache and weakness in the right arm. Although an order for admission to the neurological care unit was written, the client was not transported until 3 hours later. After the client was in the unit, the nurses called one physician regarding the client's status. Another physician returned the call 90 minutes later. Three hours later, the nurses called to report a change in neurological status. A STAT computed tomography scan was ordered, which revealed a massive brain hemorrhage. The nurses were cited for the following:

1. Delay in transferring the client to the neurological unit
2. Failure to advocate for the client

The client presented with an acute neurological problem requiring admission to an intensive care unit where appropriate observation and interventions were available. A delay in transfer may lead to delay in appropriate treatment. According to the ANA standards of care for neuroscience nurses (2002), nurses need to assess the client's changing neurological status accurately and advocate for the client. In this instance, the court stated that the

nurses should have been more assertive in attempting to reach the physician and request a prompt medical evaluation. The court sided with the family, agreeing with the plantiff's medical expert's conclusion that the client's death was related to improper management by the nursing staff.

If a Problem Arises

When served with a summons or complaint, people often panic, allowing fear to overcome reason.

First, simply answer the complaint. Failure to do this may result in a default judgment, causing greater distress and difficulties.

Second, many things can be done to protect oneself if named in a lawsuit. Legal representation can be obtained to protect personal property. Never sign any documents without consulting the malpractice insurance carrier or a legal representative. If you are personally covered by malpractice insurance, notify the company immediately, and follow their instructions carefully.

Institutions usually have lawyers to defend themselves and their employees. Whether or not you are personally insured, contact the legal department of the institution where the act took place. Maintain a file of all papers, proceedings, meetings, and telephone conversations about the case. Do not withhold any information from your attorneys, even if that information can be harmful to you. A pending or ongoing legal case should not be discussed with coworkers or friends.

Let the attorneys and the insurance company help decide how to handle the difficult situation. They are in charge of damage control. Concealing information usually causes more damage than disclosing it.

Sometimes, nurses believe they are not being adequately protected or represented by the attorneys from their employing institution. If this happens, consider hiring a personal attorney who is experienced in malpractice. This information can be obtained through either the state bar association or the local trial lawyers association.

Anyone has the right to sue; however, that does not mean that there is a case. Many negligence and malpractice courses find in favor of the health-care providers, not the client or the client's family. The following case demonstrates this situation:

The Supreme Court of Arkansas heard a case that originated from the Court of Appeals in Arkansas. A client died in a single car motor vehicle accident shortly after undergoing an outpatient colonoscopy performed under conscious sedation. The family sued the center for performing the procedure and permitting the client to drive home. The court agreed that sedation should not be admininstered without the confirmation of a designated driver for later. It also agreed that an outpatient facility needs to have directives stating that nurses and physicians may not admininster sedation unless transportation is available for later. However, the court ruled physicians and nurses may rely on information from the client. If the client states that someone will be available for transportation after the procedure, sedation may be administered. The second aspect of the case revolved around the client's insistence on leaving the facility and driving himself. When a client leaves against medical advice, the health-care personnel have a legal duty to warn and strongly advise the client against the highly dangerous action. However, nurses and physicians do not have a legal right to restrain the client physically, keep his clothes, or take away car keys. Nurses are not obligated to call a taxi, call the police, admit the client to the hospital, or personally escort the client home if the client insists on leaving. Clients have some

responsibility for their own safety (Young v. GastroIntestinal Center, Inc., 2005). *In this case, the nurses acted appropriately. They adhered to the standard of practice, documented that the client stated that someone would be available to transport him home, and filled the duty to warn.*

Professional Liability Insurance

We live in a litigious society. Although there are a variety of opinions on the issue, in today's world nurses need to consider obtaining professional liability insurance (Aiken, 2004). Various forms of professional liability insurance are available. These policies have been developed to protect nurses against personal financial losses if they are involved in a medical malpractice suit. If a nurse is charged with malpractice and found guilty, the employing institution has the right to sue the nurse to reclaim damages. Professional malpractice insurance protects the nurse in these situations.

End-of-Life Decisions and the Law

When a heart ceases to beat, a client is in a state of cardiac arrest. In health-care institutions and in the community, it is common to begin cardiopulmonary resuscitation (CPR) when cardiac arrest occurs. In health-care institutions, an elaborate mechanism is put into action when a client "codes." Much controversy exists concerning when these mechanisms should be used and whether individuals who have no chance of regaining full viability should be resuscitated.

Do Not Resuscitate Orders

A do not resuscitate (DNR) order is a specific directive to health-care personnel not to initiate CPR measures. Only a physician can write a DNR order, usually after consulting with the client or family. Other members of the health-care team are expected to comply with the order. Clients have the right to request a DNR order. However, they may make this request without a full understanding of what it really means. Consider the following example:

When Mrs. Vincent, 58 years old, was admitted to the hospital for a hysterectomy, she stated, "I want to be made a DNR." The nurse, concerned by the statement, questioned Mrs. Vincent's understanding of a DNR order. The nurse asked her, "Do you mean that if you are walking down the hall after your surgery and your heart stops beating, you do not want the nurses or physicians to do anything? You want us to just let you die?" Mrs. Vincent responded with a resounding, "No, that is not what I mean. I mean if something happens to me and I won't be able to be the way I am now, I want to be a DNR!" The nurse then explained the concept of a DNR order.

New York state has one of the most complete laws regarding DNR orders for acute and long-term care facilities. The New York law sets up a hierarchy of surrogates who may ask for a DNR status for incompetent clients. The state has also ordered that all health-care facilities ask clients their wishes regarding resuscitation (Guido, 2001). The ANA advocates that every facility have a written policy regarding the initiation of such orders (ANA, 1992). The client or, if the client is unable to speak for himself or herself, a family member or guardian should make clear the client's preference for either having as much as possible done or withholding treatment (see the next section, Advance Directives). Elements to include in a DNR order are listed in Box 3-3.

Advance Directives

The legal dilemmas that may arise in relation to DNR orders often require court decisions. For this reason, in 1990 Senator John Danforth of Missouri and Senator Daniel Moynihan of New York introduced the Patient Self-Determination Act to address questions regarding life-sustaining treatment. The act was created to allow people the opportunity to make decisions about treatment in advance of a time when they might become unable to participate in the decision-making process.

Through this mechanism, families can be spared the burden of having to decide what the family member would have wanted.

Federal law requires that health-care institutions that receive federal money (from Medicare, for example) inform clients of their right to create advance directives. The Patient Self-Determination Act (S.R. 13566) provides guidelines for developing advance directives concerning what will be done for individuals if they are no longer able to participate actively in making decisions about care options. The act states that institutions must:

- **Provide information to every client.** On admission, all clients must be informed in writing of their rights under state law to accept or refuse medical treatment while they are competent to make decisions about their care. This includes the right to execute advance directives.
- **Document.** All clients must be asked whether they have a living will or have chosen a durable power of attorney for health care (also known as a health-care surrogate). The response must be indicated on the medical record, and a copy of the documents, if available, should be placed on the client's chart.
- **Educate.** Nurses, other health-care personnel, and the community need to understand what the Patient Self-Determination Act and state laws regarding advance directives require.
- **Be respectful of clients' rights.** All clients are to be treated with respectful care regardless of their decision regarding life-prolonging treatments.
- **Have cultural humility.** Recognize that culture affects clients' decisions regarding end-of-life care. Nurses should familiarize themselves with the cultural and spiritual beliefs of their clients in order to deliver culturally sensitive care.

Living Will and Durable Power of Attorney for Health Care (Health-Care Surrogate)

The two most common forms of advance directives are living wills and durable power of attorney for health care (health-care surrogate).

A living will is a legally executed document that states an individual's wishes regarding the use of life-prolonging medical treatment in the event that he or she is no longer competent to make informed treatment decisions on his or her own behalf and is suffering from a terminal condition (Catalano, 2000; Flarey, 1991).

---

box 3-3

Elements to Include in a DNR Order

- Statement of the institution's policy that resuscitation will be initiated unless there is a specific order to withhold resuscitative measures
- Statement from the client regarding specific desires
- Description of the client's medical condition to justify a DNR order
- Statement about the role of family members or significant others
- Definition of the scope of the DNR order
- Delineation of the roles of various caregivers

American Nurses Association. (1992). Position statement on nursing care and do not resuscitate decisions. Washington, DC: ANA.

A condition is considered terminal when, to a reasonable degree of medical certainty, there is little likelihood of recovery or the condition is expected to cause death. A terminal condition may also refer to a persistent vegetative state characterized by a permanent and irreversible condition of unconsciousness in which there is (1) absence of voluntary action or cognitive behavior of any kind and (2) an inability to communicate or interact purposefully with the environment (Hickey, 2002).

Another form of advance directive is the health-care surrogate. Chosen by the client, the health-care surrogate is usually a family member or close friend. The role of the health-care surrogate is to make the client's wishes known to medical and nursing personnel. Imperative in the designation of a health-care surrogate is a clear understanding of the client's wishes should the need arise to know them.

In some situations, clients are unable to express themselves adequately or competently, although they are not terminally ill. For example, clients with advanced Alzheimer's disease or other forms of dementia cannot communicate their wishes; clients under anesthesia are temporarily unable to communicate; and the condition of comatose clients does not allow for expression of health-care wishes. In these situations, the health-care surrogate can make treatment decisions on the behalf of the client. However, when a client regains the ability to make his or her own decisions and is capable of expressing them effectively, he or she resumes control of all decision making pertaining to medical treatment (Reigle, 1992). Nurses and physicians may be held accountable when they go against a client's wishes regarding DNR orders and advance directives.

In the case *Wendland v. Sparks* (1998), the physician and nurses were sued for "not initiating CPR." In this case, the client had been in the hospital for more than 2 months for lung disease and multiple myeloma. Although improving at the time, during the hospitalization she had experienced three cardiac arrests. Even after this, the client had not requested a DNR order. Her family had not discussed this either. After one of the arrests, the client's husband had told the physician that he wanted his wife placed on artificial life support if it was necessary (Guido, 2001). The client had a fourth cardiac arrest. One nurse went to obtain the crash cart, and another went to get the physician who happened to be in the area. The physician checked the heart rate, pupils, and respirations and stated, "I just cannot do it to her." (Guido, 2001, p. 158). She ordered the nurses to stop the resuscitation, and the physician pronounced the death of the client. The nurses stated that if they had not been given a direct order they would have continued their attempts at resuscitation. "The court ruled that the physician's judgment was faulty and that the family had the right to sue the physician for wrongful death" (Guido, 2001, p. 158). The nurses were cleared in this case because they were following a physician's order.

Nursing Implications

The Patient Self-Determination Act does not specify who should discuss treatment decisions or advance directives with clients. Because directives are often implemented on nursing units, however, nurses need to be knowledgeable about living wills and health-care surrogates and be prepared to answer questions that clients may have about directives and the forms used by the health-care institution.

As client advocates, the responsibility for creating an awareness of individual rights often falls on nurses. It is the responsibility of the health-care institution to educate personnel about the policies of the institution so that nurses and others involved in client care can inform health-care consumers of their choices. Nurses who are unsure of the policies in their health-care institution should contact the appropriate department.

Legal Implications of Mandatory Overtime

Although mostly a workplace and safety issue, there are legal implications to mandatory overtime. Due to nursing shortages, there has been an increased demand by hospitals forcing nurses to work overtime (ANA, 2000). Overtime causes physical and mental fatigue, increased stress, and decreased concentration. Subsequently, these conditions lead to medical errors such as failure to assess appropriately, report, document, and administer medications safely. This practice of overtime ignores other responsibilities nurses have outside of their professional lives, which affects their mood, motivation, and productivity (Vernarec, 2000).

Forced overtime causes already fatigued nurses to deliver nursing care that may be less than optimum, which in turn may lead to negligence and malpractice. This can result in the nurse losing his or her license and perhaps even facing a wrongful death suit due to an error in judgment.

Nurses practice under state or provincial (Canada) nurse practice acts. These state that nurses are held accountable for the safety of their clients Once a nurse accepts an assignment for the client, that nurse becomes liable under his or her license.

Many states are working to create legislation restricting mandatory overtime for nurses.

Licensure

Licensure is defined by the National Council of State Boards of Nursing as the "process by which an agency of state government grants permission to an individual to engage in a given profession upon finding that the applicant has attained the essential degree of competency necessary to perform a unique scope of practice" (NCSBN, 2007). Licenses are given by a government agency to allow an individual to engage in a professional practice and use a specific title. State boards of nursing issue nursing licenses, thus limiting practice to a specific jurisdiction (Blais, Hayes, Kozier, & Erb, 2006).

Licensure can be mandatory or permissive. Permissive licensure is a voluntary arrangement whereby an individual chooses to become licensed to demonstrate competence. However, the license is not required to practice. Mandatory licensure requires a nurse to be licensed in order to practice. In the United States and Canada, licensure is mandatory.

Qualifications for Licensure

The basic qualification for licensure requires graduation from an approved nursing program. In the United States, states may add additional requirements, such as disclosures regarding health or medications that could affect practice. Most states require disclosure of criminal conviction.

Licensure by Examination

A major accomplishment in the history of nursing licensure was the creation of the Bureau of State Boards of Nurse Examiners. The formation of this agency led to the development of an identical examination in all states. The original examination, called the State Board Test Pool Examination, was created by the testing department of the National League for Nursing. This was done through a collaborating

contract with the state boards. Initially, each state determined its own passing score; however, the states did adopt a common passing score. The examination is called the NCLEX-RN and is used in all states and territories of the United States. This test is prepared and administered through a testing company, Pearson Professional Testing of Minnesota (Ellis & Hartley, 2004).

NCLEX-RN

The NCLEX-RN is administered through computerized adaptive testing (CAT). Candidates must register to take the examination at an approved testing center in their area. Because of a large test bank, CAT permits a variety of questions to be administered to a group of candidates. Candidates taking the examination at the same time may not necessarily receive the same questions. Once a candidate answers a question, the computer analyzes the response and then chooses an appropriate question to ask next. If the question was answered correctly, the following question may be more difficult; if the question was answered incorrectly, the next question may be easier.

The minimum number of questions is 75, and the maximum is 265. Although the maximum amount of time for taking the examination is 5 hours, candidates who do well or those who are not performing well may finish as soon as 1 hour. The test ends once the analysis of the examination clearly determines that the candidate has successfully passed, has undoubtedly failed, has answered the maximum number of questions, or has reached the time limit (NCSBN, 2007). The computer scores the test at the time it is taken; however, candidates are not notified of their status at the time of completion. The information first goes to the testing service, which in turn notifies the appropriate state board. The state board notifies the candidate of the examination results.

Nursing practice requires the application of knowledge, skills, and abilities (NCSBN, 2007). The items are written to Bloom's taxonomy and are organized around client needs to reflect the candidates' ability to make nursing decisions regarding client care through application and analysis of information. The examination is organized into four major client need categories. Two of these categories, safe and effective care and physiological needs, include subdivisions (NCSBN, 2007). Integrated processes incorporate "nursing process, caring, communication and documentation and teaching/learning" (NCSBN, 2007, p. 3). Table 3-2 summarizes the categories and subcategories.

Previously, all questions were written in a multiple-choice format. In 2003, alternative formats were introduced. These alternative-format questions include fill-in-the-blank; multiple-response answers; "hot spots" that require the candidate to identify an area on a picture, graph, or chart; and drag and drop (NCSBN, 2007, p. 49). More information on alternative formats can be found on the NCSBN Web site: www.ncsbn.org.

Preparing for the NCLEX-RN

There are several ways to prepare for the NCLEX-RN. Some candidates attend review courses; others view videos and DVDs, whereas others review books. These methods assist in reviewing information that was learned during education. Everyone needs to decide what works best for himself or herself. It is helpful to take practice tests, because it familiarizes one with the computer and the examination format. The NCSBN offers an on-line NCLEX-RN study program.

To prepare for the NCLEX, take time to look at the test blueprint provided by the NCSBN. This gives candidates a comprehensive overview of the types of questions to expect on the examination. Candidates can review alternative test formats by accessing pearsonvue.com/nclex/ Some test taking tips follow:

- Be positive. Remind yourself that you worked hard to reach this milestone and how prepared you are to take the licensure examination.

- Turn negative thoughts into positive ones. Rather than saying, "I hope I pass," tell yourself, "I know I will do well."
- Acknowledge your feelings regarding the NCLEX. It is fine to admit that you are anxious; however, use your positive thoughts to control the anxiety.
- Also use diaphragmatic breathing (deep breathing) to control anxiety. Deep breathing augments the relaxation response of the body. Use this method at the beginning of the test or if you encounter a question that you find confusing.
- Control the situation by making a list of the items you may need to take the test. Pack them in a bag several days before, and keep them in a place where you will remember to take them.
- Eat well, and get a good night's sleep before the test. Avoid foods high in sugar and caffeine. Contrary to popular belief, caffeine interferes with your ability to concentrate. Eat complex carbohydrates and protein to maintain your blood glucose level.
- Several days before you are scheduled to take the test, travel to the test site along the same route at the time you plan to go. Have an alternate itinerary just in case there is a disruption in your route. This will alleviate any unnecessary stress in arriving at the examination site.
- Leave early, and give yourself plenty of time to get to your destination. Arriving early also gives a sense of control.
- Finally, remember your own basic needs. Testing centers tend to be cold. Pack a jacket or sweater. Check with the testing center to see if you are allowed water or snacks.

Licensure Through Endorsement

Nurses licensed in one state may obtain a license in another state through the process of endorsement. Each application is considered independently and is granted a license based on the rules and regulations of the state.

States differ in the number of continuing education credits required, legal requirements, and other educational requirements. Some states require that nurses meet the current criteria for licensure at the time of application, whereas others may grant the license based on the criteria in effect at the time of the original licensure (Ellis & Hartley, 2004). When applying for a license through endorsement, a nurse should always contact the board of nursing for the state and find out the exact requirements for

table 3-2

Major Categories and Subcategories of Client Needs

Category	Subcategories
Safe Effective Care Environment	Management of Care
	Safety and Infection Control
Health Promotion and Maintenance	
Psychosocial Integrity	
Physiological Integrity	Basic Care and Comfort
	Pharmacological and Parenteral Therapies
	Reduction of Risk Potential
	Physiological Adaptation

Adapted from NCSBN NCLEX-RN test plan (NCSBN, 2007, pp. 3–4.)

licensure. This information can usually be found on the board of nursing Web site for that particular state.

Multistate Licensure

The concept of multistate licensure allows a nurse licensed in one state to practice in additional states without obtaining additional licenses. NCSBN created a Multistate Licensure Compact that permits this practice. States that belong to the compact have passed legislation adopting the terms of this agreement and are known as party states. The nurse's home state is the state where he or she lives and received his or her original license. Renewal of the license is completed in the home state.

A nurse can hold only one home-state license. If the nurse moves to another state that belongs to the compact, the nurse applies for licensure within that state based on residency. The nurse is expected to follow the guidelines for nursing practice for that new state. The multistate licensure applies only to a basic registered nurse license, not to advanced practice. More information on multistate licensure can be found on the NCSBN Web site.

Disciplinary Action

State boards of nursing maintain rules and regulations for the practice of nursing. Violation of these regulations results in disciplinary actions as delineated by these boards. Issues of primary concern include but are not limited to the following:

- Falsifying documents to obtain a license
- Being convicted of a felony
- Practicing while under the influence of drugs or alcohol
- Functioning outside the scope of practice
- Engaging in child or elder abuse

Nurses convicted of a felony or found guilty in a malpractice action may find themselves before their state board of nursing or, in Canada, the provincial or territorial regulatory body.

Disciplinary action may include but is not limited to the suspension or revocation of a nursing license, mandatory fines, and mandatory continuing education. For more information regarding the regulations that guide nursing practice, consult the board of nursing in your state or, in Canada, your provincial or territorial regulatory body.

Conclusion

Nurses need to understand the legalities involved in the delivery of safe health care. It is important to know the standards of care established within your institution and the rules and regulations in the nurse practice acts of your state, province, or territory because these are the standards to which you will be held accountable. Health-care consumers have a right to quality care and the expectation that all information regarding diagnosis and treatment will remain confidential. Nurses have an obligation to deliver quality care and respect client confidentiality. Caring for clients safely and avoiding legal difficulties require nurses to adhere to the expected standards of care and document changes in client status carefully. Licensure helps to ensure that health-care consumers are receiving competent and safe care from their nurses.

Study Questions

1. How do federal laws, court decisions, and state boards of nursing affect nursing practice? Give an example of each.

2. Obtain a copy of the nurse practice act in your state. What are some of the penalties for violation of the rules and regulations?

3. The next time you are on your clinical unit, look at the nursing documentation done by several different staff members. Do you believe it is adequate? Explain your rationale.

4. How does your institution handle medication errors?

5. If a nurse is found to be less than proficient in the delivery of safe care, how should the nurse manager remedy the situation?

6. Describe the where appropriate standards of care may be found. Explain whether each is an example of an internal or external standard of care.

7. Explain the importance of federal agencies in setting standards of care in health-care institutions.

8. What is the difference between consent and informed consent?

9. Look at the forms for advance directives and DNR policies in your institution. Do they follow the guidelines of the Patient Self-Determination Act?

10. What should a practicing nurse do to stay out of court? What should a nurse not do?

11. What impact would a law that prevents mandatory overtime have on nurses, nursing care, and the health-care industry?

Case Study to Promote Critical Reasoning

Mr. Evans, 40 years old, was admitted to the medical-surgical unit from the emergency department with a diagnosis of acute abdomen. He had a 20-year history of Crohn's disease and had been on prednisone, 20 mg, every day for the past year. Three months ago he was started on the new biological agent, etanercept, 50 mg, subcutaneously every week. His last dose was 4 days ago. Because he was allowed nothing by mouth (NPO), total parenteral nutrition was started through a triple-lumen central venous catheter line, and his steroids were changed to Solu-Medrol, 60 mg, by intravenous (IV) push every 6 hours. He was also receiving several IV antibiotics and medication for pain and nausea.

Over the next 3 days, his condition worsened. He was in severe pain and needed more analgesics. One evening at 9 p.m., it was discovered that his central venous catheter line was out. The registered nurse notified the physician, who stated that a surgeon would come in the morning to replace it. The nurse failed to ask the physician what to do about the IV steroids, antibiotics, and fluid replacement; the client was still NPO. She also failed to ask about the etanercept. At 7 a.m., the night nurse noticed that the client had had no urinary output since 11 p.m. the night before. She failed to report this information to the day shift.

The client's physician made rounds at 9 a.m. The nurse for Mr. Evans did not discuss the fact that the client had not voided since 11 p.m., did not request orders for alternative delivery of the steroids and antibiotics, and did not ask about administering the etanercept. At 5 p.m. that evening, while Mr. Evans was having a computed tomography scan, his blood pressure dropped to 70 mm Hg, and because no one was in the scan room with him, he coded. He was transported to the ICU and intubated. He developed severe sepsis and acute respiratory distress syndrome.

1. List all the problems you can find with the nursing care in this case.

2. What were the nursing responsibilities in reporting information?

3. What do you think was the possible cause of the drop in Mr. Evans' blood pressure and his subsequent code?

4. If you worked in risk management, how would you discuss this situation with the nurse manager and the staff?

References

Aiken, T.D. (2004). *Legal, Ethical and Political Issues in Nursing,* 2nd ed. Philadelphia: FA Davis.

American Nurses Association (ANA) 2000. http://www. nursingworld.org/MainMenuCategories/ANAMarketplace/ ANAPeriodicals/TAN/2000/JanFebShortStaffing.aspx

American Nurses Association (ANA). (1998). Legal aspects of standards and guidelines for clinical nursing practice. Washington, DC: ANA.

American Nurses Association (ANA). (2004). Nursing: Scope and standards of practice. Pub 03SSNP. Washington, DC: ANA.

American Nurses Association (ANA). (1992). Position statement on nursing care and do not resuscitate decisions. Washington, DC: ANA.

American Nurses Association (ANA). (2002). Scope and standards of neuroscience nursing practice. Pub NNS22. Washington, DC: ANA.

Balas, M., Scott, L., & Rogers, A. (2004). The prevalence and nature of errors and near errors reported by hospital staff nurses. *Applied Nursing Research, 17*(4), 224–230.

Beckman, J.P. (1995). *Nursing Malpractice: Implications for Clinical Practice and Nursing Education.* Seattle: Washington University Press.

Bernzweig, E.P. (1996). *The Nurse's Liability for Malpractice: A Programmed Text,* 6th ed. St. Louis: C.V. Mosby.

Black, H.C. (2004). In Gardner, B.A. (ed.). *Black's Law Dictionary,* 8th ed. St. Paul: West Publishing.

Blais, K.K., Hayes, J.S., Kozier, B., et al. (2006). *Professional Nursing Practice: Concepts and Perspectives,* 5th ed. Upper Saddle River, N.J.: Prentice-Hall.

Canadian Nurses Association. Canadian registered nurse examination. Retrieved on December 20, 2005, from www. cna-aiic.ca

Catalano, J.T. (2000). *Nursing Now! Today's Issue, Tomorrow's Trends,* 2nd ed. Philadelphia: FA Davis.

Charters, K.G. (2003). HIPAA's latest privacy rule. *Policy, Politics & Nursing Practice, 4*(1), 75–78.

Cushing, M. (1999). *Nursing Jurisprudence.* Upper Saddle River, N.J.: Prentice-Hall.

Ellis, J.R., & Hartley, C.L. (2004). *Nursing in Today's World: Trends, Issues and Management,* 8th ed. Philadelphia: Lippincott, Williams & Wilkins.

Flarey, D. (1991). Advanced directives: In search of self-determination. *Journal of Nursing Administration, 21*(11), 17.

Giese v. Stice. 567 NW 2d 156 (Nebraska, 1997).

Guido, G.W. (2001). *Legal and Ethical Issues in Nursing,* 3rd ed. Upper Saddle River, N.J.: Prentice-Hall.

Hickey, J. (2002). *Clinical Practice of Neurological and Neurosurgical Nursing,* 5th ed. Philadelphia: Lippincott, Williams and Wilkins.

Kozier, B., Erb, G., Blais, K., et al. (1995). *Fundamentals of Nursing: Concepts, Process and Practice,* 15th ed. Menlo Park, Calif.: Addison-Wesley.

National Council of State Boards of Nursing. (2005). Fast facts about alternative item formats and the NCLEX examination. Retrieved on December 27, 2005, from www.ncsbn.org

National Council of State Boards of Nursing. (2004). Nursing regulation. Retrieved on December 16, 2005, from www.ncsbn.org

National Council of State Boards of Nursing. (2007). 2007 NCLEX-RN test plan. Retrieved on October 30, 2008, from www.ncsbn.org

Northrop, C.E., & Kelly, M.E. (1987). *State of New Jersey v. Winter.* Legal Issues in Nursing. St. Louis: CV Mosby.

Patient Self-Care Determination Act. (1989). S.R. 13566, Congressional Record.

Prosser, W.L., & Keeton, D. (1984). *The Law of Torts,* 5th ed. St. Paul: West Publishing.

Reigle, J. (1992). Preserving patient self-determination through advance directives. *Heart Lung, 21*(2), 196–198.

Taylor, C., Lillils, C., & LeMone, P. (2008). *Fundamentals of Nursing: The Art and Science of Nursing Care.* Philadelphia: Lippincott, Williams & Wilkins.

Tovar v. Methodist Healthcare. (2005). S.W. 3d WL 3079074 (Texas App., 2005).

Vernarec, E. (2000). Just say no to mandatory overtime. *RN 63*(12), 69–72.

Wendland v. Sparks. (1998). 574 N.W. 2d 327 (Iowa, 1998).

Young v. GastroIntestinal Center, Inc. (2005). S.W. 3d WL 675751 (Arkansas, 2005).

chapter **4**

Questions of Values and Ethics

◉ ○ ○ ○ ○ ○ ○ ○ ○ ○

OBJECTIVES

After reading this chapter, the student should be able to:

- Discuss the way values are formed.
- Differentiate between personal ethics and professional ethics.
- Compare and contrast various ethical theories.
- Discuss virtue ethics.
- Apply the seven basic ethical principles to an ethical issue.
- Analyze the impact that sociocultural factors have on ethical decision making by nursing personnel.
- Discuss the influence organizational ethics have on nursing practice.
- Identify an ethical dilemma in the clinical setting.
- Discuss current ethical issues in health care and possible solutions.

It is 1961. In a large metropolitan hospital, ten health-care professionals are meeting to consider the cases of three individuals. Ironically, the cases have something in common. Larry Jones, age 66, Irma Kolnick, age 31, and Nancy Roberts, age 10, are all suffering from chronic renal failure and need hemodialysis. Equipment is scarce, the cost of the treatment is prohibitive, and it is doubtful that treatment will be covered by health insurance. The hospital is able to provide this treatment to only one of these individuals. Who shall live, and who shall die? In a novel of the same name, Noah Gordon called this decision-making group The Death Committee (Gordon, 1963). Today, such groups are referred to as ethics committees.

In previous centuries, health-care practitioners had neither the knowledge nor the technology to prolong life. The main function of nurses and physicians was to support patients through times of illness, help them toward recovery, or keep them comfortable until death. There were few "who shall live, and who shall die?" decisions.

The polio epidemic that raged through Europe and the United States during 1947–1948 initiated the development of units for patients on manual ventilation (the "iron lung"). At this time, Danish physicians invented a method of manual ventilation by using a tube placed in the trachea of polio patients. This was the beginning of mechanical ventilation as we know it today.

During the 1950s, the development of mechanical ventilation required more intensive nursing care and patient observation. The care and monitoring of patients proved to be more efficient when they were kept in a single care area; hence the term *intensive care.* The late 1960s brought greater technological advances, especially in the care of patients seriously ill with cardiovascular disease. These new therapies and monitoring methods made the intensive care unit possible (aacn.org, 2006).

Health care now can keep alive people who would die without intervention. The development of new drugs and advances in biomechanical technology permit physicians and nurses to challenge nature. This progress also brings new, perplexing questions. The ability to prolong life has created some heartbreaking situations for families and terrible ethical dilemmas for health-care professionals. How is the decision made when to turn off the life support machines that are keeping someone's

son or daughter alive after, for example, a motor vehicle accident? Families and professionals face some of the most difficult ethical decisions at times like this. How is death defined? When does it occur? Perhaps these questions need to be asked: "What is life? Is there ever a time when life is no longer worth living?"

Health-care professionals have looked to philosophy, especially the branch that deals with human behavior, for resolution of these issues. The field of biomedical ethics (or, simply, bioethics), a subdiscipline of ethics—the philosophical study of morality—has evolved. In essence, bioethics is the study of medical morality, which concerns the moral and social implications of health care and science in human life (Mappes & DeGrazia, 2005).

To understand biomedical ethics, the basic concepts of values, belief systems, ethical theories, and morality are defined, followed by a discussion of the resolution of ethical dilemmas in health care.

Values

Webster's New World Dictionary (2000) defines *values* as the "estimated or appraised worth of something, or that quality of a thing that makes it more or less desirable, useful." Values, then, are judgments about the importance or unimportance of objects, ideas, attitudes, and attributes. Values become a part of a person's conscience and worldview. They provide a frame of reference and act as pilots to guide behaviors and assist people in making choices.

Values and Moral Reasoning

Reasoning entails the use of abstractions to think creatively for the purpose of answering questions, solving problems, and formulating a plan that determine actions (Butts & Rich, 2008). Reasoning allows individuals to think for themselves and to not accept the beliefs and judgments of others at face value. Moral reasoning relates to reasoning centered around moral and/or ethical issues. Different values, viewpoints, and methods of moral reasoning have developed over time. Older worldviews have now emerged in modern history, such as the emphasis on virtue ethics or a focus on what type of person one would like to become (Butts & Rich). Virtue ethics are discussed later in this chapter.

Value Systems

A value system is a set of related values. For example, one person may value (believe to be important) societal aspects of life, such as money, objects, and status. Another person may value more abstract concepts, such as kindness, charity, and caring. Values may vary significantly, based on an individual's culture and religious upbringing. An individual's system of values frequently affects how he or she makes decisions. For example, one person may base a decision on cost, and another person placed in the same situation may base the decision on a more abstract quality, such as kindness. There are different categories of values:

■ *Intrinsic values* are those related to sustaining life, such as food and water (Steele & Harmon, 1983).
■ *Extrinsic values* are not essential to life. Things, people, and ideas, such as kindness, understanding, and material items, are extrinsically valuable.
■ *Personal values* are qualities that people consider valuable in their private lives. Such concepts as strong family ties and acceptance by others are personal values.
■ *Professional values* are qualities considered important by a professional group. Autonomy, integrity, and commitment are examples of professional values.

People's behaviors are motivated by values. Individuals take risks, relinquish their own comfort and security, and generate extraordinary efforts because of their values (Edge & Groves, 2005). Patients with traumatic brain injury may overcome tremendous barriers because they value independence. Race-car drivers may risk death or other serious injury because they value competition and winning.

Values also generate the standards by which people judge others. For example, someone who values work over leisure activities will look unfavorably on the coworker who refuses to work throughout the weekend. A person who believes that health is more important than wealth would approve of spending money on a relaxing vacation or perhaps joining a health club rather than putting the money in the bank.

Often people adopt the values of individuals they admire. For example, a nursing student may begin to value humor after observing it used effectively with patients. Values provide a guide for decision making and give additional meaning to life. Individuals develop a sense of satisfaction when they work toward achieving values that they believe are important.

How Values Are Developed

Values are learned (Wright, 1987). Values can be taught directly, incorporated through societal norms, and modeled through behavior. Children learn by watching their parents, friends, teachers, and religious leaders. Through continuous reinforcement, children eventually learn about and then adopt values as their own. Because of the values they hold dear, people often make great demands on themselves, ignoring the personal cost. For example:

> *David grew up in a family in which educational achievement was highly valued. Not surprisingly, he adopted this as one of his own values. At school, he worked very hard because some of the subjects did not come easily to him. When his grades did not reflect his great effort, he felt as though he had disappointed his family as well as himself. By the time David reached the age of 15, he had developed severe migraine headaches.*

Values change with experience and maturity. For example, young children often value objects, such as a favorite blanket or stuffed animal. Older children are more likely to value a particular event, such as a scouting expedition. As they enter adolescence, they may value peer opinion over the opinions of their parents. Young adults often value certain ideals, such as beauty and heroism. The values of adults are formed from all of these experiences as well as from learning and thought.

The number of values that people hold is not as important as what values they consider important. Choices are influenced by values. The way people use their own time and money, choose friends, and pursue a career are all influenced by values.

Values Clarification

Values clarification is deciding what one believes is important. It is the process that helps people become aware of their values. Values play an important role in everyday decision making. For this reason, nurses need to be aware of what they do and do not value. This process helps them to behave in a manner that is consistent with their values.

Both personal and professional values influence nurses' decisions. Understanding one's own values simplifies solving problems, making decisions, and developing better relationships with others when one begins to realize how others develop their values. Raths, Harmin, and Simon (1979) suggested using a three-step model of choosing, prizing, and acting, with seven substeps, to identify one's own values (Box 4-1).

You may have used this method when making the decision to go to nursing school. For some people, nursing is a first career; for others, it is a second career. Using the model in Box 4-1, the valuing process is analyzed:

1. **Choosing.** After researching alternative career options, you freely chose nursing school. This choice was most likely influenced by such factors as educational achievement and abilities, finances, support and encouragement from others, time, and feelings about people.
2. **Prizing.** Once the choice was made, you were satisfied with it and told your friends about it.
3. **Acting.** *You* have entered school and begun the journey to your new career. Later in your career, you may decide to return to school for a bachelor's or master's degree in nursing.

As you progressed through school, you probably started to develop a new set of values—your professional values. Professional values are those established as being important in your practice. These values include caring, quality of care, and ethical behaviors.

Belief Systems

Belief systems are an organized way of thinking about why people exist in the universe. The purpose of belief systems is to explain such issues as life and death, good and evil, and health and illness. Usually these systems include an ethical code that specifies appropriate behavior. People may have a personal belief system, may participate in a religion that provides such a system, or both.

Members of primitive societies worshiped events in nature. Unable to understand the science of weather, for example, early civilizations believed these events to be under the control of someone or something that needed to be appeased, and they developed rituals and ceremonies to appease these unknown entities. They called these entities gods and believed that certain behaviors either pleased or angered the gods. Because these societies associated certain behaviors with specific outcomes, they created a belief system that enabled them to function as a group.

As higher civilizations evolved, belief systems became more complex. Archeology has provided evidence of the religious practices of ancient civilizations (Wack, 1992). The Aztec, Mayan, Incan, and Polynesian cultures each had a religious belief system comprised of many gods and goddesses for the same functions. The Greek, Roman, Egyptian, and Scandinavian societies believed in a hierarchy of gods and goddesses. Although given different names by different cultures, it is very interesting that most of the deities had similar purposes. For example, Zeus was the Greek king of the gods, and Thor was the Norse god of thunder. Both used a thunderbolt as their symbol. Sociologists believe that these religions developed to explain what was then unexplainable. Human beings have a deep need to create order from chaos and to have logical explanations for events. Religion explains theologically what objective science cannot.

Along with the creation of rites and rituals, religions also developed codes of behaviors, or ethical codes. These codes contribute to the social order. There are rules regarding how to treat family members, neighbors, the young, and the old. Many religions also developed rules regarding marriage, sexual practices, business practices, property ownership, and inheritance.

The advancement of science certainly has not made belief systems any less important. In fact, the technology explosion has created an even greater need for these systems. Technological advances often place people in situations that justify religious convictions rather than oppose them. Many religions, particularly Christianity, focus on the will of

---

box 4-1

Values Clarification

Choosing
1. Choosing freely
2. Choosing from alternatives
3. Deciding after giving consideration to the consequences of each alternative

Prizing
4. Being satisfied about the choice
5. Being willing to declare the choice to others

Acting
6. Making the choice a part of one's worldview and incorporating it into behavior
7. Repeating the choice

Adapted from Raths, L.E., Harmon, M., & Simmons, S.B. (1979). Values and Teaching. *New York: Charles E. Merrill.*

a supreme being, and technology, for example, is considered a gift that allows health-care personnel to maintain the life of a loved one. Other religions, such as certain branches of Judaism, focus on free choice or free will, leaving such decisions in the hands of humankind. Many Jewish leaders believe that if genetic testing indicates, for instance, that an infant will be born with a disease such as Tay-Sachs, which causes severe suffering and ultimately death, an abortion may be an acceptable option.

Belief systems often help survivors in making decisions and living with them afterward. So far, more questions than answers have emerged from these technological advances. As science explains more and more previously unexplainable phenomena, people need beliefs and values to guide their use of this new knowledge.

Morals and Ethics

Although the terms *morals* and *ethics* are often used interchangeably, *ethics* usually refers to a standardized code as a guide to behaviors, whereas *morals* usually refers to an individual's own code for acceptable behavior.

Morals

Morals arise from an individual's conscience. They act as a guide for individual behavior and are learned through instruction and socialization. You may find, for example, that you and your patients disagree on the acceptability of certain behaviors, such as premarital sex, drug use, or gambling. Even in your nursing class, you will probably encounter some disagreements because each of you has developed a personal code that defines acceptable behavior.

Ethics

Ethics is the part of philosophy that deals with the rightness or wrongness of human behavior. It is also concerned with the motives behind behaviors. *Bioethics,* specifically, is the application of ethics to issues that pertain to life and death. The implication is that judgments can be made about the rightness or goodness of health-care practices.

Ethical Theories

Several ethical theories have emerged to justify moral principles (Guido, 2001). *Deontological theories* take their norms and rules from the duties that individuals owe each other by the goodness of the

commitments they make and the roles they take upon themselves. The term *deontological* comes from the Greek word *deon* (duty). This theory is attributed to the 18th-century philosopher Immanuel Kant (Kant, 1949). Deontological ethics considers the intention of the action, not the consequences of the action. In other words, it is the individual's good intentions or goodwill (Kant, 1949) that determines the worthiness or goodness of the action.

Teleological theories take their norms or rules for behaviors from the consequences of the action. This theory is also called *utilitarianism*. According to this concept, what makes an action right or wrong is its utility, or usefulness. Usefulness is considered to be the amount of happiness the action carries. "Right" encompasses actions that have good outcomes, whereas "wrong" is composed of actions that result in bad outcomes. This theory had its origins with David Hume, a Scottish philosopher. According to Hume, "Reason is and ought to be the slave of the passions" (Hume, 1978, p. 212). Based on this idea, ethics depends on what people want and desire. The passions determine what is right or wrong. However, individuals who follow teleological theory disagree on how to decide on the "rightness" or "wrongness" of an action (Guido, 2001) because individual passions differ.

Principalism is an arising theory receiving a great deal of attention in the biomedical ethics community. This theory integrates existing ethical principles and tries to resolve conflicts by relating one or more of these principles to a given situation. Ethical principles actually influence professional decision making more than ethical theories.

Ethical Principles

Ethical codes are based on principles that can be used to judge behavior. Ethical principles assist decision making because they are a standard for measuring actions. They may be the basis for laws, but they themselves are not laws. Laws are rules created by a governing body. Laws can operate because the government has the power to enforce them. They are usually quite specific, as are the punishments for disobeying them. Ethical principles are not confined to specific behaviors. They act as guides for appropriate behaviors. They also take into account the situation in which a decision must be made. Ethical principles speak to the essence or fundamentals of the law rather than to the exactness of the law (Macklin, 1987). Here is an example:

Mrs. Van Gruen, 82 years old, was admitted to the hospital in acute respiratory distress. She was diagnosed with aspiration pneumonia and soon became septic, developing adult respiratory distress syndrome. She had a living will, and her attorney was her designated health-care surrogate. Her competence to make decisions was uncertain because of her illness. The physician presented the situation to the attorney, indicating that without a feeding tube and tracheostomy Mrs. Van Gruen would die. According to the laws governing living wills and health-care surrogates, the attorney could have made the decision to withhold all treatments. However, he believed he had an ethical obligation to discuss the situation with his client. The client requested that the tracheostomy and the feeding tube be inserted, which was done.

In some situations, two or more principles may conflict with each other. Making a decision under these circumstances is very difficult. Following are several of the ethical principles that are most important to nursing practice—autonomy, nonmaleficence, beneficence, justice, confidentiality, veracity, and accountability—and a discussion of some of the ethical dilemmas that nurses encounter in clinical practice.

Autonomy

Autonomy is the freedom to make decisions for oneself. This ethical principle requires that nurses respect patients' rights to make their own choices about treatment. Informed consent before treatment, surgery, or participation in research is an example. To be able to make an autonomous choice, individuals need to be informed of the purpose, benefits, and risks of the procedures to which they are agreeing. Nurses accomplish this by providing information and supporting patients' choices.

Closely linked to the ethical principle of autonomy is the legal issue of competence. A patient needs to be deemed competent in order to make a decision regarding treatment options. When patients refuse treatment, health-care personnel and family members who think differently often question the patient's "competence" to make a decision. Of note is the fact that when patients agree with health-care treatment decisions, rarely is their competence questioned (AACN News, 2006).

Nurses are often in a position to protect a patient's autonomy. They do this by ensuring that others do not interfere with the patient's right to proceed with a decision. If a nurse observes that a patient has insufficient information to make an appropriate choice, is being forced into a decision, or is unable to understand the consequences of the choice, then the nurse may act as a patient advocate to ensure the principle of autonomy.

Sometimes nurses have difficulty with the principle of autonomy because it also requires respecting another's choice, even if the nurse disagrees with it. According to the principle of autonomy, a nurse cannot replace a patient's decision with his or her own, even when the nurse honestly believes that the patient has made the wrong choice. A nurse can, however, discuss concerns with patients and make sure patients have thought about the consequences of the decision they are about to make.

Nonmaleficence

The ethical principle of nonmaleficence requires that no harm be done, either deliberately or unintentionally. This rather complicated word comes from Latin roots: *non*, which means not; *male* (pronounced mah-leh), which means bad; and *facere*, which means to do.

The principle of nonmaleficence also requires that nurses protect from danger individuals who are unable to protect themselves because of their physical or mental condition. An infant, a person under anesthesia, and a person with Alzheimer's disease are examples of people with limited ability to protect themselves. Nurses are ethically obligated to protect their patients when the patients are unable to protect themselves.

Often, treatments meant to improve patient health lead to harm. This is not the intention of the nurse or of other health-care personnel, but it is a direct result of treatment. Nosocomial infections as a result of hospitalization are harmful to patients. The nurses did not deliberately cause the infection. The side effects of chemotherapy or radiation therapy may result in harm. Chemotherapeutic agents cause a decrease in immunity that may result in a severe infection, whereas radiation may burn or damage the skin. For this reason, many patients opt not to pursue treatments.

The obligation to do no harm extends to the nurse who for some reason is not functioning at an optimal level. For example, a nurse who is impaired by alcohol or drugs is knowingly placing patients at risk. Other nurses who observe such behavior have an ethical obligation to protect patients according to the principle of nonmaleficence.

Beneficence

The word "beneficence" also comes from Latin: *bene,* which means well, and *facere,* which means to do.

The principle of beneficence demands that good be done for the benefit of others. For nurses, this means more than delivering competent physical or technical care. It requires helping patients meet all their needs, whether physical, social, or emotional. Beneficence is caring in the truest sense, and caring fuses thought, feeling, and action. It requires knowing and being truly understanding of the situation and the thoughts and ideas of the individual (Benner & Wrubel, 1989).

Sometimes physicians, nurses, and families withhold information from patients for the sake of beneficence. The problem with doing this is that it does not allow competent individuals to make their own decisions based on all available information. In an attempt to be beneficent, the principle of autonomy is violated. This is just one of many examples of the ethical dilemmas encountered in nursing practice. For instance:

Mrs. Chung has just been admitted to the oncology unit with ovarian cancer. She is scheduled to begin chemotherapy treatment. Her two children and her husband have requested that the physician ensure that Mrs. Chung not be told her diagnosis because they believe she would not be able to cope with it. The information is communicated to the nursing staff. After the first treatment, Mrs. Chung becomes very ill. She refuses the next treatment, stating that she did not feel sick until she came to the hospital. She asks the nurse what could possibly be wrong with her that she needs a medicine that makes her sick when she does not feel sick. Only people who get cancer medicine get this sick! Mrs. Chung then asks the nurse, "Do I have cancer?"

As the nurse, you understand the order that the patient not be told her diagnosis. You also understand your role as a patient advocate.

1. To whom do you owe your duty: the family or the patient?
2. How do you think you may be able to be a patient advocate in this situation?

3. What information would you communicate to the family members, and how can you assist them in dealing with their mother's concerns?

Justice

The principle of justice obliges nurses and other health-care professionals to treat every person equally regardless of gender, sexual orientation, religion, ethnicity, disease, or social standing (Edge & Groves, 2005). This principle also applies in the work and educational setting. Everyone should be treated and judged by the same criteria according to this principle. Here is an example:

Mr. Johnson, found on the street by the police, was admitted through the emergency room to a medical unit. He was in deplorable condition: his clothes were dirty and ragged, he was unshaven, and he was covered with blood. His diagnosis was chronic alcoholism, complicated by esophageal varices and end-stage liver disease. Several nursing students overheard the staff discussing Mr. Johnson. The essence of the conversation was that no one wanted to care for him because he was dirty and smelly and brought this condition on himself. The students, upset by what they heard, went to their instructor about the situation. The instructor explained that every individual has a right to good care despite his or her economic or social position. This is the principle of justice.

The concept of *distributive justice* necessitates the fair allocation of responsibilities and advantages, especially in a society where resources may be limited (Davis, Arokar, Liaschenko, & Drought, 1997). Health-care costs have increased tremendously over the years, and access to care has become a social and political issue. In order to understand distributive justice, certain concepts need to be addressed: need, individual effort, ability to pay, contribution to society, and age (Davis, et al., p. 53).

Age has become an extremely controversial issue as it leads to quality-of-life questions, particularly technological care at the end of life. The other issue regarding age revolves around technology in neonatal care. How do health-care providers place value on one person's quality of life over that of another? Should millions of dollars be spent preserving the life of an 80-year-old man who volunteers in his community, plays golf twice a week, and teaches reading to underprivileged children, or should that money be spent on a 26-week-old fetus that will most likely require intensive therapies and treatments for a lifetime, adding up to more millions of health-care dollars? In the social and business world, welfare payments are based on need, and jobs and promotions are usually distributed on an individual's contributions and achievements. Is it possible to apply these measures to health-care allocations?

Philosopher John Rawls addressed the issues of justice as fairness and justice as the foundation of social structures. According to Rawls, the idea of the original position should be used to negotiate the principles of justice. The original position based on Kant's social contract theory presents a hypothetical situation in which individuals act as a trustee for the interests of all individuals. The individuals, known as negotiators, are knowledgeable in the areas of sociology, political science, and economics. However, they are placed under certain limitations referred to as the *veil of ignorance.* These limitations represent the moral essentials of original position arguments.

The veil of ignorance eliminates information about age, gender, socioeconomic status, and religious convictions from the issues. Once this information is unavailable to the negotiators, the vested interests of involved parties disappear. According to Rawls, in a just society the rights protected by justice are not issues for political bargaining or subject to the calculations of social interests. Simply put, everyone has the same rights and liberties.

Fidelity

The principle of fidelity requires loyalty. It is a promise that the individual will fulfill all commitments made to himself or herself and to others. For nurses, fidelity includes the professional's loyalty to fulfill all responsibilities and agreements expected as part of professional practice. Fidelity is the basis for the concept of accountability—taking responsibility for one's own actions (Shirey, 2005).

Confidentiality

The principle of confidentiality states that anything said to nurses and other health-care providers by their patients must be held in the strictest confidence. Confidentiality presents both a legal and an ethical issue. Exceptions exist only when patients give permission for the release of information or when the law requires the release of specific information. Sometimes, just sharing information

without revealing an individual's name can be a breach in confidentiality if the situation and the individual are identifiable. It is important to realize that what seems like a harmless statement can become harmful if other people can piece together bits of information and identify the patient.

Nurses come into contact with people from different walks of life. Within communities, people know other people who know other people, and so on. Individuals have lost families, jobs, and insurance coverage because nurses shared confidential information and others acted on that knowledge (AIDS Update Conference, 1995).

In today's electronic environment, the principle of confidentiality has become a major concern. Many health-care institutions, insurance companies, and businesses use electronic media to transfer information. These institutions store sensitive and confidential information in computer databases. These databases need to have security safeguards to prevent unauthorized access. Health-care institutions have addressed the situation through the use of limited access, authorization passwords, and security tracking systems. However, even the most secure system is vulnerable and can be accessed by an individual who understands the complexities of computer systems.

Veracity

Veracity requires nurses to be truthful. Truth is fundamental to building a trusting relationship. Intentionally deceiving or misleading a patient is a violation of this principle. Deliberately omitting a part of the truth is deception and violates the principle of veracity. This principle often creates ethical dilemmas. When is it permissible to lie? Some ethicists believe it is never appropriate to deceive another individual. Others think that if another ethical principle overrides veracity, then lying is permissible. Consider this situation:

Ms. Allen has just been told that her father has Alzheimer's disease. The nurse practitioner wants to come into the home to discuss treatment. Ms. Allen refuses, saying that the nurse practitioner should under no circumstances tell her father the diagnosis. She explains to the practitioner that she is sure he will kill himself if he learns that he has Alzheimer's disease. She bases this concern on statements he has made regarding this disease. The nurse practitioner replies that medication is available that might help her father. However, it is available only through a research study being conducted at a nearby university. To participate in the research, the patient must be informed of the purpose of the study, the medication to be given and its side effects, and follow-up procedures. Ms. Allen continues to refuse to allow her father to be told his diagnosis because she is certain he will commit suicide.

The nurse practitioner faces a dilemma: does he abide by Ms. Allen's wishes based on the principle of beneficence, or does he abide by the principle of veracity and inform his patient of the diagnosis. What would you do?

Accountability

Accountability is linked to fidelity and means accepting responsibility for one's actions. Nurses are accountable to their patients and to their colleagues. When providing care to patients, nurses are responsible for their actions, good and poor. If something was not done, do not chart or tell a colleague that it was. An example of violating accountability is the story of Anna:

Anna was a registered nurse who worked nights on an acute care unit. She was an excellent nurse, but as the acuity of the patients' conditions increased, she was unable to keep up with both patients' needs and the technology, particularly intravenous (IV) lines. She began to chart that all the IVs were infusing as they should, even when they were not. Each morning, the day shift would find that the actual infused amount did not agree with what the paperwork showed. One night, Anna allowed an entire liter to be infused in 2 hours into a patient with congestive heart failure. When the day staff came on duty, they found the patient expired, the bag empty, and the tubing filled with blood. Anna's IV sheet showed 800 mL left in the bag. It was not until a lawsuit was filed that Anna took responsibility for her behavior.

The idea of a standard of care evolves from the principle of accountability. Standards of care provide a rule for measuring nursing actions.

Ethical Codes

A code of ethics is a formal statement of the rules of ethical behavior for a particular group of individuals. A code of ethics is one of the hallmarks of a profession. This code makes clear the behavior expected of its members.

The Code of Ethics for Nurses with Interpretive Statements provides values, standards, and principles to help nursing function as a profession. The original code was developed in 1985. In 1995 the American Nurses Association Board of Directors and the Congress on Nursing Practice initiated the Code of Ethics Project (ANA, 2002). The code may be viewed online at nursingworld.org

Ethical codes are subject to change. They reflect the values of the profession and the society for which they were developed. Changes occur as society and technology evolve. For example, years ago no thought was given to do not resuscitate (DNR) orders or withholding food and fluids. Technological advances have since made it possible to keep people in a kind of twilight life, comatose and unable to participate in living in any way, but nevertheless making DNR and withholding very important issues in health care. Technology has increased knowledge and skills, but the ability to make decisions regarding care is still guided by the principles of autonomy, nonmaleficence, beneficence, justice, confidentiality, fidelity, veracity, and accountability.

Virtue Ethics

Virtue ethics focuses on virtues, or moral character, rather than on duties or rules that emphasize the consequences of actions. Take the following example:

Norman is driving along the road and finds a crying child sitting by a fallen bicycle. It is obvious that the child needs assistance. From one ethical standpoint (utilitarianism), helping the child will increase Norman's personal feelings of "doing good." The deontological stance states that by helping, Norman is behaving in accordance with a moral rule such as "Do unto others...." Virtue ethics looks at the fact that helping the person would be charitable or benevolent.

Plato and Aristotle are considered the founders of virtue ethics. Its roots can be found in Chinese philosophy. During the 1800s virtue ethics disappeared, but in the late 1950s it reemerged as an Anglo-American philosophy. Neither deontology nor utilitarianism considered the virtues of moral character and education and the question: "What type of person should I be, and how should I live" (Hooker, 2000; Driver, 2001). Virtues include such qualities as honesty, generosity, altruism, and reliability. They are concerned with many other elements as well, such as emotions and emotional reactions, choices, values, needs, insights, attitudes, interests, and expectations. To embrace a virtue means that you are a person with a certain complex way of thinking. Nursing has practiced virtue ethics for many years.

Nursing Ethics

Up to this point, the ethical principles discussed apply to ethics for nurses; however, nurses do not customarily find themselves enmeshed in the biomedical ethical decision-making processes that gain the attention of the news media. However, the ethical principles that guide nursing practice are rooted in the philosophy and science of health care and are considered a subcategory of bioethics (Butts & Rich, 2008).

Nursing ethics deals with the experiences and needs of nurses and nurses' perceptions of their experiences (Varcoe, et al., 2004). It is viewed from the perspective of nursing theory and practice (Johnstone, 1999). Relationships are the center of nursing ethics. These relationships focus on ethical issues that impact nurses and their patients.

Organizational Ethics

Organizational ethics focus on the workplace and are aimed at the organizational level. Every organization, even one with hundreds of thousands of employees, consists of individuals. Each individual makes his and her own decisions about how to behave in the workplace. Each person has the opportunity to make the organization a more or less ethical place. These individual decisions can have a powerful effect on the lives of many others in the organization as well as in the surrounding community. Shirey (2005) explains that employees need to experience uniformity between what the organization states and what it practices.

Research conducted by the Ethics Research Center concluded the following:

- If positive outcomes are desired, ethical culture is what makes the difference;
- Leadership, especially senior leadership, is the most critical factor in promoting an ethical culture; and
- In organizations that are trying to strengthen their culture, formal program elements can help to do that (Harned, 2005, p. 1).

When looking for a professional position, it is important to consider the organizational culture.

What are the values and beliefs of the organization? Do they blend with yours, or are they in conflict with your value system? To find out this information, look at the organization's mission, vision, and value statements. Speak with other nurses who work in the organization. Do they see consistency between what the organization states and what it actually expects from the employees? For example, if an organization states that it collaborates with the nurses in decision making, do nurses sit on committees that have input into the decision-making process?

Ethical Issues on the Nursing Unit

Organizational ethics refer to the values and expected behaviors entrenched within the organizational culture. The nursing unit represents a subculture of the organization. Ideally, the nursing unit should mirror the ethical atmosphere and culture of the organization. This requires the individuals that comprise the unit to hold the same values and model the expected behaviors.

Conflicts of the values and ethics among individuals who work together on the unit often create issues that result in moral suffering for some nurses. Moral suffering occurs when nurses experience a feeling of uneasiness or concern regarding behaviors or circumstances that challenge their own moral beliefs and values. These situations may be the result of unit policies, physicians' orders that the nurse believes may not be beneficial for the patient, professional behaviors of colleagues, or family attitudes about the patient.

Perhaps one of the most disconcerting ethical issues nurses on the unit face is the one that challenges their professional values and ethics. Friendships often emerge from work relationships, and these friendships may interfere with judgments. Similarly, strong negative feelings may cloud a nurse's ability to view a situation fairly and without prejudice. Take the following example:

Addie and Jamie attended nursing school together and developed a strong friendship. They work together on the pediatric surgical unit of a large teaching hospital. Jamie made a medication error that caused a problem, resulting in a child having to be transferred to the intensive care unit. Addie realized what had happened and confronted Jamie. Jamie begged her not to say anything. Addie knew the error should be reported, but how would this affect her long time friendship with Jamie? Taking this situation to the other extreme, if a friendship had not been involved, would Addie react the same way?

When working with others, it is important to hold true to your personal values and morals. Practicing virtue ethics, i.e., "doing the right thing," may cause difficulty due to the possible consequences of the action. Nurses should support each other but not at the expense of patients or each other's professional duties. There are times when not acting virtuously may cause a colleague more harm.

Ethical Dilemmas

What is a dilemma? The word *dilemma* is of Greek derivation. A lemma was an animal resembling a ram and having two horns. Thus came the saying "stuck on the horns of a dilemma." The story of Hugo illustrates a hypothetical dilemma, with a touch of humor:

One day, Hugo, dressed in a bright red cape, walked through his village into the countryside. The wind caught the corners of the cape, and it was whipped in all directions. As he walked down the dusty road, Hugo happened to pass by a lemma. Hugo's bright red cape caught the lemma's attention. Lowering its head, with its two horns poised in attack position, the animal began to chase Hugo down the road. Panting and exhausted, Hugo reached the end of the road, only to find himself blocked by a huge stone wall. He turned to face the lemma, which was ready to charge. A decision needed to be made, and Hugo's life depended on this decision. If he moved to the left, the lemma would gore his heart. If he moved to the right, the lemma would gore his liver. No matter what his decision, Hugo would be "stuck on the horns of the lemma."

Like Hugo, nurses are often faced with difficult dilemmas. Also, as Hugo found, an ethical dilemma can be a choice between two serious alternatives.

An ethical dilemma occurs when a problem exists that forces a choice between two or more ethical principles. Deciding in favor of one principle will violate the other. Both sides have goodness and badness to them, but neither decision satisfies all the criteria that apply. Ethical dilemmas also have the added burden of emotions. Feelings of anger, frustration, and fear often override rationality in the decision-making process. Consider the case of Mr. Sussman:

Mr. Sussman, 80 years old, was admitted to the neuroscience unit after suffering left hemispheric

bleeding. He had a total right hemiplegia and was completely nonresponsive, with a Glasgow Coma Scale score of 8. He had been on IV fluids for 4 days, and the question was raised of placing a percutaneous endoscopic gastrostomy (PEG) tube for enteral feedings. The older of the two children asked what the chances of recovery were. The physician explained that Mr. Sussman's current state was probably the best he could attain but that "miracles happen every day" and stated that tests could help in determining the prognosis. The family asked that these tests be performed. After the results were in, the physician explained that the prognosis was grave and that IV fluids were insufficient to sustain life. The PEG tube would be a necessity if the family wished to continue with food and fluids. After the physician left, the family asked the nurse, Gail, who had been with Mr. Sussman during the previous 3 days, "If this was your father, what would you do?" This situation became an ethical dilemma for Gail as well.

If you were Gail, what would you say to the family? Depending on your answer, what would be the possible principles that you might violate?

Resolving Ethical Dilemmas Faced by Nurses

Ethical dilemmas can occur in any aspect of life, personal or professional. This section focuses on the resolution of professional dilemmas. The various models for resolving ethical dilemmas consist of 5 to 14 sequential steps. Each step begins with the complete understanding of the dilemma and concludes with the evaluation of the implemented decision.

The nursing process provides a helpful mechanism for finding solutions to ethical dilemmas. The first step is assessment, including identification of the problem. The simplest way to do this is to create a statement that summarizes the issue. The remainder of the process evolves from this statement (Box 4-2).

Assessment

Ask yourself, "Am I directly involved in this dilemma?" An issue is not an ethical dilemma for nurses unless they are directly involved or have been asked for their opinion about a situation. Some nurses involve themselves in situations even when their

box 4-2

Questions to Help Resolve Ethical Dilemmas

- What are the medical facts?
- What are the psychosocial facts?
- What are the patient's wishes?
- What values are in conflict?

opinion has not been solicited. This is generally unwarranted, unless the issue involves a violation of the professional code of ethics.

Nurses are frequently in the position of hearing both sides of an ethical dilemma. Often, all that is wanted is an empathetic listener. At other times, when guidance is requested, nurses can help people work through the decision-making process (remember the principle of autonomy).

Collecting data from all the decision makers helps identify the reasoning process being used by these individuals as they struggle with the issue. The following questions assist in the information-gathering process:

- *What are the medical facts?* Find out how the physicians, physical and occupational therapists, dietitians, and nurses view the patient's condition and treatment options. Speak with the patient, if possible, and determine his or her understanding of the situation.
- *What are the psychosocial facts?* In what emotional state is the patient right now? The patient's family? What kind of relationship exists between the patient and his or her family? What are the patient's living conditions? Who are the individuals who form the patient's support system? How are they involved in the patient's care? What is the patient's ability to make medical decisions about his or her care? Do financial considerations need to be taken into account? What does the patient value? What does the patient's family value? The answers to these questions will provide a better understanding of the situation. Ask more questions, if necessary, to complete the picture. The social facts of a situation also include institutional policies, legal aspects, and economic factors. The personal belief systems of physicians and other health-care professionals also influence this aspect.
- *What are the cultural beliefs?* Cultural beliefs play a major role in ethical decisions. Some cultures do

not allow surgical interventions as they fear that the "life force" may escape. Many cultures forbid organ donation. Other cultures focus on the sanctity of life, thereby requesting all methods for sustaining life be used regardless of the futility.

- *What are the patient's wishes?* Remember the ethical principle of autonomy. With very few exceptions, if the patient is competent, his or her decisions take precedence. Too often, the family's or physician's worldview and belief system overshadow those of the patient. Nurses can assist by maintaining the focus on the patient. If the patient is unable to communicate, try to discover whether the individual has discussed the issue in the past. If the patient has completed a living will or designated a health-care surrogate, this will help determine the patient's wishes. By interviewing family members, the nurse can often learn about conversations in which the patient has voiced his or her feelings about treatment decisions. Through guided interviewing, the nurse can encourage the family to tell anecdotes that provide relevant insights into the patient's values and beliefs.
- *What values are in conflict?* To assess values, begin by listing each person involved in the situation. Then identify the values represented by each person. Ask such questions as, "What do you feel is the most pressing issue here?" and "Tell me more about your feelings regarding this situation." In some cases, there may be little disagreement among the people involved, just a different way of expressing beliefs. In others, however, a serious value conflict may exist.

Planning

For planning to be successful, everyone involved in the decision must be included in the process. Thompson and Thompson (1992) listed three specific and integrated phases of this planning:

1. *Determine the goals of treatment.* Is cure a goal, or is the goal to keep the patient comfortable? Is life at any cost the goal, or is the goal a peaceful death at home? These goals need to be patient-focused, reality-centered, and attainable. They should be consistent with current medical treatment and, if possible, be measurable according to an established period.
2. *Identify the decision makers.* As mentioned earlier, nurses may or may not be decision makers in

these health-related ethical dilemmas. It is important to know who the decision makers are and what their belief systems are. When the patient is a capable participant, this task is much easier. However, people who are ill are often too exhausted to speak for themselves or to ensure that their voices are heard. When this happens, the patient needs an advocate. Family, friends, spiritual advisers, and nurses often act as advocates. A family member may need to be designated as the primary decision maker, a role often called the *health-care surrogate.*

The creation of living wills, establishment of advance directives, and appointment of a health-care surrogate while a person is still healthy often ease the burden for the decision makers during a later crisis. Patients can exercise autonomy through these mechanisms, even though they may no longer be able to communicate their wishes directly. When these documents are not available, the information gathered during the assessment of social factors helps identify those individuals who may be able to act in the patient's best interest.

3. *List and rank all the options.* Performing this task involves all the decision makers. It is sometimes helpful to begin with the least desired choice and methodically work toward the preferred treatment choice that is most likely to lead to the desired outcome. Asking all participating parties to discuss what they believe are reasonable outcomes to be attained with the use of available medical treatment often helps in the decision process. By listening to others in a controlled situation, family members and health-care professionals discover that they actually want the same result as the patient but had different ideas about how to achieve their goal.

Implementation

During the implementation phase, the patient or the surrogate (substitute) decision maker(s) and members of the health-care team reach a mutually acceptable decision. This occurs through open discussion and sometimes negotiation. An example of negotiation follows:

Elena's mother has metastatic ovarian cancer. She and Elena have discussed treatment options. Her physician suggested the use of a new chemotherapeutic agent that has demonstrated success in many cases. But Elena's mother emphatically states that she has "had enough" and prefers to spend her remaining time doing whatever she chooses. Elena wants her mother to try the drug. To resolve the dilemma, the oncology nurse practitioner and the physician talk with Elena and her mother. Everyone reviews the facts and expresses their feelings about the situation. Seeing Elena's distress, Elena's mother says, "OK, I will try the Taxol for a month. If there is no improvement after this time, I want to stop all treatment and live out the time I have with my daughter and her family." All agreed that this was a reasonable decision.

The role of the nurse during the implementation phase is to ensure that communication does not break down. Ethical dilemmas are often emotional issues, filled with guilt, sorrow, anger, and other strong emotions. These strong feelings can cause communication failures among decision makers. Remind yourself, "I am here to do what is best for this patient."

Keep in mind that an ethical dilemma is not always a choice between two attractive alternatives. Many are between two unattractive, even unpleasant, choices. Elena's mother's options did not include the choice she really wanted: good health and a long life.

Once an agreement is reached, the decision makers must accept it. Sometimes, an agreement is not reached because the parties cannot reconcile their conflicting belief systems or values. At other times, caregivers are unable to recognize the worth of the patient's point of view. Occasionally, the patient or the surrogate may make a request that is not institutionally or legally possible. In some cases, a different institution or physician may be able to honor the request. In other cases, the patient or surrogate may request information from the nurse regarding illegal acts. When this happens, the nurse should ask the patient and family to consider the consequences of their proposed actions. It may be necessary to bring other counselors into the discussion (with the patient's permission) to negotiate an agreement.

Evaluation

As in the nursing process, the purpose of evaluation in resolving ethical dilemmas is to determine whether the desired outcomes have occurred. In the case of Mr. Sussman, some of the questions that could be posed by Gail to the family are as follows:

- "I have noticed the amount of time you have been spending with your father. Have you observed any changes in his condition?"
- "I see Dr. Washburn spoke to you about the test results and your father's prognosis. How do you feel about the situation?"
- "Now that Dr. Washburn has spoken to you about your father's condition, have you considered future alternatives?"

Changes in patient status, availability of medical treatment, and social facts may call for reevaluation of a situation. The course of treatment may need to be altered. Continued communication and cooperation among the decision makers are essential.

Another model, the MORAL model created by Thiroux (1977) and refined for nursing by Halloran (1982), is gaining popularity. The MORAL acronym reminds nurses of the sequential steps needed for resolving an ethical dilemma. This ethical decision-making model is easily implemented in all patient care settings (Box 4-3).

Current Ethical Issues

During fall 1998, Dr. Jack Kevorkian (sometimes called Dr. Death in the media) openly admitted that at the patient's request, he gave the patient a lethal dose of medication, causing death. His statement raised the consciousness of the American people and the health-care system about the issues of euthanasia and assisted suicide. Do individuals have the right to consciously end their own lives when they are suffering from terminal conditions? If they are unable to perform the act themselves, should others assist them in ending their lives? Should assisted suicide be legal? There are no answers to these difficult questions, and patients and their families face these same questions every day.

---

box 4-3

The Moral Model

M: Massage the dilemma

O: Outline the option

R: Resolve the dilemma

A: Act by applying the chosen option

L: Look back and evaluate the complete process, including actions taken

---

More recently, the Terri Schiavo case gained tremendous media attention, probably becoming the most important case of clinical ethics in more than a decade. Her illness and death created a major medical, legal, theological, ethical, political, and social controversy. The case brought to the forefront the deep divisions and fears that reside in society regarding life and death, the role of the government and courts in life decisions, and the treatment of disabled persons. Many aspects of this case will never be clarified; however, many questions raised by this case need to be addressed for future ethical decision making. Some of these are:

1. What is the true definition of a persistent vegetative state?
2. How is cognitive recovery determined?
3. What role do the courts play when there is a family dispute? Who has the right to make decisions when an individual is married?
4. What are the duties of surrogate decision makers? (Hook & Mueller, 2005)

The primary goal of nursing and other health-care professions is to keep people alive and well or, if this cannot be done, to help them live with their problems and die peacefully. To accomplish this, health-care professionals struggle to improve their knowledge and skills so they can care for their patients, provide them with some quality of life, and help return them to wellness. The costs involved in achieving this goal can be astronomical.

Questions are being raised more and more often about who should receive the benefits of this technology. Managed care and the competition for resources are also creating ethical dilemmas. Other difficult questions, such as who should pay for care when the illness may have been due to poor health-care practices such as smoking or substance abuse, are also being debated.

Practice Issues Related to Technology

Genetics and the Limitations of Technology

In issues of technology, the principles of beneficence and nonmaleficence may be in conflict. A specific technology administered with the intention of "doing good" may result in enormous suffering. Causing this type of torment is in direct conflict with the idea of "do no harm" (Burkhardt & Nathaniel, 2007). At times, this is an accepted consequence, such as in the use of chemotherapy. However, the ultimate outcome in this case is that recovery is expected. In situations in which little or no improvement is expected, the issue of whether the good outweighs the bad prevails. Suffering induced by technology may include physical, spiritual, and emotional components for the patient and the families.

Today, many infants who have low birth weight or birth defects, who not so long ago would have been considered unable to live, are maintained on machines in highly sophisticated neonatal units. This process may keep babies alive only to die several months later or may leave them with severe chronic disabilities. Children with chronic disabilities require additional medical, educational, and social services. These services are expensive and often require families to travel long distances to obtain them (Urbano, 1992).

Genetic diagnosis and gene therapy present new ethical issues for nursing. *Genetic diagnosis* is a process that involves analyzing parents or an embryo for a genetic disorder. This is usually done before in vitro fertilization for couples who run a high risk of conceiving a child with a genetic disorder. The embryos are tested, and only those that are free of genetic flaws are implanted.

Genetic screening is used as a tool to determine whether couples hold the possibility of giving birth to a genetically impaired infant. Testing for the most common genetic disorders has become an expected standard of practice of health-care providers caring for women who are planning to become pregnant or who are pregnant. Couples are encouraged to seek out information regarding their genetic health history in order to identify the possibilities of having a child with a genetic disorder. If a couple has one child with a genetic disorder, genetic specialists test the parents or the fetus for the presence of the gene.

Genetic screening leads to issues pertaining to reproductive rights. It also opens new issues. What is a disability versus a disorder, and who decides this? Is a disability a disease, and does it need to be cured or prevented? The technology is also used to determine whether individuals are predisposed to certain diseases, such as breast cancer or Huntington's chorea. This has created additional ethical issues regarding genetic screening. For example:

Bianca, 33 years old, is diagnosed with breast cancer. She has two daughters, ages 6 and 4 years. Bianca's mother and grandmother had breast cancer. Neither

survived more than 5 years post treatment. Bianca undergoes a lumpectomy followed by radiation and chemotherapy. Her cancer is found to be nonhormonally-dependent. Due to her age and family history, Bianca's oncologist recommends that she see a geneticist and have genetic testing for the BRCA-1 *and* BRCA-2 *genes. Bianca makes an appointment to discuss the testing. She meets with the nurse who has additional education in genetics and discusses the following questions: "If I am positive for the genes, what are my options? Should I have a bilateral mastectomy with reconstruction?" "Will I be able to get health insurance coverage, or will the companies consider this to be a preexisting condition?" "What are the future implications for my daughters?"*

If you were the nurse, how would you address these concerns?

Genetic engineering is the ability to change the genetic structure of an organism. Through this process, researchers have created disease-resistant fruits and vegetables and certain medications, such as insulin. This process theoretically allows for the genetic alteration of embryos, eliminating genetic flaws and creating healthier babies. This technology enables researchers to make a brown-haired individual blonde, to change brown eyes to blue, and to make a short person taller. Imagine being able to "engineer" your child. Imagine, as Aldous Huxley did in *Brave New World* (1932), being able to create a society of perfect individuals: "We also predestine and condition. We decant our babies as socialized human beings, as Alphas or Epsilons, as future sewage workers or future . . . he was going to say future World controllers but correcting himself said future directors of Hatcheries, instead" (p. 12).

The ethical implications pertaining to genetic technology are profound. For example, some questions raised by the Human Genome Project relate to:

■ Fairness in the use of the genetic information.
■ Privacy and confidentiality of obtained genetic information.
■ Genetic testing of an individual for a specific condition due to family history. Should testing be performed if no treatment is available? Should parents have the right to have minors tested for adult-onset diseases? Should parents have the right to use gene therapy for genetic enhancement?

The Human Genome Project is dedicated to mapping and identifying the genetic composition of humans. Scientists hope to identify and eradicate many of the genetic disorders affecting individuals. Initiated in 1990, the Human Genome Project was projected to be a 13-year effort coordinated by the U.S. Department of Energy and the National Institutes of Health. However, because of swift technological advances, in February 2001 the scientists announced they had cracked the human genetic code and accomplished the following goals (Human Genome Project Information, 2002):

- Identified all of the genes in human DNA.
- Determined the sequences of the three billion chemical bases that make up human DNA
- Stored this information in databases
- Developed tools for data analysis
- Addressed the ethical, legal, and social issues that may arise from the project.

Rapid advances in the science of genetics and its applications present new and complex ethical and policy issues for individuals, health-care personnel, and society. Economics come into play because, currently, only those who can afford the technology have access to it. Efforts need to be directed toward creating standards that identify the uses for genetic data and the protection of human rights and confidentiality. This is truly the new frontier.

Stem Cell Use and Research

Over the last several years, issues regarding stem cell research and stem cell transplant technology have come to the forefront of ethical discussion. Stem cell research shows promise in possibly curing neurological disorders such as Parkinson's disease, spinal cord injury, and dementia. Questions have been raised regarding the moral and ethical issues of using stem cells from fetal tissue for research and the treatment of disease. Stem cell transplants have demonstrated success in helping cancer patients recover and giving them a chance for survival when traditional treatments have failed.

A new business has emerged from this technology as companies now store fetal cord blood for future use if needed. This blood is collected at the time of delivery and may be used for the infant and possibly future siblings if necessary. The cost for this service is high, which limits its availability to only those who can afford the process.

When faced with the prospect of a child who is dying from a terminal illness, some parents have resorted to conceiving a sibling in order to obtain the stem cells for the purpose of using them to save the first child. Nurses who work in pediatrics and pediatric oncology units may find themselves dealing with this situation. It is important for nurses to examine their own feelings regarding these issues and understand that, regardless of their personal beliefs, the family is in need of sensitivity and the best nursing care.

A primary responsibility of nursing is to help patients and families cope with the purposes, benefits, and limitations of the new technologies. Hospice nurses and critical care nurses help patients and their families with end-of-life decisions. Nurses will need to have knowledge about the new genetic technologies because they will fill the roles of counselors and advisers in these areas. Many nurses now work in the areas of in vitro fertilization and genetic counseling.

Professional Dilemmas

Most of this chapter has dealt with patient issues, but ethical problems may involve leadership and management issues as well. What do you do about an impaired coworker? Personal loyalties often cause conflict with professional ethics, creating an ethical dilemma. For this reason, most nurse practice acts now address this problem and require the reporting of impaired professionals and providing rehabilitation for them.

Other professional dilemmas may involve working with incompetent personnel. This may be frustrating for both staff and management. Regulations created to protect individuals from unjustified loss of position and the enormous amounts of paperwork, remediation, and time that must be exercised to terminate an incompetent health-care worker often make management look the other way.

Employing institutions that provide nursing services have an obligation to establish a process for the reporting and handling of practices that jeopardize patient safety (ANA, 1994). The behaviors of incompetent staff place patients and other staff members in jeopardy; eventually, the incompetency may lead to legal action that may have been avoidable if a different approach had been taken.

Conclusion

Ethical dilemmas are becoming more common in the changing health-care environment. More questions are being raised, and fewer answers are available. New guidelines need to be developed to assist in finding more answers. Technology has provided enormous power to alter the human organism and to keep the human organism alive, but economics may force answers to the questions of what living is and when people should be allowed to die. Will society become the brave new world of Aldous Huxley? Again and again the question is raised, "Who shall live, and who shall die?" What is *your* answer?

Study Questions

1. What is the difference between intrinsic and extrinsic values? Make a list of your intrinsic values.

2. Consider a decision you made recently that was based on your values. How did you make your choice?

3. Describe how you could use the valuing process of choosing, prizing, and acting in making the decision considered in Question 2.

4. Which of your personal values would be primary if you were assigned to care for a microcephalic infant whose parents have decided to withhold all food and fluids?

5. The parents of the microcephalic infant in Question 4 confront you and ask, "What would you do if this were your baby?" What do you think would be most important for you to consider in responding to them?

6. Your friend is single and feels that her "biological clock is ticking." She decides to undergo in vitro fertilization using donor sperm. She tells you that she has researched the donor's background extensively and wants to show you the "template" for her child. She asks for your professional opinion about this situation. How would you respond? Identify the ethical principles involved.

7. Over the past several weeks, you have noticed that your closest friend, Jimmy, has been erratic and has been making poor patient-care decisions. On two separate occasions, you quietly intervened and "fixed" his errors. You have also noticed that he volunteers to give pain medications to other nurses' patients, and you see him standing very close to other nurses when they remove controlled substances from the medication distribution center. Today you watched him go to the center immediately after another colleague and then saw him go into the men's room. Within about 20 minutes his behavior had changed completely. You suspect that he may be taking controlled substances. You and Jimmy have been friends for more than 20 years. You grew up together and went to nursing school together. You realize that if you approach him, you may jeopardize this close friendship that means a great deal to you. Using the MORAL ethical decision-making model, devise a plan to resolve this dilemma.

Case Study to Promote Critical Reasoning

Andy is assigned to care for a 14-year-old girl, Amanda, admitted with a large tumor located in the left groin area. During an assessment, Amanda shares her personal feelings with Andy. She tells him that she feels "different" from her friends. She is ashamed of her physical development because all her girlfriends have "breasts" and boyfriends. She is very flat-chested and embarrassed. Andy listens attentively to Amanda and helps her focus on some of her positive attributes and talents.

A CT scan is ordered and reveals that the tumor extends to what appears to be the ovary. A gynecological surgeon is called in to evaluate the situation. An ultrasonic-guided biopsy is performed. It is discovered that the tumor is an enlarged lymph node and that the "ovary" is actually a testis. Amanda has both male and female gonads.

When this information is given to Amanda's parents, they do not want her to know. They feel that she was raised as "their daughter." They ask the surgeon to remove the male gonads and leave only the female gonads. That way, "Amanda will never need to know." The surgeon refuses to do this. Andy believes that the parents should discuss the situation with Amanda as they are denying her choices. The parents are adamant about Amanda not knowing anything. Andy returns to Amanda's room, and Amanda begins asking all types of questions regarding the tests and the treatments. In answering, Andy hesitates, and Amanda picks up on this, demanding that he tell her the truth.

1. How should Andy respond?

2. What are the ethical principles in conflict?

3. What are the long-term effects of Andy's decision?

References

AIDS Update Conference. (1995). Hollywood Memorial Hospital, Hollywood, Fla.

American Association of Critical Care Nurses (AACN). At loggerheads: Questioning patient autonomy. Retrieved on January 11, 2006, from aacn.org/AACN/aacnnews.nsf/GetArticle/ArticleThree184?

American Nurses Association (ANA). (2002). Code of Ethics Project. Washington, DC: ANA.

American Nurses Association (ANA). (1994). Guidelines on Reporting Incompetent, Unethical, or Illegal Practices. Washington, DC: ANA.

Benner, P., & Wrubel, J. (1989). *The Primacy of Caring: Stress and Coping in Health and Illness.* Menlo Park, Calif.: Addison Wesley.

Burkhardt, M.A., & Nathaniel, A.K. (2007). *Ethics and Issues in Contemporary Nursing.* Albany, N.Y.: Delmar.

Butts, J. B., & Rich, K. L. (2008). *Nursing Ethics: Across the Curriculum and Into Practice,* 2nd ed. Boston: Jones & Bartlett.

Davis, A.J., Arokar, M.A., Liaschenko, J., & Drought, T.S. (1997). *Ethical Dilemmas and Nursing Practice,* 4th ed. Stamford, Conn.: Appleton & Lange.

Driver, J. (2001). *Uneasy Virtue.* New York: Cambridge University Press.

Edge, R.S., & Groves, J.R. (2005). *The Ethics of Healthcare: A Guide for Clinical Practice.* 3rd ed. Albany, N.Y.: Thomson–Delmar Learning.

Gordon, N. (1963). *The Death Committee.* New York: Fawcett Crest.

Guido, G.W. (2001). *Legal and Ethical Issues in Nursing,* 3rd ed. Saddle River, N.J.: Prentice-Hall.

Halloran, M.C. (1982). Rational ethical judgments utilizing a decision-making tool. *Heart Lung,* 11(6), 566–570.

Harned, P. (2005). National business ethics survey, 2005. Ethics Today Online, 4(2). Retrieved on January 13, 2005, from ethics.org/today/et_current. html pres

Hook, C.C., & Mueller, P.S. (2005). The Terri Schiavo saga: The making of a tragedy and lessons learned. Retrieved on April 20, 2006, from mayoclinicproceedings.com/inside.asp?AID=1054&UID=8934

Hooker, B. (2000). *Ideal Code, Real World.* Oxford, U.K.: Oxford University Press.

Human Genome Project. Retrieved on July 19, 2002, from ornl.gov/hgmis/about

Hume, D. (1978). A treatise of human nature. In Johnson, O.A. *Ethics,* 4th ed. New York: Holt, Rinehart, and Winston, p. 212.

Huxley, A. (1932). *Brave New World.* New York: Harper Row Publishers.

Johnstone, M.J. (1999). *Bioethics: A nursing perspective,* 3rd ed. Sydney, Australia: Harcourt Saunders.

Kant, I. (1949). *Fundamental Principles of the Metaphysics of Morals.* New York: Liberal Arts.

Macklin, R. (1987). *Mortal Choices: Ethical Dilemmas in Modern Medicine.* Boston: Houghton Mifflin.

Mappes, T.A., & DeGrazia, D. (2005). *Biomedical Ethics,* 6th ed. St. Louis: McGraw-Hill.

Raths, L.E., Harmin, M., & Simon, S.B. (1979). *Values and Teaching.* New York: Charles E. Merrill.

Shirey, M.R. (2005). Ethical climate in nursing practice: The leader's role. *Journal of Nursing Administration,* 7(2), 59–67.

Steele, S.M., & Harmon, V. (1983). *Values Clarification in Nursing.* New York: Appleton-Century-Crofts.

Thiroux, J. (1977). *Ethics: Theory and Practice.* Philadelphia: MacMillan.

Thompson, J., & Thompson, H. (1992). *Bioethical Decision Making for Nurses.* New York: Appleton-Century-Crofts.

Urbano, M.T. (1992). *Preschool Children with Special Health-Care Needs.* San Diego: Singular Publishing.

Varcoe, C., Doane, G., Pauly, B., Rodney, P., et al. (2007). *Journal of Advanced Nursing,* 45(3), 316–325.

Wack, J. (1992). *Sociology of Religion.* Chicago: University of Chicago Press.

Webster's New World Dictionary. (2000). New York: Simon & Schuster.

Wright, R.A. (1987). *Human Values in Health Care.* St. Louis: McGraw-Hill.

Organizations, Power, and Empowerment

○●○ ○ ○ ○ ○ ○ ●○ ○ ○ ○

The subjects of this chapter—organizations, power, and empowerment—are not as remote from a nurse's everyday experience as you may first think. It is difficult to focus on these "big picture" factors when caught up in the busy day-to-day work of a staff nurse, but they have an effect on your practice as you will see in this chapter. Consider two scenarios, which are analyzed later in the chapter.

Were the disappointments experienced by Hazel Rivera and the critical care department staff predictable? Could they have been avoided? Without a basic understanding of organizations and of the part that power plays in health-care institutions, people are doomed to be continually surprised by the responses to their well-intentioned efforts. As you read this chapter, you will learn why Hazel Rivera and the critical care department staff were disappointed.

This chapter begins by looking at some of the characteristics of the organizations in which nurses work and how these organizations operate. Then it focuses on the subject of power within organizations: what it is, how it is obtained, and how nurses can become empowered.

Understanding Organizations

One of the attractive features of nursing as a career is the wide variety of settings in which nurses can work. From rural migrant health clinics to organ transplant units, nurses' skills are needed wherever there are concerns about people's health. Relationships with patients may extend for months or years, as they do in school health or in nursing homes, or they may be brief and never repeated, as often happens in doctors' offices, operating rooms, and emergency departments.

Types of Health-Care Organizations

Although some nurses work as independent practitioners, as consultants, or in the corporate world, most nurses are employed by health-care

---

Scenario 1

In school, Hazel Rivera had always received high praise for the quality of her nursing care plans. "Thorough, comprehensive, systematic, holistic—beautiful!" was the comment she received on the last one she wrote before graduation.

Now Hazel is a staff nurse on a busy orthopedic unit. Although her time to write comprehensive care plans during the day is limited, Hazel often stays after work to complete them. Her friend Carla refuses to stay late with her. "If I can't complete my work during the shift, then they have given me too much to do," she said.

At the end of their 3-month probationary period, Hazel and Carla received written evaluations of their progress and comments about their value to the organization. To Hazel's surprise, her friend Carla received a higher rating than she did. Why? ■

Scenario 2

The nursing staff of the critical care department of a large urban hospital formed an evidence-based practice group about a year ago. They had made many changes in their practice based on reviews of the research on several different procedures, and they were quite pleased with the results.

"Let's look at the bigger picture next month," their nurse manager suggested. "We should consider the research on different models of patient care. We might get some good ideas for our unit." The staff nurses agreed. It would be a nice change to look at the way they organized patient care in their department.

The nurse manager found a wealth of information on different models for organizing nursing care. One research study about a model for caring for the chronically critically ill (Rudy, et al., 1995) particularly interested them because they had had many patients in that category.

Several nurses volunteered to form an ad hoc committee to design a similar unit for chronically critically ill patients within their critical care department. When the plan was presented, both the nurse manager and the staff thought it was excellent. The nurse manager offered to present the plan to the vice president for nursing. The staff eagerly awaited the vice president's response.

The nurse manager returned with discouraging news. The vice president did not support their concept and said that, although they were free to continue developing the idea, they should not assume that it would ever be implemented. What happened? ■

organizations. These organizations can be classified into three types on the basis of their sponsorship and financing:

1. **Private not-for-profit.** Many health-care organizations were founded by civic, charitable, or religious groups. Some have been in existence for generations. Many hospitals, long-term care facilities, home-care services, and community agencies began this way. Although they need money to pay their staff and expenses, they do not have to generate a profit.
2. **Publicly supported.** Government-operated service organizations range from county public health departments to complex medical centers, such as those operated by the Veterans Administration, a federal agency.
3. **Private for-profit.** Increasing numbers of health-care organizations are operated for profit like any other business. These include large hospital and nursing home chains, health maintenance organizations, and many freestanding centers that provide special services, such as surgical and diagnostic centers.

The differences between these categories have become blurred for several reasons:

- All compete for patients, especially for patients with health-care insurance or the ability to pay their own health-care bills.
- All experience the effects of cost constraints.
- All may provide services that are eligible for government reimbursement, particularly Medicaid and Medicare funding, if they meet government standards.

Organizational Characteristics

The size and complexity of many health-care organizations make them difficult to understand. One way to begin is to find a metaphor or image that describes their characteristics. Morgan (1997) suggested using animals or other familiar images to describe an organization. For example, an aggressive organization that crushes its competitors is like a bull elephant, whereas a timid organization in danger of being crushed by that bull elephant is like a mouse. Using images, an organization adrift without a clear idea of its future in a time of crisis could be described as a rudderless boat on a stormy sea, whereas an organization with its sights set clearly on exterminating its competition could be described as a guided missile.

Organizational Culture

People seek stability, consistency, and meaning in their work. To achieve this, some type of culture will develop within an organization (Schein, 2004). An organizational culture is an enduring set of shared values, beliefs, and assumptions (Cameron & Quinn, 2006). It is taught (often indirectly or unconsciously) to new employees as the "right way" or "our way" to assess patient needs, provide care, and relate to fellow caregivers. As with the cultures of societies and communities, it is easy to observe the superficial aspects of an organization's culture, but much of it remains hidden from the casual observer. Edgar Schein, a well-known scholar of organizational culture, divided the various aspects of organizational culture into three levels:

1. **Artifact level:** visible characteristics such as patient room layout, patient record forms, etc.
2. **Espoused beliefs:** stated, often written, goals; philosophy of the organization
3. **Underlying assumptions:** unconscious but powerful beliefs and feelings, such as a commitment to cure every patient, no matter the cost (Schein, 2004)

Organizational cultures differ a great deal. Some are very traditional, preserving their customary ways of doing things even when these processes no longer work well. Others, in an attempt to be progressive, chase the newest management fad or buy the latest high-technology equipment. Some are warm, friendly, and open to new people and new ideas. Others are cold, defensive, and indifferent or even hostile to the outside world (Tappen, 2001). These very different organizational cultures have a powerful effect on the employees and the people served by the organization. Organizational culture shapes people's behavior, especially their responses to each other, which is a particularly important factor in health care.

Culture of Safety

The way in which a health-care organization's operation affects patient safety has been a subject of much discussion. The shared values, attitudes, and behaviors that are directed to preventing or minimizing patient harm have been called the culture of safety (Vogus & Sutcliffe, 2007). The following are important aspects of an organization's culture of safety:

- Willingness to acknowledge mistakes
- Vigilance in detecting and eliminating error-prone situations

- Openness to questioning existing systems and to changing them to prevent errors (Armstrong & Laschinger, 2006; Vogus & Sutcliffe, 2007).

It is not easy to change an organization's culture. In fact, Hinshaw (2008) points out we are trying to create a culture of safety at a particularly difficult time, given the shortages of nurses and other resources within the health-care system (Connaughton & Hassinger, 2007). Nurses who are not well prepared, not valued by their employer or colleagues, not involved in decisions about organizing patient care, and are fatigued due to excessive workloads are certainly more likely to be error-prone. For example, increased workload and stress have been found to increase adverse events by as much as 28% (Weissman, et al., 2007; Redman, 2008). Clearly, organizational factors can contribute either to an increase in errors or to protecting patient safety.

Care Environments

There is also much concern about the environment in which care is provided, an issue that is closely related to patient safety. Patients have lower risk of failure to rescue and death in better care environments (see Aiken, et al., 2008). What constitutes a better care environment? Collegial relationships with physicians, skilled nurse managers with high levels of leadership ability, emphasis on staff development, and quality of care are important factors. Mackoff and Triolo (2008) offer a similar list of factors that contribute to excellence and longevity (low turnover) of nurse managers:

- *Excellence:* always striving to be better, refusing to accept mediocrity
- *Meaningfulness:* being very clear about the purpose of the organization (for example, serving the poor, healing the environment, protecting abused women)
- *Regard:* understanding the work people do and valuing it
- *Learning and growth:* providing mentors, guidance, opportunities to grow and develop

Identifying an Organization's Culture

The culture of an organization is intangible; you cannot see it or touch it, but you will recognize it when you bump up against it. To find out what the culture of an organization is when you are applying for a new position or trying to familiarize yourself with your new workplace, you can ask several people who work there or are familiar with the organization to describe it in just a few words. You can also ask about workload and decision making, and you can ask for examples of nursing impact on patient safety.

Does it matter in what type of organization you work? The answer, emphatically, is yes. For example, the extreme value placed on "busyness" in hospitals, i.e., being seen doing something at all times, leads to manager actions such as floating a staff member to a "busier" unit if she or he is found reading new research or looking up information on the Web (Scott-Findley & Golden-Biddle, 2005). Even more important, a hospital with a positive work environment is not only a better place for nurses to work but also safer for patients.

Once you have grasped the totality of an organization in terms of its overall culture, you are ready to analyze it in a little more detail, particularly its goals, structure, and processes.

Organizational Goals

Try answering the following question:

Question: The primary goal of any health-care organization is to keep people healthy, restore them to health, or assist them in dying as comfortably as possible. True or false?

Answer: False. The statement is only partially correct. Most health-care organizations have several goals.

What other goals might a health-care organization have? Following are some examples:

- **Survival.** Organizations have to maintain their own existence. Many health-care organizations are cash-strapped, causing them to limit hiring, streamline work, and reduce costs, putting enormous pressure on remaining staff (Roark, 2005). The survival goal is threatened when, for example, reimbursements are reduced, competition increases, the organization fails to meet standards, or patients are unable to pay their bills (Trinh & O'Connor, 2002).
- **Growth.** Chief executive officers (CEOs) typically want their organizations to grow by expanding into new territories, adding new services, and bringing in new patients.
- **Profit.** For-profit organizations are expected to return some profit to their owners. Not-for-profit organizations have to be able to pay their bills

and to avoid slipping into too much debt. This is sometimes difficult to accomplish.

- **Status.** The leaders or owners of many health-care organizations also want to be known as the best in their field; for example, by having the best open-heart surgeon, providing "the best nursing care in the world" (Frusti, Niesen, & Campion, 2003, p. 34), providing gourmet meals, or having the most attractive birthing rooms in town.
- **Dominance.** Some organizations also want to drive others out of the health-care business or acquire them, surpassing the goal of survival and moving toward dominance of a particular market by driving out the competition.

These additional goals are not discussed in public as often as the first, more lofty statement of goals in the true-or-false question. However, they still drive an organization, especially the way an organization handles its finances and treats its employees.

These goals may have profound effects on every one of the organization's employees, nurses included. For example, return to the story of Hazel Rivera. Why did she receive a less favorable rating than her friend Carla?

After comparing ratings with those of her friend Carla, Hazel asked for a meeting with her nurse manager to discuss her evaluation. The nurse manager explained the rating: Hazel's care plans were very well done, and the nurse manager genuinely appreciated Hazel's efforts to make them so. The

problem was that Hazel had to be paid overtime for this work according to the union contract, and this reduced the amount of overtime pay the nurse manager had available when the patient care load was especially high. "The corporation is very strict about staying within the budget," she said. "In fact, my rating is higher when I don't use up all of my budgeted overtime hours." When Hazel asked what she could do to improve her rating, the nurse manager offered to help her streamline the care plans and manage her time better so that the care plans could be done during her shift.

Structure

The Traditional Approach

Almost all health-care organizations have a hierarchical structure of some kind (Box 5-1). In a traditional hierarchical structure, employees are ranked from the top to the bottom, as if they were on the steps of a ladder (Fig. 5.1). The number of people on the bottom rungs of the ladder is almost always much greater than the number at the top. The president or CEO is usually at the top of this ladder; the housekeeping and maintenance crews are usually at the bottom. Nurses fall somewhere in the middle of most health-care organizations, higher than the cleaning people, aides, and technicians, but lower than physicians and administrators. The organizational structure of a small ambulatory care center in a horizontal form is illustrated in Figure 5.2.

box 5-1

What Is a Bureaucracy?

Although it seems as if everyone complains about "the bureaucracy," not everyone is clear about what a bureaucracy really is. Max Weber defined a *bureaucratic organization* as having the following characteristics:

- **Division of labor.** Specific parts of the job to be done are assigned to different individuals or groups. For example, nurses, physicians, therapists, dietitians, and social workers all provide portions of the health care needed by an individual.
- **Hierarchy.** All employees are organized and ranked according to their level of authority within the organization. For example, administrators and directors are at the top of most hospital hierarchies, whereas aides and maintenance workers are at the bottom.
- **Rules and regulations.** Acceptable and unacceptable behavior and the proper way to carry out various tasks are defined, often in writing. For example, procedure books, policy manuals, bylaws, statements, and memos prescribe many types of behavior, from acceptable isolation techniques to vacation policies.
- **Emphasis on technical competence.** People with certain skills and knowledge are hired to carry out specific parts of the total work of the organization. For example, a community mental health center has psychiatrists, social workers, and nurses to provide different kinds of therapies and clerical staff to do the typing and filing. Some bureaucracy is characteristic of the formal operation of every organization, even the most deliberately informal, because it promotes smooth operations within a large and complex group of people.

Adapted from Weber, M. (1969). Bureaucratic organization. In Etzioni, A. (ed.). Readings on Modern Organizations. Englewood Cliffs, N.J.: Prentice-Hall.

CEO

Administrators

Managers (also medical staff)

Staff nurses

Technicians
(including LPNs)

Aides; housekeeping;
maintenance

Figure 5.1 The organizational ladder.

The people at the top of the ladder have authority to issue orders, spend the organization's money, and hire and fire people. Much of this authority is delegated to people below them, but they retain the right to reverse a decision or regain control of these activities whenever they deem necessary.

The people at the bottom have little authority but do have other sources of power. They usually play no part in deciding how money is spent or who will be hired or fired but are responsible for carrying out the directions from people above them on the ladder. If there was no one at the bottom, the work would not get done.

Some amount of bureaucracy is characteristic of the formal operation of every organization, even the most deliberately informal, because it promotes smooth operations within a large and complex group of people.

More Innovative Structures

There is much interest in restructuring organizations, not only to save money but also to make the best use of a health-care organization's most valuable resource: its people. This begins with hiring the right people. It also involves providing them with the resources they need to function and the kind of leadership that can inspire the staff and unleash their creativity (Rosen, 1996).

Increasingly, people recognize that organizations need to be both efficient and adaptable. Organizations need to be prepared for uncertainty, for rapid changes in their environment, and for quick, creative responses to these challenges. In addition, they need to provide an internal climate that not only allows but also motivates employees to work to the best of their ability. They need to stop thinking of the managers

as the brains of the organization and employees as the muscle (Parker & Gadbois, 2000, p. 428).

Innovative organizations have adapted an increasingly *organic* structure that is more dynamic, more flexible, and less centralized than the static traditional hierarchical structure (Yourstone & Smith, 2002). In these organically structured organizations, decisions are made by the people who will implement them, not by their bosses.

The organic network emphasizes increased flexibility of the organizational structure, decentralized decision making, and autonomy for working groups or teams. Rigid unit structures are reorganized into autonomous teams that consist of professionals from different departments and disciplines. Each team is given a specific task or function (e.g., intravenous team, a hospital infection control team, a child protection team in a community agency). The teams are responsible for their own self-correction and self-control, although they may also have a designated leader. Together, team members make decisions about work assignments and how to deal with problems that arise. In other words, the teams supervise and manage themselves.

Supervisors, administrators, and support staff have different functions in an organic network. Instead of spending their time observing and controlling other people's work, they become planners and resource people. They are responsible for providing the conditions required for the optimal functioning of the teams, and they are expected to ensure that the support, information, materials, and funds needed to do the job well are available to the teams. They also act as coordinators between the teams so that the teams are cooperating rather than blocking each other, working toward the same goals, and not duplicating effort.

Organic networks have been compared with spider plants, with a central cluster and offshoots of smaller clusters (Morgan, 1997). Each cluster represents a discipline (e.g., nursing, social work, occupational therapy) or a service (e.g., psychiatry, orthopedics). For example, Figure 5.3 shows an organic network for a wellness center. Each cluster represents a separate set of services. A patient might use just one or all of them to develop a personal plan for wellness. Staff members may move from one cluster to another, or the entire configuration of interconnected clusters may be reorganized as the organization shapes and is shaped by the environment.

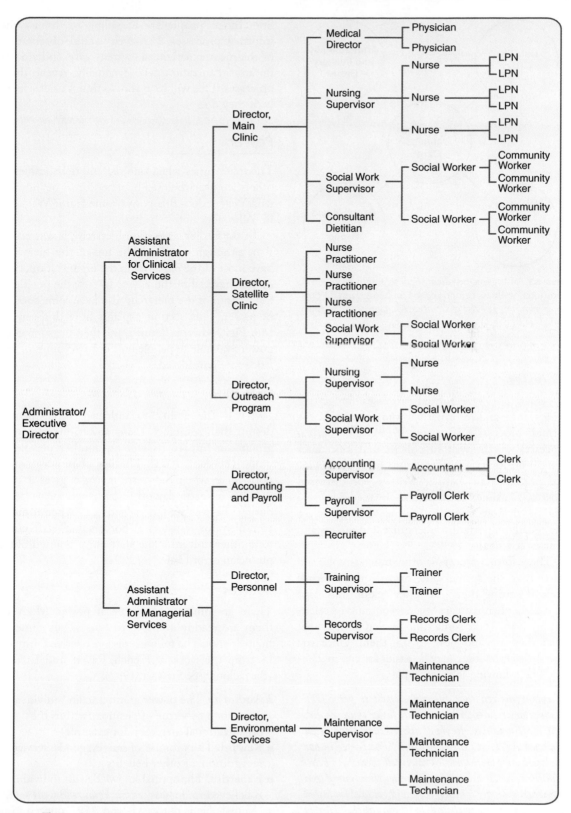

Figure 5.2 Table of organization of an ambulatory care center. (Adapted from DelBueno, D.J. [1987]. An organizational checklist. *Journal of Nursing Administration*, 17[5], 30–33.)

Figure 5.3 An organic organizational structure for a non-traditional wellness center. (Based on Morgan, A. [1993]. *Imaginization: The Art of Creative Management.* Newbury Park, Calif.: Sage.)

Processes

Organizations have formal processes for getting things done and informal ways to get around the formal processes (Perrow, 1969). The *formal* processes are the written policies and procedures that all health-care organizations have. The *informal* processes are neither written nor discussed most of the time. They exist in organizations as a kind of "shadow" organization that is harder to see but equally important to recognize and understand (Purser & Cabana, 1999).

The informal process is often much simpler and faster than the formal one. Because the informal ways of getting things done are seldom discussed (and certainly not a part of a new employee's orientation), it may take some time for you to figure out what they are and how to use them. Once you know they exist, they may be easier for you to identify. The following is an example:

> *Jocylene noticed that Harold seemed to get STAT laboratory results on his patients faster than she did. At lunch one day, Jocylene asked Harold why that happened. "That's easy," he said. "The people in our lab feel unappreciated. I always tell them how helpful they are. Also, if you call and let them know that the specimens are coming, they will get to them faster. They can't monitor their e-mail constantly." Harold has just explained an informal process to Jocylene.*

Sometimes, people are unwilling to discuss the informal processes. However, careful observation of the most experienced "system-wise" individuals in an organization will eventually reveal these processes. This will help you do things as efficiently as they do.

Power

There are times when one's attempts to influence others are overwhelmed by other forces or individuals. Where does this power come from? Who has it? Who does not?

In the earlier section on hierarchy, it was noted that, although people at the top of the hierarchy have most of the *authority* in the organization, they do not have all of the *power*. In fact, the people at the bottom of the hierarchy also have some sources of power. This section explains how this can be true. First, power is defined, and then the sources of power available to people on the lower rungs of the ladder are considered.

Definition

Power is the ability to influence other people despite their resistance. Using power, one person or group can impose its will on another person or group (Haslam, 2001). The use of power can be positive, as when the nurse manager gives a staff member an extra day off in exchange for working during the weekend, or negative, as when a nurse administrator transfers a "bothersome" staff nurse to another unit after the staff nurse pointed out a physician error (Talarico, 2004).

Sources

There are numerous sources of power. Many of them are readily available to nurses, but some of them are not. The following is a list derived primarily from the work of French, Raven, and Etzioni (Barraclough & Stewart, 1992):

- **Authority.** The power granted to an individual or a group by virtue of position (within the organizational hierarchy, for example)
- **Reward.** The promise of money, goods, services, recognition, or other benefits
- **Expertise.** The special knowledge an individual is believed to possess; as Sir Francis Bacon said, "Knowledge is power" (Bacon, 1597, quoted in Fitton, 1997, p. 150)

■ **Coercion.** The threat of pain or of harm, which may be physical, economic, or psychological

There is power at the bottom of the organizational ladder as well as at the top. Patients also have sources of power (Bradbury-Jones, Sambrook, & Irvine, 2007). Various groups of people in a health-care organization have different types of power available to them:

■ *Managers* are able to reward people with salary increases, promotions, and recognition. They can also cause economic or psychological pain for the people who work for them, particularly through their authority to evaluate and fire people but also through their responsibility for making assignments, allowing days off, and so on.
■ *Patients* at first appear to be relatively powerless within the health-care organization. However, if patients refused to use the services of a particular organization, that organization would eventually cease to exist. Patients can reward health-care workers by praising them to their supervisors. They can also cause problems by complaining about them.
■ *Assistants and technicians* may also appear to be relatively powerless because of their low positions in the hierarchy. Imagine, how-ever, how the work of the organization (e.g., hospital, nursing home) would be impeded if all the nursing aides failed to appear one morning.
■ *Nurses* have expert power and authority over licensed practical nurses, aides, and other per-sonnel by virtue of their position in the hierar-chy. They are critical to the operation of most health-care organizations and could cause considerable trouble if they refused to work, another source of nurse power.

Fralic (2000) offered a good example of the power of information that nurses have always had: Florence Nightingale showed very graphically in the 1800s that wherever her nurses were, far fewer died, and wherever they were not, many more died. Think of the power of that information. Immediately, people were saying, "What would you like, Miss Nightingale? Would you like more money? Would you like a school of nursing? What else can we do for you?" She had solid data, she knew how to collect it, and she knew how to interpret and distribute it in terms of things that people valued (p. 340).

Empowering Nurses

This final section looks at several ways in which nurses, either individually or collectively, can maxi-mize their power and increase their feelings of empowerment.

Power is the actual or potential actual ability to "recognize one's will even against the resistance of others," according to Max Weber (quoted in Mondros & Wilson, 1994, p. 5). *Empowerment* is a psychological state, a feeling of competence, con-trol, and entitlement. Given these definitions, it is possible to be powerful and yet not feel empow-ered. *Power* refers to ability, and *empowerment* refers to feelings. Both are of importance to nurs-ing leaders and managers.

Feeling empowered includes the following:

■ **Self-determination.** Feeling free to decide how to do your work
■ **Meaning.** Caring about your work, enjoying it, and taking it seriously
■ **Competence.** Confidence in your ability to do your work well
■ **Impact.** Feeling that people listen to your ideas, that you can make a difference (Spreitzer & Quinn, 2001)

The following contribute to nurse empowerment:

■ **Decision-making.** Control of nursing practice within an organization
■ **Autonomy.** Ability to act on the basis of one's knowledge and experience (Manojlovich, 2007)
■ **Manageable workload.** Reasonable work assign-ments
■ **Reward and recognition.** Appreciation received for a job well done
■ **Fairness.** Consistent, equitable treatment of all staff (Spence, Laschinger, & Finegan, 2005)

The opposite of empowerment is *disempower-ment*. Inability to control one's own practice leads to frustration and sometimes failure. Work over-load and lack of meaning, recognition, or reward produce emotional exhaustion and burnout (Spence, Laschinger, & Finegan, 2005). Nurses, like most people, want to have some power and to feel empowered. They want to be heard, to be recognized, to be valued, and to be respected. They do not want to feel unimportant or insignificant to society or to the organization in which they work.

Participation in Decision Making

Actions can be taken by managers and higher-level administrators to empower nursing staff. The amount of power available to or exercised by a given group (e.g., nurses) *within* an organization can vary considerably from one organization to the next. Three sources of power are particularly important in health-care organizations:

- **Resources.** The money, materials, and human help needed to accomplish the work
- **Support.** Authority to take action without having to obtain permission
- **Information.** Patient care expertise and knowledge about the organization's goals and activities of other departments

In addition, nurses also need access to *opportunities*: opportunities to be involved in decision making, to be involved in vital functions of the organization, to grow professionally, and to move up the organizational ladder (Sabiston & Laschinger, 1995). Without these, employees cannot be empowered (Bradford & Cohen, 1998). Nurses who are part-time, temporary, or contract employees are less likely to feel empowered than full-time permanent employees, who generally feel more secure in their positions and connected to the organization (Kuokkanen & Katajisto, 2003).

Shared Governance

In shared governance, staff nurses are included in the highest levels of decision making within the nursing department through representation on various councils that govern practice and management issues. These councils set the standard for staffing, promotion, and so forth. In many cases, a change in the organizational culture is necessary before shared governance can work (Currie & Loftus-Hills, 2002).

Genuine sharing of decision making is difficult to accomplish, partly because managers are reluctant to relinquish control or to trust their staff members to make wise decisions. Yet genuine empowerment of the nursing staff cannot occur without this sharing. Having some control over one's work and the ability to influence decisions are essential to empowerment (Manojlovich & Laschinger, 2002). For example, if staff members do not control the budget for their unit, they cannot implement a decision to replace aides with registered nurses without approval from higher-level management. If they want increased autonomy in decision making about the care of individual patients, they cannot do so if opposition by another group, such as the physicians, is given greater credence by the organization's administration.

Return to the example of the staff of the critical care department (Scenario 2). Why did the vice president for nursing tell the nurse manager that the plan would not be implemented?

Actually, the vice president for nursing thought the plan had some merit. He believed that the proposal to implement a nurse-managed model of care for the chronically critically ill could save money, provide a higher quality of patient care, and result in increased nursing staff satisfaction. However, the critical care department was the centerpiece of the hospital's agreement with a nearby medical school. In this agreement, the medical school provided the services of highly skilled intensivists in return for the learning opportunities afforded their students. In its present form, the nurses' plan would not allow sufficient autonomy for the medical students, a situation that would not be acceptable to the medical school. The vice president knew that the board of trustees of the hospital believed their affiliation with the medical school brought a great deal of prestige to the organization and that they would not allow anything to interfere with this relationship.

"If shared governance were in place here, I think we could implement this or a similar model of care," he told the nurse manager.

"How would that work?" she asked.

"If we had shared governance, the nursing practice council would review the plan and, if they approved it, forward it to a similar medical practice council. Then committees from both councils would work together to figure out a way for this to benefit everyone. It wouldn't necessarily be easy to do, but it could be done if we had real collegiality between the professions. I have been working toward this model but haven't convinced the rest of the administration to put it into practice yet. Perhaps we could bring this up at the next nursing executive meeting. I think it is time I shared my ideas on this subject with the rest of the nursing staff."

In this case, the organizational goals and processes existing at the time the nurses developed their proposal did not support their idea. However, the vice president could see a way for it to be accomplished in the future. Implementation of real shared governance would make it possible for the critical care nurses to accomplish their goal.

Professional Organizations

Although the purposes of the American Nurses Association and that of other professional organizations are discussed in Chapter 15, these organizations are considered here specifically in terms of how they can empower nurses.

A collective voice, expressed through these organizations, can be stronger and more easily heard than one individual voice. By joining together in professional organizations, nurses make their viewpoint known and their value recognized. The power base of nursing professional organizations is derived from the number of members and their expertise in health matters.

Why there is power in numbers may need some explanation. Large numbers of active, informed members of an organization represent large numbers of potential voters to state and national legislators, most of whom wish to be remembered favorably in forthcoming elections. Large groups of people also have a "louder" voice: they can write more letters, speak to more friends and family members, make more telephone calls, and generally attract more attention than small groups can.

Professional organizations can empower nurses in a number of ways:

- Collegiality, the opportunity to work with peers on issues of importance to the profession
- Commitment to improving the health and well-being of the people served by the profession
- Representation at the state or province and national level when issues of importance to nursing arise
- Enhancement of nurses' competence through publications and continuing education
- Recognition of achievement through certification programs, awards, and the media

Collective Bargaining

Like professional organizations, collective bargaining uses the power of numbers, in this case for the purpose of equalizing the power of employees and employer to improve working conditions, gain respect, increase job security, and have greater input into collective decisions (empowerment) and pay increases (Tappen, 2001). When people join for a common cause, they can often exert more power than when they attempt to bring about change individually. Large numbers of people have the potential to cause more psychological or economic pain than an individual can. For example, the resignation of one nursing assistant or one nurse may cause a temporary problem, but it is usually resolved rather quickly by hiring another individual. If 50 or 100 aides or nurses resign, however, the organization can be paralyzed and will have much more difficulty replacing these essential workers. Collective bargaining takes advantage of this power in numbers.

An effective collective bargaining contract can provide considerable protection to employees. However, the downside of collective bargaining (as with most uses of coercive power) is that it may encourage conflict rather than cooperation between employees and managers, an "us" against "them" environment (Haslam, 2001). Many nurses are also concerned about the effect that going out on strike might have on their patients' welfare and on their own economic security. Most administrators and managers prefer to operate within a union-free environment (Hannigan, 1998).

Research Example

Can nurse managers empower their staff? The answer is yes, according to nurse researchers who surveyed 537 staff nurses in two large hospitals. Fostering autonomy and showing confidence in the staff were especially empowering. Empowered staff worked more effectively and had lower levels of job-related tension. (Laschinger, H.K.S., Wong, C., McMahon, L., & Kaufman, C. (1999). Leader behavior impact on staff nurse empowerment, job tension, and work effectiveness. *Journal of Nursing Administration,* 29[5], 28–39.)

Enhancing Expertise

Most health-care professionals, including nurses, are empowered to some extent by their own professional knowledge and competence. You can take steps to enhance your own competence, thereby increasing your own sense of empowerment (Fig. 5.4)

- Participate in interdisciplinary team conferences and patient-centered conferences on your unit.
- Attend continuing education offerings to enhance your expertise.
- Attend local, regional, and national conferences sponsored by relevant nursing and specialty organizations.

Participate in interdisciplinary conferences

Attend continuing education offerings

Attend professional organization meetings

Read books and journals related to your nursing practice

Problem-solve and brainstorm with colleagues

Return to school to earn a higher degree

Figure 5.4 How to increase your expert power.

- Read journals and books in your specialty area.
- Participate in nursing research projects related to your clinical specialty area.
- Discuss with colleagues in nursing and other disciplines how to handle a difficult clinical situation.
- Observe the practice of experienced nurses.
- Return to school to earn a bachelor's degree and higher degrees in nursing.

You can probably think of more, but this list at least gives you some ideas. You can also share the knowledge and experience you have gained with other people. This means not only using your knowledge to improve your own practice but also communicating what you have learned to your colleagues in nursing and in other health-care professions. It also means letting your supervisors know that you have enhanced your professional competence. You can share your knowledge with your patients, empowering them as well. You may even reach the point at which you have learned more about a particular subject than most nurses have and want to write about it for publication.

Conclusion

Although most nurses are employed by health-care organizations, too few nurses have taken the time to analyze the operation of their employing health-care organizations and the effect it has on their practice. Understanding organizations and the power relationships within them will increase the effectiveness of your leadership.

Study Questions

1. Describe the organizational characteristics of a facility in which you currently have a clinical assignment. Include the following: the type of organization, the organizational culture, how the organization is structured, and the formal and informal goals and processes of the organization.

2. Define power, and describe how power affects the relationships between people of different disciplines (e.g., nursing, medicine, physical therapy, housekeeping, administration, finance, social work) in a health-care organization.

3. Discuss ways in which nurses can become more empowered. How can you use your leadership skills to do this?

Case Study to Promote Critical Reasoning

Tanya Washington will finish her associate's degree nursing program in 6 weeks. Her preferred clinical area is pediatric oncology, and she hopes to become a pediatric nurse practitioner one day. Tanya has received two job offers, both from urban hospitals with large pediatric populations. Because several of her friends are already employed by these facilities, she asked them for their thoughts.

"Central Hospital is a good place to work," said one friend. "It is a dynamic, growing institution, always on the cutting edge of change. Any new idea that seems promising, Central is the first to try it. It's an exciting place to work."

"City Hospital is also a good place to work," said her other friend. "It is a strong, stable institution where traditions are valued. Any new idea must be carefully evaluated before it is adapted. It's been a pleasure to work there."

1. How would the organizational culture of each hospital affect a new graduate?

2. Which organizational culture do you think would be best for a new graduate, Central's or City's?

3. Would your answer differ if Tanya were an experienced nurse?

4. What do you need to know about Tanya before deciding which hospital would be best for her?

5. What else would you like to know about the two hospitals?

References

Aiken, L.H., Clarke, S.P., Sloane, D.M., Lake, C.T., et al. (2008). Effects of hospital care environments on patient mortality and nurse outcomes. *Journal of Nursing Administration, 38*(5), 223-229.

Armstrong, K.J., & Laschinger, H. (2006). Structural empowerment, magnet hospital characteristics, and patient safety culture. *Journal of Nursing Care Quality,* 21(2), 124–132.

Barraclough, R.A., & Stewart, R.A. (1992). Power and control: Social science perspectives. In Richmond, V.P., & McCroskey, J.C. (eds.). *Power in the classroom: Communication, control and concern.* Hillsdale, N.J.: Lawrence Erlbaum.

Bradbury-Jones, C., Sambrook, S., & Irvine, F. (2007). Power and empowerment in nursing: A fourth theoretical approach. *Journal of Advanced Nursing, 62*(2), 258–266.

Bradford, D.L., & Cohen, A.R. (1998). *Power up: Transforming organizations through shared leadership.* New York: John Wiley & Sons.

Cameron, K., Quinn, R. (2006). *Diagnosing and changing organizational culture.* San Francisco: Jossey-Bass.

Connaughton, M.J., & Hassinger, J. (2007). Leadership character: Antidote to organizational fatigue. *Journal of Nursing Administration,* 37(10), 464–470.

Currie, L., & Loftus-Hills, A. (2002). The nursing view of clinical governance. *Nursing Standard,* 16(27), 40–44.

DelBueno, D.J. (1987). An organizational checklist. *Journal of Nursing Administration,* 17(5), 30–33.

Fitton, R.A. (1997). *Leadership: Quotations from the world's greatest motivators.* Boulder, Colo.: Westview Press.

Fralic, M.F. (2000). What is leadership? *Journal of Nursing Administration,* 30(7/8), 340–341.

Frusti, D.K., Niesen, K.M., & Campion, J.K. (2003). Creating a culturally competent organization. *Journal of Nursing Administration,* 33(1), 33–38.

Hannigan, T.A. (1998). *Managing tomorrow's high-performance unions.* Westport, Conn.: Greenwood Publishing.

Haslam, S.A. (2001). *Psychology in organizations.* Thousand Oaks, Calif.: Sage.

Hinshaw, A.S. (2008). Navigating the perfect storm: Balancing a culture of safety with workforce. *Nursing Research,* 57(1S), S4–10.

Kuokkanen, L., & Katajisto, J. (2003). Promoting or impeding empowerment? *Journal of Nursing Administration,* 33(4), 209–215.

Laschinger, H.K., & Finegan, J. (2005). Empowering nurses for work engagement and health in hospital settings. *Journal of Nursing Administration,* 35(10), 439–441.

Laschinger, H.K.S., Wong, C., McMahon, L., & Kaufman, C. (1999). Leader behavior impact on staff nurse empowerment, job tension, and work effectiveness. *Journal of Nursing Administration,* 29(5), 28–39.

Mackoff, B.L., & Triolo, P.K. (2008). Why do nurses, managers stay? Building a model of engagement: Part 2: Cultures of engagement. *Journal of Nursing Administration,* 38(4), 166–171.

Manojlovich, M. (2007). Power and empowerment in nursing: Looking backward to inform the future. *New Hampshire Nursing News,* 14–16.

Manojlovich, M., & Laschinger, H.K. (2002). The relationship of empowerment and selected personality characteristics to nursing job satisfaction. *Journal of Nursing Administration,* 32(11), 586–595.

Mondros, J.B., & Wilson, S.M. (1994). *Organizing for power and empowerment.* New York: Columbia University Press.

Morgan, A. (1997). *Images of organization.* Thousand Oaks, Calif.: Sage.

Morgan, A. (1993). *Imagination: The art of creative management.* Newbury Park, Calif.: Sage.

Parker, M., & Gadbois, S. (2000). Building community in the healthcare workplace. *Journal of Nursing Administration,* 30(9), 426–431.

Perrow, C. (1969). The analysis of goals in complex organizations. In Etzioni, A. (ed.). *Readings on modern organizations.* Englewood Cliffs, N.J.: Prentice-Hall.

Purser, R.E., & Cabana, S. (1999). *The self-managing organization.* New York: Free Press (Simon & Schuster).

Redman, R.W. (2008). Symposium in tribute to a nursing leader: Ada Sue Hinshaw. *Nursing Research,* 51(15), S1–S3.

Roark, D.C. (2005). Managing the healthcare supply chain. *Nursing Management,* 36(2), 36–40.

Rosen, R.H. (1996). *Leading people: Transforming business from the inside out.* New York: Viking Penguin.

Rudy, E.B., Daly, B.J., Douglas, S., Montenegro, H.D., et al. (1995). Patient outcomes for the chronically critically ill: Special care unit versus intensive care unit. *Nursing Research,* 44, 324–331.

Sabiston, J.A., & Laschinger, H.K.S. (1995). Staff nurse work empowerment and perceived autonomy. *Journal of Nursing Administration,* 28(9), 42–49.

Schein, E.H. (2004). *Organizational Culture and Leadership.* New York: Jossey-Bass.

Scott-Findley, S., & Golden-Biddle, K. (2005). Understanding how organizational culture shapes research use. *Journal of Nursing Administration,* 35(7/8), 359–365.

Spreitzer, G.M., & Quinn, R.E. (2001). *A Company of Leaders.* San Francisco: Jossey-Bass.

Talarico, K.M. (2004, April 27) A look at power in nursing. *Vital Signs,* 6–7, 21.

Tappen, R.M. (2001). *Nursing leadership and management: Concepts and practice,* 4th ed. Philadelphia: FA Davis.

Trinh, H.Q., & O'Connor, S.J. (2002). Helpful or harmful? The impact of strategic change on the performance of U.S. urban hospitals. *Health Services Research,* 37(1), 145–171.

Vogus, T.J., & Sutcliffe, K.M. (2007). The safety organizing scale: Development and validation of a behavioral measure of safety culture in hospital nursing units. *Medical Care,* 45(1), 56–54.

Weber, M. (1969). Bureaucratic organization. In Etzioni, A. (ed.). *Readings on modern organizations.* Englewood Cliffs, N.J.: Prentice-Hall.

Weissman, J.S., Rothschild, J.M., Bendavid, E., Sprivulis, P., et al. (2007). Hospital workload and adverse events. *Medical Care, 45*(5), 448–455.

Yourstone, S.A., & Smith, H.L. (2002). Managing system errors and failures in health care organizations: Suggestions for practice and research. *Health Care Management Review, 27*(1), 50–61.

2 *unit*

Working Within the Organization

chapter 6

Getting People to Work Together

⊙ ○ ○ ○ ○ ○ ○ ○ ○ ○ ○

OBJECTIVES

After reading this chapter, the student should be able to:

- Describe the basic listening sequence and principles for effective communication.
- Identify barriers to effective communication.
- Discuss strategies for communication with colleagues and patients in health-care settings.
- Provide positive and negative feedback in a constructive manner.
- Respond to feedback in a constructive manner.
- Evaluate the conduct of performance appraisals.
- Participate in formal peer review.

Claude has been working on a busy oncology floor for several years. He usually has a caseload of six to eight patients on his shift, and he believes that he provides safe, competent care. While Claude was on his way to medicate a patient suffering from osteosarcoma, a colleague called to him, "Claude, come with me, please." Claude responded, "I need to medicate Mr. J. in Room 203. I will come right after that. Where will you be?" "Never mind!" his colleague answered. "I'll find someone who's more helpful. Don't ask me for help in the future." This was not the response Claude had expected. He thought he had expressed both an interest in his patient and a willingness to help his colleague. What was the problem?

After Claude gave Mr. Juniper his pain medication, he went back to his colleague. "Sonja, what's the matter?" he asked. Sonja replied, "Mrs. Vero fell in the bathroom. I needed someone to stay with her while I got her walker." "Why didn't you tell me it was urgent?" asked Claude. "I was so upset that I wasn't thinking about what else you were doing," answered Sonja. Claude added, "And I didn't ask you why you needed me. I guess we need to work on our communication, don't we?"

In the busy and sometimes chaotic world of nursing practice, nurses work continuously with all sorts of people. This variety makes the job dynamic and challenging. Just when things appear to have settled down, something happens that requires immediate attention. Busy people need to communicate effectively with each other. This chapter helps new nurses communicate effectively with their colleagues and work with people in all kinds of activities, even those that are filled with multiple demands and constant change.

Communication

People often assume that communication is simply giving information to another person. Communication involves the spoken word as well as the nonverbal message, the emotional state of people involved, and the cultural background that affects their interpretation of the message (Fontaine & Fletcher, 2002). Superficial listening often results in misinterpretation of the message. An individual's attitude also influences what is heard and how the message is interpreted. Active listening is necessary to pick up all these levels of meaning in a communication.

It is important for nurses to observe nonverbal behavior when communicating with colleagues and patients and to try to make their own nonverbal behavior congruent with their verbal communications. Telling people you understand their problem when you appear thoroughly confused or inattentive is an example of incongruence between verbal and nonverbal communication.

The Basic Listening Sequence

Listening is the most critical of all communication skills. To be a good listener, one needs to listen for both the information (content) and emotion (feelings) conveyed. A good listener also shows attentiveness through eye contact and body language and gives the speaker some feedback to indicate that what is being said is understood (Rees, 2005) (Box 6-1). Contrast this to the poor listener who interrupts, misinterprets what is said, or misses it entirely due to inattention (Rees, 2005).

Principles for Effective Communication

To communicate effectively with others, consider the following principles (Table 6-1).

1. Be sure that the message is understood. Ask for feedback from the receiver to clarify any confusion. Bring focus to the interaction. Repeating key words or phrases as questions or using open-ended questions can accomplish this. For example: "You have been telling me that Susan is not providing safe care to her patients. Can you tell me specifically what you have identified as unsafe care?"

---

box 6-1

Basic Listening Sequence

Listen to the:
- Information
- Emotion

Demonstrate attentiveness through:
- Eye contact
- Body language

Verify understanding by:
- Asking occasional questions
- Repeating important points
- Summarizing

Adapted from Rees, F. (2005). 25 Activities for Developing Team Leaders. San Francisco: Pfeiffer.

table 6-1

Principles for Effective Communication	
Principle One	Aim for clarity and focus.
Principle Two	Use direct and exact language.
Principle Three	Encourage feedback.
Principle Four	Acknowledge the contributions of others.
Principle Five	Use the most direct channels of communication available.

Tappen, R.M. (2001). Nursing Leadership and Management: Concepts and Practice (4th ed.). Philadelphia: FA Davis, with permission.

2. Use direct and exact language. In both written and spoken messages, use language that is easily understood by all involved.
3. Encourage feedback. This is the best way to help people understand each other and work together better. Remember, though, that feedback may not be complimentary. This is discussed later in the chapter.
4. Acknowledge the contributions of others. Everyone wants to feel that he or she has worth.
5. Use the most direct channel of communication available. The greater the number of individuals involved in filtering a message, the less likely the message will be received correctly. Just as in an old children's game, messages sent through a number of senders become more and more distorted. Information that is controversial or distressing should definitely be delivered in person so that the receiver can ask questions or receive further clarification. A memo delivered "To all nursing staff" in which cutbacks in staffing are announced would deliver a message very different from that in a meeting in which staff are allowed to talk and ask questions.

Assertiveness in Communication

Assertive behaviors allow people to stand up for themselves and their rights without violating the rights of others. Several authors have stated that nurses lack assertiveness, claiming that nurses would rather be silent than voice opinions that may result in confrontation (Tappen, 2001). Assertiveness is different from aggressiveness. People use aggressive behaviors to force their wishes or ideas on others. In assertive communication, an individual's position

is stated clearly and firmly, using "I" statements. For example:

> *The nurse manager noticed that Steve's charting has been of lower quality than expected during the past few weeks. She approached Steve and said, "JCAHO surveyors are coming in several months. I have been reviewing records and noticed that on several of your charts some pertinent information is missing. I have scheduled time today and tomorrow from 1:00 to 2:00 in the afternoon for us to review the charts. This allows you time to make the necessary corrections and return the charts to me."*

By using "I" statements, the nurse manager is confronting the issue without being accusatory. Assertive communication always requires congruence between verbal and nonverbal messages. Had she shaken her finger close to Steve's face or used a loud voice, the nurse manager might think she was being assertive when in fact her manner would have been aggressive.

There is a misconception that people who communicate assertively always get what they want. Being assertive involves both rights and responsibilities. Assertive communicators have the right to speak up, but they must also be prepared to listen to the response.

Barriers to Effective Communication in the Workplace

People are often unwilling or unable to accept responsibility or to perform a specific task because they do not fully understand what is expected of them. Professional nurses are required to communicate patient information to other members of the nursing team. Although this may sound easy, there are many potential barriers to communication. These barriers may be physical, psychological, semantic, or even gender-related.

Physical Barriers

Physical barriers to communication include extraneous noise, too much activity in the area where the communication is taking place, and physical separation of the people trying to engage in verbal interaction.

Psychological Barriers

Psychological "noise," such as increased anxiety, may interfere with the ability to pay attention to the other speaker. Social values, emotions, judgments, and cultural influences also impede communication. Previous life experiences and preconceived ideas about other cultures also influence how people communicate.

Semantic Barriers

Semantic refers to the meaning of words. Sometimes, no matter how great the effort, the message just does not get across. For example, words such as *neat, cool,* and *bad,* may convey meanings other than those intended. Many individuals have learned English as a second language and therefore understand only the literal meaning of certain words. For example, to many people, *cool* means interesting, unique, or clever (e.g., "This is a cool way to find the vein."). To someone for whom the word *cool* refers only to temperature (e.g., "It is cool outside."), the preceding statement would make very little sense.

Gender Barriers

Men and women develop dissimilar communication skills and are inclined to communicate differently. Often, they give different meanings to conveyed information or feelings. This may be related to psychosocial development. Boys learn to use communication as a way to negotiate and to develop independence, whereas girls use communication to confirm, minimize disparities, and create or strengthen closeness (Blais, Hayes, Kozier, & Erb, 2002).

Communication With Colleagues

Information Systems and E-Mail

Computerized Systems

Communication through the use of computer technology is rapidly growing in nursing practice. A study conducted by KPMG–Peat Marwick of health-care systems that used bedside terminals found that medication errors and use of patient call bells decreased and nurse productivity increased. The use of electronic patient records allows health-care providers to retrieve and distribute patient information precisely and quickly. Decisions regarding patient care can be made more efficiently with less waiting time. Information systems in many organizations also provide opportunities to access current, high-quality clinical and research data to support evidence-based practice. Unfortunately, these rich resources are still underutilized by most nurses (Dee, 2005). Additional benefits of computerized systems for health-care applications are listed in Box 6-2 (Arnold & Pearson, 1992; Hebda, Czar, & Mascara, 1998).

E-Mail

Today, most institutions use e-mail. Using e-mail competently and effectively requires writing skills; the same communication principles apply to both e-mail and letter writing. Remember, when communicating by e-mail, you are not only making an impression but also leaving a written record (Shea, 2000).

The rules for using e-mail in the workplace are somewhat different than for using e-mail among friends. Much of the humor and wit found in personal e-mail is not appropriate for the work setting. Professional e-mail may remain informal. However, the message must be clear, concise, and courteous. Think about what you need to say before you write it. Then write it, read it, and reread it. Once you are satisfied that the message is clear and concise, send it.

Many executives read personal e-mail sent to them, which means that it is often possible to contact them directly. Many systems make it easy to send e-mail to everyone at the health-care institution. For this reason, it is important to keep e-mail professional. Remember the "chain of command": always go through the proper channels.

The fact that you have the capability to send e-mail instantly to large groups of people does not necessarily make sending it a good idea. Be careful if you have access to an all-company mailing list. It is easy to send an e-mail throughout the system

---

box 6-2

Potential Benefits of Computer-Based Patient Information Systems

- Increased hours for direct patient care
- Patient data accessible at bedside
- Improved accuracy and legibility of data
- Immediate availability of all data to all members of the team
- Increased safety related to positive patient identification, improved standardization, and improved quality
- Decreased medication errors
- Increased staff satisfaction

Adapted from Arnold, J., & Pearson, G. (eds.). (1992). Computer Applications in Nursing Education and Practice. N.Y.: National League for Nursing.

without intending this to happen. Consider the following example:

A respiratory therapist and a department administrator at a large health-care institution were engaged in a relationship. They started sending each other personal notes over the company e-mail system. One day, one of them accidentally sent one of these notes to all the employees at the health-care institution. Both were fired. The moral of this story is simple: Do not send anything by e-mail that you would not want published on the front page of a national newspaper or hear on your favorite radio station tomorrow morning.

Although voice tone cannot be "heard" in e-mail, the use of certain words and writing styles indicates emotion. A rude tone in an e-mail message may provoke extreme reactions. Follow the "rules of netiquette" (Shea, 2000) when communicating through e-mail. Some of these rules are listed in Box 6-3.

Reporting Patient Information

Change-of-Shift Report

It is important to understand exactly how your day at work will begin. Regardless of which shift an individual works, some things never change. Nurses traditionally give one another a "report." The change-of-shift report has become the accepted method of communicating patient care needs from one nurse to another. In the report, pertinent information related to events that occurred is given to the individuals responsible for providing continuity of care (Box 6-4). Although historically the report has been given face to face, there are newer ways to share information. Many health-care institutions use audiotape and computer printouts as mechanisms

for sharing information. These mechanisms allow the nurses from the previous shift to complete their tasks and those coming on duty to make inquiries for clarification as necessary.

The report should be organized, concise, and complete, with relevant details. Not every unit uses the same system for giving a change-of-shift report. The system is easily modified according to the pattern of nursing care delivery and the types of patients serviced. For example, many intensive care units, because of their small size and the more acute needs of their patients, use walking rounds as a means for giving the report. This system allows nurses to discuss the current patient status and to set goals for care for the next several hours. Together, the nurses gather objective data as one nurse ends a shift and another begins. This way, there is no confusion as to the patient's status at shift change. This same system is often used in emergency departments and labor and delivery units. Larger patient care units may find the "walking report" time-consuming and an inefficient use of resources.

It is helpful to take notes or create a worksheet while listening to the report. A worksheet helps

---

box 6-3

Rules of Netiquette

1. If you were face-to-face, would you say this?
2. Follow the same rules of behavior online that you follow when dealing with individuals personally.
3. Send information only to those individuals who need it.
4. Avoid flaming; that is, sending remarks intended to cause a negative reaction.
5. Do not write in all capital letters; this suggests anger.
6. Respect other people's privacy.
7. Do not abuse the power of your position.
8. Proofread your e-mail before sending it.

Adapted from Shea, V. (2000). Netiquette. San Rafael, Calif.: Albion.

---

box 6-4

Information for Change-of-Shift Report

- Identify the patient, including the room and bed numbers.
- Include the patient diagnosis.
- Account for the presence of the patient on the unit. If the patient has left the unit for a diagnostic test, surgery, or just to wander, it is important for the oncoming staff members to know the patient is off the unit.
- Provide the treatment plan that specifies the goals of treatment. Note the goals and the critical pathway steps either achieved or in progress. Personalized approaches can be developed during this time and patient readiness for those approaches evaluated. It is helpful to mention the patient's primary care physician. Include new orders and medications and treatments currently prescribed.
- Document patient responses to current treatments. Is the treatment plan working? Present evidence for or against this. Include pertinent laboratory values as well as any negative reactions to medications or treatments. Note any comments the patient has made regarding the hospitalization or treatment plan that the oncoming staff members need to address.
- Omit personal opinions and value judgments about patients as well as personal/confidential information not pertinent to providing patient care. If you are using computerized information systems, make sure you know how to present the material accurately and concisely.

organize the work for the day (Fig. 6.1). As specific tasks are mentioned, the nurse coming on duty makes a note of the activity in the appropriate time slot. Medications and treatments can also be added.

Any changes from the previous day are noted, particularly when the nurse is familiar with the patient. Recording changes counteracts the tendency to remember what was done the day before and

Name_____ Room #_____ Allergies _____

0700	0800	0900	1000	1100	1200	1300	1400	1500	1600	1700	1800

Name_____ Room #_____ Allergies _____

0700	0800	0900	1000	1100	1200	1300	1400	1500	1600	1700	1800

Name_____ Room #_____ Allergies _____

0700	0800	0900	1000	1100	1200	1300	1400	1500	1600	1700	1800

Figure 6.1 Organization and time management schedule for patient care.

repeat it, often without checking for new orders. During the day, the worksheet acts as a reminder of the tasks that have been completed and of those that still need to be done.

Reporting skills improve with practice. When presenting information in a report, certain details must be included. Begin the report by identifying the patient and the admitting as well as current diagnoses. Include the expected treatment plan and the patient's responses to the treatment. For example, if the patient has had multiple antibiotics and a

reaction occurred, this information is important to relay to the next nurse. Value judgments and personal opinions about the patient are inappropriate (Fig. 6.2).

Team Conferences

Members of a team share information through verbal and written communication in an interdisciplinary team conference. The team conference begins by stating the patient's name, age, and diagnoses. Each member of an interdisciplinary team

Room # _____ Patient Name _____ Diagnoses _____

Diet _____ Activity_____

1900	0100
2000	0200
2100	0300
2200	0400
2300	0500
2400	0600

Figure 6.2 Patient information report.

then explains the goal of his or her discipline, the interventions, and the outcome. Effectiveness of treatment, development of new interventions, and setting new goals are discussed. The key to a successful interdisciplinary conference is presenting information in a clear, concise manner and ensuring input from all disciplines and levels of care providers, from unlicensed assistive personnel to physicians.

Communicating With Other Disciplines

Breakdowns in verbal and written communication among health-care providers present a major concern in the health-care delivery system. The Joint Commission (www.jcaho.org) attributes a high percentage of sentinel events to be related to poor communication among health-care providers. In many settings, nurses act as patient care managers. Integration, coordination, and communication among all disciplines that are delivering care to a specific patient ultimately are the responsibility of the nurse care manager. Nurses often find themselves in the particularly advantageous position to observe the patient's responses to treatments. For example:

> *Mr. Richards is a 75-year-old man who was in a motor vehicle accident with closed head trauma. He had right-sided weakness and dysphagia. The speech therapy, physical therapy, and social services departments were called in to see Mr. Richards. A speech therapist was working with Mr. Richards to assist him with swallowing. He was to receive pureed foods for the second day. The RN assigned an LPN to feed Mr. Richards. The LPN reported that although Mr. Richards had done well the previous day, he had difficulty swallowing today. The RN immediately notified the speech therapist, and a new treatment plan was developed.*

Communicating With the Health-Care Provider

The function of professional nurses in relation to their patients' health-care providers is to communicate changes in the patient's condition, share other pertinent information, discuss modifications of the treatment plan, and clarify orders. This can be stressful for a new graduate who still has some role insecurity. Using good communication skills and having the necessary information at hand are helpful when discussing patient needs.

Before calling a health-care provider, make sure that all the information you need is available. The provider may want more clarification. If you are calling to report a drop in a patient's blood pressure, be sure to have the list of the patient's medications, laboratory results, vital signs, and blood pressure trends, together with a general assessment of the patient's present status.

Sometimes when a nurse calls a physician or health-care provider, the physician does not return the call. It is important to document all health-care provider contacts in the patient's record. Many units keep calling logs. In the log, enter the health-care provider's name, the date, the time, the reason for the call, and the time the health-care provider returns the call.

SBAR

In response to the number of patients who die from or confront a preventable adverse event during hospitalization, health-care institutions have been challenged to improve patient safety standards. This challenge forced health-care institutions to look at the causes of most sentinel events within their environments. SBAR, developed by experts at Kaiser Permanente, one of the largest health-care systems, is an abbreviation for *S*ituation, *B*ackground, *A*ssessment, and *R*ecommendation (Haig, Sutton, & Whittingdon, 2006). It provides a framework for communicating critical patient information in a systemized and organized fashion. The SBAR method focuses on the immediate situation so that decisions regarding patient care may be made quickly and safely.

Although originally established to be used as an "escalation tool," to be implemented when a rapid change in patient status occurs or is imminent, many institutions have decided to implement the method as a standard for shift report and other coordinating communications (Haig, Sutton, & Whittingdon; www.rwjf.org, 2008). The use of the SBAR format helps to standardize a communication system to effectively transmit needed information to provide safe and effective patient care. Table 6-2 defines the steps of the SBAR communication model.

The implementation of SBAR as a communication technique has demonstrated such success that the Institute for Healthcare Improvement recommends its use as a standard for communicating between and among health-care providers. The Joint Commission is now requiring it as a standard for

table 6-2

SBAR (Situation, Background, Assessment, Recommendation)

Elements	Description	Example
Situation	Brief description of the existing situation	Critical laboratory value that needs to be addressed (critical blood gas value, International Normalized ratio [INR], etc.)
Background	Medical, nursing, or family information that is significant to the care and/or patient condition	Patient admitted with a pulmonary embolus and on heparin therapy, receiving oxygen at 4 L via nasal cannula; what steps have been taken
Assessment	Recent assessment data that indicate the most current clinical state of the patient	Vital signs, results of laboratory values, lung sounds, mental status, pulse oximetry results, electrocardiogram results
Recommendation	Information for future interventions and/or activities	Monitor patient Change heparin dose Repeat INR Repeat computed tomography or ventilation-perfusion scan

communicating patient information for hand-off reporting (Haig, Sutton & Whittingdon, 2006; IHI, 2006).

Health-Care Provider Orders

Professional nurses are responsible for accepting, transcribing, and implementing health-care provider orders. The two main types of orders are *written* and *telephone*. *Written orders* are dated and placed on the appropriate institutional form. *Telephone orders* are given from the health-care provider directly to the nurse by telephone. Many health-care institutions are moving to maintaining the electronic medical record (EMR) and away from verbal orders as the health-care provider is present and can enter the order on the appropriate form in the patient's record. A telephone order needs to be written on the appropriate institutional form, the time and date noted, and the form signed as a telephone order by the nurse.

Most institutions require the physician to cosign the order within 24 hours. When receiving a telephone order, repeat it back to the physician for confirmation. If the health-care provider is speaking too rapidly, ask him or her to speak more slowly. Then repeat the information for confirmation.

Professionalism and a courteous attitude by all parties are necessary to maintain collegial relationships with physicians and other health-care professionals. One nurse explained their importance as follows:

RN satisfaction simply is not about money. A major factor is how well nurses feel supported in their work. Do people listen to us—our managers, upper management, human resources? Being able to communicate with each other—to be able to speak directly with your peers, physicians, or managers in a way that is nonconfrontational—is really important to having good working relationships and to providing good care. You need to have mutual respect. (Quoted by Trossman, 2005, p. 1.)

Communicating With Patients and Their Families

Communicating with patients and their families occupies a major portion of the nurse's day. Nurses teach patients and their families about medications and the patient's condition, clarify the treatment plan, and explain procedures. To do this effectively, nurses need to use communication skills and recognize the barriers to communication.

The health-care consumer may enter the setting in a highly emotional state. Nurses need to recognize the signs of an anxious or angry patient and promptly intervene to defuse the situation before it escalates. Practicing good listening skills and showing interest in the patient often helps.

Short-term stays and early-morning admissions on the day of surgery make patient teaching a challenge. The nurse must complete the admission requirements, surgical checklists, and preoperative teaching within a short time. Time for postoperative teaching is also shortened. It is important for the nurse to communicate clearly and concisely what will be done and what is expected of the patient. Allow time for questions and clarifications.

For many patients, a written preoperative and/or postoperative teaching guide helps to clarify the instructions.

Feedback

Why Do People Need Feedback?

In good weather, Herbert usually played basketball with his kids after dinner. Yesterday, however, he told them he was too tired. This evening, he said the same thing. When they urged him to play anyway, he snapped at them and told them to leave him alone.

"Herbert!" his wife exclaimed, "Why did you do that?"

"I don't know," he responded. "I'm just so tense these days. My annual review was supposed to be today, but my nurse manager was out sick. I have no idea what she is going to say. I can't think about anything else."

Had Herbert's nurse manager been providing informal feedback to staff on a regular basis, Herbert would have known his rating. He would have had a good idea about what his strengths and weaknesses were and would not be afraid of an unpleasant surprise during the review. He would also be looking forward to the opportunity to review his accomplishments and make plans with his manager for further developing his skills. He still would have been disappointed that she was unavailable, but he would not have been as distressed by it.

The process of giving and receiving evaluative feedback is an essential leadership responsibility. Done well, it is very helpful, promoting growth and increasing employee satisfaction. Done poorly, as in Herbert's case, it can be stressful, even injurious. This section considers the do's and don't's of giving and receiving feedback, how to share positive and negative evaluative comments with coworkers, and how people can respond constructively when they receive negative comments.

We all need feedback because it is difficult for us to see ourselves as others see us. Curiously, competent people generally underestimate their ability and focus on their shortcomings, and incompetent people generally fail to recognize their incompetence (Channer & Hope, 2001). The following are just a few of the reasons that evaluative feedback is so important:

- **Reinforces constructive behavior.** Positive feedback lets people know which behaviors are

the most productive and encourages continuation of those behaviors.
- **Discourages unproductive behavior.** Correction of inappropriate behavior begins with provision of negative feedback.
- **Provides recognition.** The power of praise (positive feedback) to motivate people is underestimated.
- **Develops employee skills.** Feedback helps people identify their strengths and weaknesses and guides them in seeking opportunities to further develop their strengths and manage their weaknesses (Rosen, 1996).

Guidelines for Providing Feedback

Done well, evaluative feedback can reinforce motivation, strengthen teamwork, and improve the quality of care given. When done poorly, evaluation can reinforce poor work habits, increase insecurity, and destroy motivation and morale (Table 6-3).

Evaluation involves making judgments and communicating these judgments to others. People make judgments all the time about all types of things. Unfortunately, these judgments are often based on opinions, preferences, and inaccurate or partial information.

Subjective, biased judgment offered as objective feedback has given evaluation a bad name. Poorly communicated feedback has an equally negative effect. Many people who are uncomfortable with evaluation have been recipients of subjective, biased, or poorly communicated evaluations.

Evaluative feedback is most effective when given immediately, frequently, and privately. To be constructive, it must be objective, based on observed behavior, and skillfully communicated. The feedback message should include the reasons

table 6-3	
Do's and Don't's of Providing Feedback	
Do	**Don't**
Include positive comments	Focus only on the negative
Be objective	Let personalities intrude
Be specific when correcting someone	Be vague
Treat everyone the same	Play favorites
Correct people in private	Correct people in front of others

Adapted from Gabor, D. (1994). Speaking Your Mind in 101 Difficult Situations. N.Y.: Stonesong Press (Simon & Schuster).

that a behavior has been judged satisfactory or unsatisfactory. If the message is negative, it should include both suggestions and support for change and improvement (Box 6-5).

Provide Both Positive and Negative Feedback

Leaders and managers often neglect to provide positive feedback. If questioned about this, they often say, "If I don't say anything, that means everything is okay." They do not realize that some people assume that everything is not okay when they receive no feedback. Others assume that no one is aware of how much effort they have made unless it is acknowledged with positive feedback.

Most people want to do their work well. They also want to know that their efforts are recognized and appreciated. Kron (1981) called positive feedback a "psychological paycheck." She pointed out that it is almost as important to people as their actual paychecks. It is a real pleasure, not only for staff members but also for their leaders and managers, to be able to share the satisfaction of a job well done with someone else. Leaders and managers should do everything they can to reward and retain their best staff members (Bowers & Lapziger, 2001). In fact, some claim that the very best managers focus on people's strengths and work around their weaknesses (DiMichele & Gaffney, 2005).

Providing negative feedback is just as necessary but probably more difficult to do well. Too often, negative feedback is critical rather than helpful. Simply telling someone that something has gone wrong or could have been done better is inadequate. Instead, make feedback a learning experience by suggesting ways to make changes or by working together to develop a strategy for improvement. It is easier to make broad, critical comments (e.g., "You're too slow.") than to describe the specific behavior that needs improvement (e.g., "Waiting in Mr. D.'s room while he cleans his dentures takes up too much of your time.") and to add a suggestion for change (e.g., "You could get your bath supplies together while he finishes.").

Unsatisfactory work must be acknowledged and discussed with the people involved. Too many managers avoid it, not wanting to hurt people's feelings (Watson & Harris, 1999). Tolerating poor work encourages its continuation.

Give Immediate Feedback

The most helpful feedback is given as soon as possible after the behavior has occurred. There are several reasons for this. Immediate feedback is more meaningful to the person receiving it. Address inappropriate behavior when it occurs, whether it is low productivity, tardiness, or other problems. Problems that are ignored often get worse. Ignoring them puts stress on others and reduces morale. Resolving them boosts productivity, lowers stress, increases retention of good staff, and ultimately results in higher-quality care (Briles, 2005).

Provide Frequent Feedback

Frequent feedback keeps motivation high. It also becomes easier with practice. If giving and receiving feedback are frequent, integral parts of team functioning, such communication will be easier to accomplish and will be less threatening. It becomes an ordinary, everyday occurrence, one that happens spontaneously and is familiar to everyone on the team.

Give Negative Feedback Privately

Giving negative feedback privately prevents unnecessary embarrassment. It avoids the possibility that those who overhear the discussion misunderstand it and draw erroneous conclusions. A good manager praises staffers in public but corrects them in private (Matejka, Ashworth, & Dodd-McCue, 1986).

Be Objective

Being objective can be very difficult. Evaluate people on the basis of job expectations and the results of their efforts (Fonville, Killian, & Tranberger, 1998). Do not compare them, favorably or unfavorably, with other staff members (Gellerman & Hodgson, 1988).

Another way to increase objectivity is to always give a reason why a behavior has been judged as good or poor. Consider the effect or outcome of the behavior in forming your conclusion. Give reasons

---

box 6-5

Tips for Providing Helpful Feedback

- Provide both positive and negative feedback.
- Give feedback immediately.
- Provide feedback frequently.
- Give negative feedback privately.
- Base feedback on observable behavior.
- Communicate effectively.
- Include suggestions for change.

for both positive and negative messages. For example, if you tell a coworker, "That was a good patient interview," you have told that person only that the interview pleased you. However, when you add, "because you asked open-ended questions that encouraged the patient to explore personal feelings," you have identified and reinforced this specific behavior that made your evaluation positive.

Finally, use broad and generally accepted standards for making judgments as much as possible rather than basing evaluation on your personal likes and dislikes. Objectivity can be increased by using standards that reflect the consensus of the team, the organization, the community, or the nursing profession. Formal evaluation is based on commonly accepted, written standards of behavior. Informal evaluation, however, is based on unwritten standards. If these unwritten standards are based on personal preferences, the evaluation will be highly subjective. The following are examples:

- A team leader who describes a female social worker as having a professional appearance because she wears muted suits instead of bright dresses to work is using a personal standard to evaluate that social worker.
- A supervisor who asks an employee to stop wearing jewelry that could get caught in the equipment used at work is applying a standard for safety in making the evaluative statement.

Base Feedback on Observable Behavior

An evaluative statement should describe observed performance, not your interpretation of another's behavior. For example, saying, "You were impatient with Mrs. G. today" is an interpretive comment. Saying, "You interrupted Mrs. G. before she finished explaining her problem" is based on observable behavior. The second statement is more specific and may be more accurate because the caregiver may have been trying to redirect the conversation to more immediate concerns rather than being impatient. The latter statement is also more likely to evoke an explanation than a defensive response.

Include Suggestions for Change

When you give feedback that indicates that some kind of change in behavior is needed, it is helpful to suggest some alternative behaviors. This is easier to do when the change is a simple one.

When complex change is needed (as with Mr. S. below), you may find that the person is aware of the problem but does not know how to solve it. In such a case, offering to engage in searching for the solution is appropriate. A willingness to listen to the other person's side of the story and assist in finding a solution indicates that your purpose is to help rather than to criticize.

Accept Feedback in Return

An evaluative statement is a form of confrontation. Any message that contains a statement about the behavior of a staff member confronts that staff member with his or her behavior. The leader who gives evaluative feedback needs to be prepared to receive feedback in return and to engage in active listening. Active listening is especially important because the person receiving the evaluation may respond with intense emotion. The following is an example of what may happen:

> You point out to Mr. S. that his clients need to be monitored more frequently. Mr. S. responds, with some agitation, that he is doing everything possible for the patients and does not have a free moment all day for one extra thing. In fact, Mr. S. tells you, he never even takes a lunch break and goes home exhausted. Active listening and problem solving aimed at relieving his overloaded time schedule are a must in this situation.

When you give negative feedback, allow time for the receiver to express his or her opinions and for problem solving. This is particularly important if the problem has been ignored or has become serious (Box 6-6).

Seeking Evaluative Feedback

It is equally important to be able to accept constructive The reasons for seeking feedback are the same as those for giving it to others. The criteria

---

box 6-6

TACTFUL Guidelines for Providing Negative Feedback

T: Think before you speak.

A: Apologize quickly if you make a mistake.

C: Converse; do not be patronizing or sarcastic.

T: Time your comments carefully.

F: Focus on behavior, not on personality.

U: Uncover hidden feelings.

L: Listen for feedback.

for evaluating the feedback you receive are also the same.

When Is Evaluative Feedback Needed?

You may find yourself in a work situation in which you receive very little feedback, or you may be getting only positive and no negative comments (or vice versa) (Box 6-7).

You also need to look for feedback when you feel uncertain about how well you are doing or whether you have interpreted the expectations of the job correctly. The following are examples of these situations:

■ You have been told that good patient care is the highest priority, but you feel frustrated by never having enough staff members to give good care.
■ You thought you were expected to do case finding and health teaching in your community, but you receive the most recognition for the number of home visits made and the completeness of your records.

Another instance in which you should request feedback is when you believe that your needs for recognition and job satisfaction have not been met adequately.

Request feedback in the form of "I" messages. If you have received only negative comments, ask, "In what ways have I done well?" If you receive only positive comments, you can ask, "In what areas do I need to improve?" If you are seeking feedback from a patient, you could ask, "How can I be of more help to you?"

Responding to Evaluative Feedback

Sometimes, it is appropriate to critically analyze the feedback you are getting. If the feedback seems totally negative or you feel threatened by receiving it, ask for further explanation. You may have misunderstood what your nurse manager intended to say.

It is hard to avoid responding defensively to negative feedback that is subjective or laced with

threats and blame. If you are the recipient of such a poorly done evaluation, however, it may help both you and your supervisor to try to guide the discussion into more constructive areas. You can ask for reasons why the evaluation was negative, on what standard it was based, what the person's expectations were, and what the person suggests as alternative behavior.

When the feedback is positive but nonspecific, you may also want to ask for some clarification so that you can learn what that person's expectations really are. Do not hesitate to seek that psychological paycheck. Tell other people about your successes; most are happy to share the satisfaction of a successful outcome or positive development in a patient's care.

Performance Appraisal

Performance appraisal is the formal evaluation of an employee by a superior, usually a manager or supervisor. To prepare an appraisal, the employee's behavior is compared with his or her job description and the standard describing how the employee is expected to perform (Hayes, 2002). Employees need to know what has to be done, how much has to be done, and when it has to be done. Evaluate actual performance, not good intentions.

Procedure

In the ideal situation, the performance appraisal begins when the employee is hired. Based on the written job description, the employee and manager discuss performance expectations and then write a set of objectives they think the employee can reasonably accomplish within a given time. The objectives should be written at a level of performance that demonstrates that some learning, refinement of skill, or advancement toward some long-range objective will have occurred. The following are examples of objectives a new staff nurse could accomplish in the first 6 months of employment:

■ Complete the staff nurse orientation program successfully.
■ Master the basic skills necessary to function as a staff nurse on the assigned unit.
■ Supervise the unlicensed assistive personnel assigned to his or her patients.

Monthly reviews of progress toward these goals help keep the new staff member on track and provide opportunities to identify needs for further orientation or extended training (Hayes, 2002; Lombardi, 2001). Six months later, the staff nurse and nurse manager sit down again and evaluate the staff nurse's performance in terms of the previously set goals. The evaluation is based on the staff nurse's self-evaluation and the nurse manager's observation of specific behaviors. New objectives for the next 6 months and plans for achieving them may be agreed on at the time of the appraisal or at a separate meeting (Beer, 1981). A copy of the performance appraisal and the new goals must be available to employees so that they can refer to them and check on their progress.

It is important to set aside adequate time for feedback and goal-setting processes. Both the staff nurse and the nurse manager bring data for use at this session. These data include a self-evaluation by the staff nurse and observations by the evaluator of the employee's activities and their outcomes. Data may also be obtained from peers and patients. Some organizations use surveys for getting this information from patients.

Most of the guidelines for providing evaluative feedback discussed earlier apply to the conduct of performance appraisals. Although not as frequent or immediate as informal feedback, formal evaluation should be just as objective, private, skillfully communicated, and growth-promoting.

Standards for Evaluation

Unfortunately, many organizations' employee evaluation procedures are far from ideal. Such procedures may be inconsistent, subjective, and even unknown to the employee in some cases. The following is a list of standards for a fair and objective employee evaluation procedure that you can use to judge your employer's procedures:

- Standards are clear, objective, and known in advance.
- Criteria for pay raises and promotions are clearly spelled out and uniformly applied.
- Conditions under which employment may be terminated are known.
- Appraisals are part of the employee's permanent record and have space for employee comments.
- Employees may inspect their own personnel file.
- Employees may request and be given a reasonable explanation of any rating and may appeal the rating if they do not agree with it.

- Employees are given a reasonable amount of time to correct any serious deficiencies before other action is taken, unless the safety of self or others is immediately threatened.

In some organizations, collective bargaining agreements are used to enforce adherence to fair and objective performance appraisals. However, collective bargaining agreements may emphasize seniority (length of service) over merit, a situation that does not promote growth or change.

Peer Review

Peer review is the evaluation of an individual's practice by his or her colleagues (peers) who have similar education, experience, and occupational status. Its purpose is to provide the individual with feedback from those who are best acquainted with the requirements and demands of that individual's position: colleagues. Peer review is directed to both *actions* (process) and the *outcomes* of actions. It also encompasses decision making (critical thinking) and technical and interpersonal skills (Mustard, 2002).

Professionals frequently observe and judge their colleagues' performance. However, many feel uncomfortable telling colleagues directly what they think of their performance, so they do not indicate their thoughts unless informal feedback is shared regularly or a formal system of peer review is established (Katzenbach & Smith, 2003). Whenever staff members meet to audit records or otherwise evaluate the quality of care they have given, they are engaging in a kind of peer review.

Formal peer review programs are often one of the last formal evaluation procedures to be implemented in a health-care organization. They increase the number of sources of feedback and contribute to a rich, comprehensive evaluation process (Guthrie & King, 2004).

Fundamentals of Peer Review

There are many possible variations of the peer review process. The observations may be shared only with the person being reviewed, with the person's supervisor, or with a review committee. The evaluation report may be written by the reviewer, or it may come from the review committee. The use of a committee defeats the purpose of peer review if the committee members are not truly peers of the individual being reviewed.

A Comprehensive Peer Review System

Peer review systems can simply be informal feedback regularly shared among colleagues, or they may be comprehensive systems that are fully integrated into the formal evaluation structure of a health-care organization. When a peer review system is fully integrated, the evaluative feedback from peers is joined with the performance appraisals by the nurse manager, and both are used to determine pay raises and promotions for individual staff nurses. This is a far more collegial approach than the hierarchical one typically used, in which employees are evaluated only by their manager.

A comprehensive peer review system begins with the development of job descriptions and performance standards for each level within the nursing staff. The job description is a very general statement, whereas the standards are specific behaviors that can be observed and recorded.

In a participative environment, the standards are developed by committees having representatives from different units and from each staff level, from the new staff nurse to top-level management. In some instances, they are very specific, quantifiable criteria, but others are likely to require professional judgment as to the quality of the care provided (Chang et al., 2002).

In some organizations, the standards may be considered the minimal qualifications for each level. In this case, additional activities and professional development are expected before promotion to the next level. The candidate for promotion to an advanced-level position prepares a promotion portfolio for review (Schultz, 1993). The promotion portfolio may include a self-assessment, peer reviews, patient surveys, a management performance appraisal, and evidence of professional growth. Such evidence can derive from participating in the quality improvement program, evaluating a new product or procedure, serving as a translator or disaster volunteer, making post-discharge visits to patients from the unit, or taking courses related to nursing.

Writing useful job descriptions and measurable standards of performance is an arduous but rewarding task. It requires clarification and explication of the work nurses actually do and goes beyond the usual generalizations. Under effective group leadership and with strong administrative support for this process, it can be a challenging and stimulating

experience. Without administrative support and guidance, however, the committee work can be frustrating when the group gets bogged down in details and disagreements.

When the job descriptions and performance standards for each level have been developed and agreed on, a procedure for their use must also be worked out. This can be done in several ways. In some organizations, an evaluation form that lists the performance standards can be completed by one or two colleagues selected by the individual staff member. In some organizations, the information from these forms is used along with the nurse manager's evaluation to determine pay raises and promotions. In others, the evaluation from one's peers is used for counseling purposes only and is not taken into consideration in determining pay raises or promotions. This second approach provides useful feedback but weakens the impact of peer review.

A different approach is the use of a professional practice committee. The committee, consisting of colleagues selected by the nursing staff, reviews the peer evaluation forms and makes its recommendations to the director of nursing or vice president for patient care services, who then makes the final decision regarding the appropriate rewards (raises, promotions, commendations) or penalties (demotion, transfer, termination of employment).

Conclusion

The responsibility for delivering and coordinating patient care is an important part of the role of the professional nurse. To accomplish this, nurses need good communication skills. Being assertive without being aggressive and conducting interactions in a professional manner enhance the relationships that nurses develop with colleagues, physicians, and other members of the interdisciplinary team.

A major focus of the national safety goals is improved communication among health-care professionals. In an effort to improve patient safety, health-care institutions have moved toward implementing a communication protocol referred to as the SBAR method. SBAR sets a specific procedure that reminds nurses how to relay information quickly and effectively to the patient's health-care provider, which ultimately leads to improved patient outcomes.

Communication skills are also part of evaluation. A comprehensive evaluation system can be an effective mechanism for improving staff skills and morale and for reducing costs by increasing staff productivity. Constructive feedback demands objectivity and fairness in dealing with each other and leadership of both staff members and management. Done well, feedback can provide many opportunities for increased professionalism and learning as well as ensure appropriate rewards for high performance levels and professionalism on the job.

Study Questions

1. This is your first position as an RN, and you are working with an LPN who has been on the unit for 20 years. On your first day she says to you, "The only difference between you and me is the size of the paycheck." Demonstrate how you would respond to this statement, using assertive communication techniques.

2. A physician orders "Vit K 10 mg IV." You realize that this is a dangerous order. How would you approach the physician?

3. A patient is admitted to the same-day surgical center for a breast biopsy. She is accompanied by her significant other, who has just had an altercation with an admissions secretary about their insurance. The patient then has to wait 30 minutes after her designated arrival time. When the nurse comes to call the patient, her significant other turns and says loudly, "What is wrong with you people? Can't you ever get anything straight? If you can't get the insurance right, and you can't get the time right, how can we expect you to get the surgery right?" How would you defuse the situation?

4. Why is feedback important? Who needs to receive feedback? Who should give feedback to health-care providers?

5. Describe the difference between constructive (helpful) and destructive (unhelpful) feedback.

6. Describe an ideal version of a 3-month performance appraisal of a new staff nurse. Why do nurse managers sometimes fail to meet this ideal when providing formal evaluative feedback? Can new staff nurses do anything to improve these procedures in their place of employment?

7. What is peer review? How is it different from other types of evaluation? Why is it important?

Case Study to Promote Critical Reasoning

Tyrell Jones is a new unlicensed assistant who has been assigned to your acute rehabilitation unit. Tyrell is a hard worker; he comes in early and often stays late to finish his work. But Tyrell is gruff with the patients, especially with the male patients. If a patient is reluctant to get out of bed, Tyrell often challenges him, saying, "C'mon, man. Don't be such a wimp. Move your big butt." Today, you overheard Tyrell telling a female patient who said she did not feel well, "You're just a phony. You like being waited on, but that's not why you're here." The woman started to cry.

1. You are the newest staff nurse on this unit. How would you handle this situation? What would happen if you ignored it?

2. If you decided that you should not ignore it, with whom should you speak? Why? What would you say?

3. Why do you think Tyrell speaks to patients this way?

References

Arnold, J., & Pearson, G. (eds.). (1992). *Computer Applications in Nursing Education and Practice.* N.Y.: National League for Nursing.

Beer, M. (1981, Winter). Performance appraisal: Dilemmas and possibilities. *Organizational Dynamics, 24.*

Blais, K.B., Hayes, J.S., Kozier, B., & Erb, G. (2002). *Professional Nursing Practice: Concepts and Perspectives,* 4th ed. Upper Saddle River, N.J.: Prentice-Hall.

Bowers, B., & Lapziger, D. (2001). *The New York Times Management Reader.* N.Y.: Times Books.

Briles, J. (2005). Steer your solution in the right direction. *Nursing Management,* 36:5, 68.

Chang, B.L., Lee, J.L., Pearson, M.L., Kahn, K.L., et al. (July/August 2002). Evaluating quality of nursing care. *Journal of Nursing Administration,* 32(7/8), 405–415.

Channer, P., & Hope, T. (2001). *Emotional Impact: Passionate Leaders and Corporate Transformation.* Hampshire, U.K.: Palgrave.

Dee, C. (2005). Making the most of nursing's electronic resources. *American Journal of Nursing,* 105:9, 79–85.

DiMichele, C., & Gaffney, L. (2005). Proactive teams yield exceptional care. *Nursing Management,* 36:5, 61.

Fontaine, K.L., & Fletcher, J.S. (2002). *Mental Health Nursing,* 5th ed. Redwood City, Calif.: Prentice-Hall.

Fonville, A.M., Killian, E.R., & Tranberger, R.E. (1998). Developing new nurse leaders. *Nurse Economics,* 16, 83–87.

Gabor, D. (1994). *Speaking Your Mind in 101 Difficult Situations.* N.Y.: Stonesong Press (Simon & Schuster).

Gellerman, S.W., & Hodgson, W.G. (1988). Cyanamid's new take on performance appraisal. *Harvard Business Review,* 88(3), 36–41.

Guthrie, V.A., & King, S.N. (2004). Feedback-Intensive Program. In McCauly, C.D., & Van Velsor, E. (eds.). *The Center for Creative Leadership Handbook of Leadership Development.* San Francisco: Jossey-Bass.

Haig, K.M., Sutton, S., & Whittingdon, J. (2006). SBAR: A shared mental model for improving communication between clinicians. *Journal on Quality and Patient Safety,* 32(3), 167-175.

Hayes, H. (Winter 2002). Employee training and job descriptions. *Maryland Medicine,* 3(1), 39–41.

Hebda, T., Czar, P., & Mascara, C. (1998). *Handbook of Informatics for Nurses and Health Care Professionals.* Menlo Park, Calif.: Addison-Wesley.

Institute for Healthcare Improvement. (2006). Using SBAR to improve communication between caregivers. Retrieved November 30, 2008, from http://www.ihi.org/IHI/Programs/AudioAndWebPrograms/WebACTIONUsingSBARtoImproveCommunication.htm?TabId=7

Katzenbach, J.R., & Smith, D.K. (2003). *The Wisdom of Teams.* N.Y.: Harper Collins.

Kron, T. (1981). *The Management of Patient Care: Putting Leadership Skills to Work.* Philadelphia: WB Saunders.

Lombardi, D.N. (2001). *Handbook for the New Health Care Manager.* San Francisco: Jossey-Bass.

Matejka, J.K., Ashworth, D.N., & Dodd-McCue, D. (1986). Discipline without guilt. *Supervisory Management,* 31(5), 34–36.

Mustard, L.W. (2002). Caring and competency. *JONA's Healthcare Law, Ethics and Regulation,* 4(2), 36–43.

Rees, F. (2005). *25 Activities for Developing Team Leaders.* San Francisco: Pfeiffer.

Robert Wood Johnson Foundation. (2008). Improving nurse-physician communication. Retrieved November 30, 2008, from http://www.rwjf.org

Rosen, R.H. (1996). *Leading People: Transforming Business From the Inside Out.* N.Y.: Viking Penguin.

Schultz, A.W. (1993). Evaluation for clinical advancement systems. *Journal of Nursing Administration,* 23(2), 13–19.

Shea, V. (2000). *Netiquette.* San Rafael, Calif.: Albion.

Tappen, R.M. (2001). *Nursing Leadership and Management: Concepts and Practice,* 4th ed. Philadelphia: FA Davis.

Trossman, S. (2005). Who you work with matters. *American Nurse,* 37:4, 1, 8. American Nurses Association.

Watson, T., & Harris, P. (1999). *The Emergent Manager.* London: Sage Publications.

chapter 7

Dealing With Problems and Conflicts

⊙ ○ ○ ○ ○ ○ ○ **○** ○ ○ ○

OBJECTIVES

After reading this chapter, the student should be able to:

- Identify common sources of conflict in the workplace.
- Guide an individual or small group through the process of problem resolution.
- Participate in informal negotiations.
- Discuss the purposes of collective bargaining.

OUTLINE

Various pressures and demands in the workplace generate problems and conflicts among people. These conflicts can interfere with the ability to work together. If the various polls and surveys of nurses are correct, there seems to be an increasing amount of hostility and unresolved conflict experienced by nurses at work (Lazoritz & Carlson, 2008; Siu, Laschinger, & Finegan, 2008;). Harassment from doctors, supervisors, managers, and colleagues can be very stressful (McVicar, 2003; Vivar, 2006). Consider Case 1, which is the first of three in this chapter that will be used to illustrate how to deal with problems and conflicts.

Conflict

There are no conflict-free work groups (Van de Vliert & Janssen, 2001). Small or large, conflicts are a daily occurrence in the life of nurses (McElhaney, 1996), and they can interfere with getting work done, as shown in Case 1.

Serious conflicts can be very stressful for the people involved. Stress symptoms—such as difficulty concentrating, anxiety, sleep disorders, and withdrawal—or other interpersonal relationship problems can occur. Bitterness, anger, and even violence can erupt in the workplace if conflicts are not resolved.

Conflict also has a positive side, however. For example, in the process of learning how to manage conflict, people can develop more open, cooperative ways of working together (Tjosvold & Tjosvold, 1995). They can begin to see each other as people with similar needs, concerns, and dreams instead of as competitors or blocks in the way of progress. Being involved in successful conflict resolution can be an empowering experience (Horton-Deutsch & Wellman, 2002).

The goal in dealing with conflict is to create an environment in which conflicts are dealt with in as cooperative and constructive a manner as possible, rather than in a competitive and destructive manner.

Many Sources of Conflict

Why do conflicts occur? Health care brings people of different ages, gender, income levels, ethnic groups, educational levels, lifestyles, and professions together for the purpose of restoring or maintaining people's

---

Case 1

Team A and Team B

Team A has stopped talking to Team B. If several members of Team A are out sick, no one on Team B will help Team A with their work. Likewise, Team A members will not take telephone messages for anyone on Team B. Instead, they ask the person to call back later. When members of the two teams pass each other in the hall, they either glare at each other or turn away to avoid eye contact. Arguments erupt when members of the two teams need the same computer terminal or another piece of equipment at the same time.

When a Team A nurse reached for a pulse oximeter at the same moment as a Team B nurse did, the second nurse said, "You've been using that all morning."

"I've got a lot of patients to monitor," was the response.

"Oh, you think you're the only one with work to do?"

"We take good care of our patients."

"Are you saying we don't?"

The nurses fell silent when the nurse manager entered the room.

"Is something the matter?" she asked. Both nurses shook their heads and left quickly.

"I'm not sure what's going on here," the nurse manager thought to herself, "but something's wrong, and I need to find out what it is right away."

We will return to this case later as we discuss workplace problems and conflicts, their sources, and how to resolve them.

health. Some conflicts are focused on issues related to the work being done; these are task-related conflicts. Others are primarily related to personal and social issues; these are relationship conflicts (Jordan & Troth, 2004). Differences of opinion over how to best accomplish this goal are a normal part of working with people of various skill levels and backgrounds (Wenckus, 1995). In addition, the workplace itself can be a generator of conflict. Following are some of the most common reasons why conflict occurs in the workplace.

Power Plays and Competition Between Groups

Nurse-physician relationships are frequent sources of conflicts (Vivar, 2006). The most common problem is disrespect, but sarcasm, finger pointing, throwing things, inappropriate language, and demeaning remarks also occur (Lazoritz & Carlson, 2008). Disagreements over professional "territory" can occur in any setting. Nurse practitioners and physicians may disagree over limitations on nurse practitioner independence. Bullying involves behavior intended to exert power over another person. Physician dominance and authoritarian management may create an environment in which bullying occurs.

In some settings nurses feel powerless, trapped by the demands of the tasks they must complete and frustrated that they cannot provide quality care (Ramos, 2006). Union-management conflicts occur regularly in some workplaces. Gender-based conflicts, including equal pay for women and sexual harassment issues, are other examples (Ehrlich, 1995).

Increased Workload

Emphasis on cost reductions has resulted in *work intensification*, a situation in which employees are required to do more in less time (Willis, Taffoli, Henderson, & Walter, 2008). Common examples are skipping lunch and unpaid overtime. This leaves many health-care workers believing that their employers are taking advantage of them (Ketter, 1994) and causes conflict if they believe others are not working as hard as they are.

Multiple Role Demands

Inappropriate task assignments (e.g., asking nurses to clean the floors as well as nurse their patients) are often the result of cost-control efforts, which

can lead to disagreements about who does what task and who is responsible for the outcome.

Threats to Safety and Security

When cost saving is emphasized and staff members face layoffs, people's economic security is threatened. This can be a source of considerable stress and tension (Qureshi, 1996; Rondeau & Wagar, 2002).

Scarce Resources

Inadequate money for pay raises, equipment, supplies, or additional help can increase competition between or among departments and individuals as they scramble to grab their share of what little there is available.

Cultural Differences

Different beliefs about how hard a person should work, what constitutes productivity, and even what it means to arrive at work "on time" can lead to problems if they are not reconciled.

Invasion of Personal Space

Crowded conditions and the constant interactions that occur at a busy nurses' station can increase interpersonal tension and lead to battles over scarce work space (McElhaney, 1996).

When Conflict Occurs

Conflicts can occur at any level and involve any number of people, including supervisors, subordinates, peers, or patients (Sanon-Rollins, 2000). On the individual level, they can occur between two people on a team, between two people in different departments, or between a staff member and a patient or family member (Box 7-1). On the group level, conflict can occur between two teams

---

box 7-1

Signs That Conflict Resolution Is Needed

- You feel very uncomfortable in a situation.
- Members of your team are having trouble working together.
- Team members stop talking with each other.
- Team members begin "losing their cool," attacking each other verbally.

Adapted from Patterson, K., Grenny, J., McMillan, R., & Surtzler, A. (18 March 2003). Crucial conversations: Making a difference between being healed and being seriously hurt. Vital Signs, 13(5), 14–15.

(as in Case 1), two departments, or two different professional groups (e.g., nurses and social workers, over who is responsible for discharge planning). On the organizational level, conflicts can occur between two organizations (e.g., when two home health agencies compete for a contract with a large hospital). The focus in this chapter is primarily on the first two levels: among individuals and groups of people within a health-care organization.

Resolving Problems and Conflicts

Win, Lose, or Draw?

Some people think about problems and conflicts that occur at work in the same way they think about a football game or tennis match: unless the score is tied at the end of the game, someone has won, and someone has lost. There are some problems in this comparison with sports competition. First, the aim of conflict resolution is to work together more effectively, not to defeat the other party. Second, the people who lose are likely to feel bad about losing. As a result, they may spend their time and energy preparing to win the next round rather than on their work.

A win-win result in which both sides gain some benefit is the best resolution (Haslan, 2001). However, sometimes the people involved cannot reach agreement (consensus) but can recognize and accept their differences and get on with their work (McDonald, 2008).

Other Conflict Resolution Myths

Many people think of what can be "won" as a fixed amount: "I get half, and you get half." This is the *fixed pie* myth of conflict resolution (Thompson & Fox, 2001). The problem is that if one side gets everything, then the other side gets nothing. Another erroneous assumption is called the *devaluation reaction*: "If the other side is getting what they want, then it has to be bad for us." These erroneous beliefs can be serious barriers to achievement of a mutually beneficial resolution of a conflict.

When disagreements first arise, *problem solving* may be sufficient. If the situation has already developed into a full conflict, however, *negotiation*, either informal or formal, of a settlement may be necessary.

Problem Resolution

The use of the problem-solving process in patient care should be familiar. The same approach can be used when staff problems occur. The goal is to find a solution to a given problem that satisfies everyone involved. The process itself, illustrated in Figure 7.1, includes identifying the issue, generating solutions, evaluating the suggested solutions, choosing what appears to be the best solution, implementing that solution, evaluating the extent to which the problem has been resolved and, finally, concluding either that the problem has been resolved or that it will be necessary to repeat the process to find a better solution.

Identify the Problem or Issue

Ask participants in the conflict what they want (Sportsman, 2005). If the issue is not highly charged or highly political, they may be able to give a direct answer. At other times, however, some discussion and exploration of the issues are necessary before the real problem emerges. "It would be nice," wrote Browne and Kelley, "if what other people were really saying was always obvious, if all their essential thoughts were clearly labeled for us . . . and if all knowledgeable people agreed about answers to important questions" (1994, p. 5). Of course, this is not what usually happens. People are often vague about what their real concern is; sometimes they are genuinely uncertain about what the real problem is. High emotion may further cloud the issue. All this needs to be sorted out so that the problem is identified clearly and a solution can be sought.

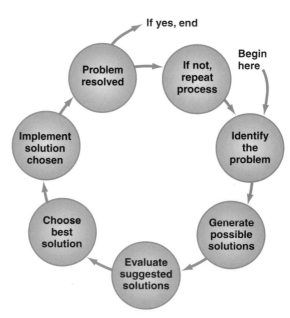

Figure 7.1 The process of resolving a problem.

Generate Possible Solutions

Here, creativity is especially important. Try to discourage people from using old solutions for new problems. It is natural for people to try to repeat something that has already worked well, but previously successful solutions may not work in the future (Walsh, 1996). Instead, encourage searching for innovative solutions (Smialek, 2001).

When an innovative solution is needed, suggest that the group take some time to *brainstorm*. Ask everyone to write down (or call out as you write on a flip chart) as many solutions as he or she can come up with (Rees, 2005). Then give everyone a chance to consider each suggestion on its own merits.

Evaluate Suggested Solutions

An open-minded evaluation of each suggestion is needed, but accomplishing this is not always easy. Some groups are "stuck in a rut," unable to "think outside the box." Other times, groups find it difficult to separate the suggestion from its source. On an interdisciplinary team, for example, the status of the person who made the suggestion may influence whether the suggestion is judged to be useful. Whose solution is most likely to be the best one: the physician's or the unlicensed assistant's? That depends. Judge the suggestion on its merits, not its source.

Choose the Best Solution

Which of the suggested solutions is most likely to work? A combination of suggestions is often the best solution.

Implement the Solution Chosen

The true test of any suggested solution is how well it actually works. Once a solution has been implemented, it is important to give it time to work. Impatience sometimes leads to premature abandonment of a good solution.

Is the Problem Resolved?

Not every problem is resolved successfully on the first attempt. If the problem has not been resolved, then the process needs to be resumed with even greater attention to what the real problem is and how it can be resolved successfully.

Consider the following situation in which problem solving was helpful (Case 2)

The nurse manager asked Ms. Deloitte to meet with her to discuss the problem. The following is a summary of their problem solving:

- **The Issue.** Ms. Deloitte wanted to take her vacation from the end of December through early January. Making the assumption that she was going to be permitted to go, she had purchased nonrefundable tickets. The policy forbids vacations from December 20 to January 5. The

---

Case 2

The Vacation

Francine Deloitte has been a unit secretary for 10 years. She is prompt, efficient, accurate, courteous, flexible, and productive—everything a nurse manager could ask for in a unit secretary. When nursing staff members are very busy, she distributes afternoon snacks or sits with a family for a few minutes until a nurse is available. There is only one issue on which Ms. Deloitte is insistent and stubborn: taking her 2-week vacation over the Christmas and New Year holidays. This is forbidden by hospital policy, but every nurse manager has allowed her to do this because it is the only special request she ever makes and because it is the only time she visits her family during the year.

A recent reorganization of the administrative structure had eliminated several layers of nursing managers and supervisors. Each remaining nurse manager was given responsibility for two or three units. The new nurse manager for Ms. Deloitte's unit refused to grant her request for vacation time at the end of December. "I can't show favoritism," she explained. "No one else is allowed to take vacation time at the end of December." Assuming that she could have the time off as usual, Francine had already purchased a nonrefundable ticket for her visit home. When her request was denied, she threatened to quit. On hearing this, one of the nurses on Francine's unit confronted the new nurse manager saying, "You can't do this. We are going to lose the best unit secretary we've ever had if you do."

former nurse manager had not enforced this policy with Ms. Deloitte, but the new nurse manager thought it fair to enforce the policy with everyone, including Ms. Deloitte.

■ **Possible Solutions**

1. Ms. Deloitte resigns.
2. Ms. Deloitte is fired.
3. Allow Ms. Deloitte to take her vacation as planned.
4. Allow everyone to take vacations between December 20 and January 5 as requested.
5. Allow no one to take a vacation between December 20 and January 5.

■ **Evaluate Suggested Solutions.** Ms. Deloitte preferred solutions 3 and 4. The new nurse manager preferred 5. Neither wanted 1 or 2. They could agree only that none of the solutions satisfied both of them, so they decided to try again.

■ **Second List of Possible Solutions**

1. Reimburse Ms. Deloitte for the cost of the tickets.
2. Allow Ms. Deloitte to take one last vacation between December 20 and January 5.
3. Allow Ms. Deloitte to take her vacation during Thanksgiving instead.
4. Allow Ms. Deloitte to begin her vacation on December 26 so that she would work on Christmas Day but not on New Year's Day.
5. Allow Ms. Deloitte to begin her vacation earlier in December so that she could return in time to work on New Year's Day.

■ **Choose the Best Solution.** As they discussed the alternatives, Ms. Deloitte said she could change the day of her flight without a penalty. The nurse manager said she would allow solution 5 on the second list if Ms. Deloitte understood that she could not take vacation time between December 20 and January 5 in the future. Ms. Deloitte agreed to this.

■ **Implement the Solution.** Ms. Deloitte returned on December 30 and worked both New Year's Eve and New Year's Day.

■ **Evaluate the Solution.** The rest of the staff members had been watching the situation very closely. Most believed that the solution had been fair to them as well as to Ms. Deloitte. Ms. Deloitte thought she had been treated fairly. The nurse manager believed both parties had found a solution that was fair to Ms. Deloitte

but still reinforced the manager's determination to enforce the vacation policy.

■ **Resolved, or Resume Problem Solving?** Ms. Deloitte, staff members, and the nurse manager all thought the problem had been solved satisfactorily.

Negotiating an Agreement Informally

When disagreement has become too big, too complex, or too heated, a more elaborate process may be required to resolve it. On evaluating Case 1, the nurse manager decided that the tensions between Team A and Team B had become so great that negotiation would be necessary.

The process of negotiation is a complex one that requires much careful thought beforehand and considerable skill in its implementation. Box 7-2 is an outline of the most essential aspects of negotiation. Case 1 is used to illustrate how it can be done.

Scope the Situation

For a strategy to be successful, it is important that the entire situation be understood thoroughly. Walker and Harris (1995) suggested asking three questions:

1. *What am I trying to achieve?* The nurse manager in Case 1 is concerned about the tensions between Team A and Team B. She wants the members of these two teams to be able to work together in a cooperative manner, which they are not doing at the present time.
2. *What is the environment in which I am operating?* The members of Teams A and B were openly hostile to each other. The overall climate of the organization, however, was benign. The nurse manager knew that teamwork was encouraged

---

box 7-2

The Informal Negotiation Process

• Scope the situation. Ask yourself:

What am I trying to achieve?
What is the environment in which I am operating?
What problems am I likely to encounter?
What does the other side want?

• Set the stage.
• Conduct the negotiation.
• Set the ground rules.
• Clarify the problem.
• Make your opening move.
• Continue with offers and counteroffers.
• Agree on the resolution of the conflict.

and that her actions to resolve the conflict would be supported by administration.

3. *What problems am I likely to encounter?* The nurse manager knew that she had allowed the problem to go on too long. Even physicians, social workers, and visitors to the unit were getting caught up in the conflict. Team members were actively encouraging other staff to take sides, making clear they thought that "if you're not with us, you're against us." This made people from other departments very uncomfortable because they had to work with both teams. The nurse manager knew that resolution of the conflict would be a relief to many people. It is important to ask one additional question in preparation for negotiations:

4. *What does the other side want?* In this situation, the nurse manager was not certain what either team really wanted. She realized that she needed this information before she could begin to negotiate.

Set the Stage

When a conflict such as the one between Teams A and B has gone on for some time, the opposing sides are often unwilling to meet to discuss the problem. If this occurs, it may be necessary to confront them with direct statements designed to open communications between the two sides to challenge them to seek resolution of the situation. At the same time, it is important to avoid any implication of blame because this provokes defensiveness rather than willingness to change.

To confront Teams A and B with their behavior toward one another, the nurse manager called them together at the end of the day shift. "I am very concerned about what I have been observing lately," she told them. "It appears to me that instead of working together, our two teams are working against each other." She continued with some examples of what she had observed, taking care not to mention names or blame anyone for the problem. She was also prepared to take responsibility for having allowed the situation to deteriorate before taking this much-needed action.

Conduct the Negotiation

As indicated earlier, conducting a negotiation requires a great deal of skill.

1. Manage the emotions. When staff members are very emotional, they have trouble thinking clearly. Acknowledging these emotions is essential to negotiating effectively (Fiumano, 2005). When faced with a highly charged situation, do not respond with added emotion. Take time out if you need to get your own feelings under control. Then find out why emotions are high (watch both verbal and nonverbal cues carefully) (Hart & Waisman, 2005), and refocus the discussion on the issues (Shapiro & Jankowski, 1998). Without effective leadership to prevent emotional outbursts and personal attacks, a mishandled negotiation can worsen a situation. With effective leadership, the conflict may be resolved (Box 7-3).

2. Set ground rules. Members of Teams A and B began flinging accusations at each other as soon as the nurse manager made her statement. The nurse manager stopped this quickly and said, "First, we need to set some ground rules for this discussion. Everyone will get a chance to speak but not all at once. Please speak for yourself, not for others. And please do not make personal remarks or criticize your coworkers. We are here to resolve this problem, not to make it worse." She had to remind the group of these ground rules several times during the meeting. Teaching others how to negotiate can create a more collaborative environment in which the negotiation will take place (Schwartz & Pogge, 2000).

3. Clarification of the problem. The nurse manager wrote a list of problems raised by team members on a chalkboard. As the list grew longer, she asked the group, "What do you

---

box 7-3

Tips for Leading the Discussion

- Create a climate of comfort.
- Let others know the purpose is to resolve a problem or conflict.
- Freely admit your own contribution to the problem.
- Begin with the presentation of facts.
- Recognize your own emotional response to the situation.
- Set ground rules.
- Do not make personal remarks.
- Avoid placing blame.
- Allow each person an opportunity to speak.
- Do speak for yourself but not for others.
- Focus on solutions.
- Keep an open mind.

Adapted from Patterson, K., Grenny, J., McMillan, R., & Surtzler, A. (18 March 2003). Crucial conversations: Making a difference between being healed and being seriously hurt. Vital Signs, 13(5), 14–15.

see here? What is the real problem?" The group remained silent. Finally, someone said, "We don't have enough people, equipment, or supplies to get the work done." The rest of the group nodded in agreement.

4. **Opening move.** Once the problem is clarified, it is time to obtain everyone's agreement to seek a way to resolve the conflict. In more formal negotiation, you may make a statement about what you wish to achieve. For example, if you are negotiating a salary increase, you might begin by saying, "I am requesting a 10% increase for the following reasons: . . ." Of course, your employer will probably make a counteroffer, such as, "The best I can do is 3%." These are the opening moves of a negotiation.

5. **Continue the negotiations.** The discussion should continue in an open, nonhostile manner. Each side's concerns may be further explained and elaborated. Additional offers and counteroffers are common. As the discussion continues, it is usually helpful to emphasize areas of agreement as well as disagreement so that both parties are encouraged to continue the negotiations (Tappen, 2001).

Agree on a Resolution of the Conflict

After much testing for agreement, elaborating each side's positions and concerns, and making offers and counteroffers, the people involved should finally reach an agreement.

The nurse manager of Teams A and B led them through a discussion of their concerns related to working with severely limited resources. The teams soon realized that they had a common concern and that they might be able to help each other rather than compete with each other. The nurse manager agreed to become more proactive in seeking resources for the unit. "We can simultaneously seek new resources and develop creative ways to use the resources we already have," she told the teams. Relationships between members of Team A and Team B improved remarkably after this meeting. They learned that they could accomplish more by working together than they had ever achieved separately.

Formal Negotiation: Collective Bargaining

There are many varieties of formal negotiations, from real estate transactions to international peace treaty negotiations. A formal negotiation process of special interest to nurses is collective bargaining, which is highly formalized because it is governed by laws and contracts called *collective bargaining agreements.*

Collective bargaining involves a formal procedure governed by labor laws, such as the National Labor Relations Act in the United States. Nonprofit health-care organizations were added to the organizations covered by these laws in 1974. Once a union or professional organization has been designated as the official bargaining agent for a group of nurses, a contract defining such important matters as salary increases, benefits, time off, unfair treatment, safety issues, and promotion of professional practice is drawn up. This contract governs employee-management relations within the organization.

Case 3 is an example of how collective bargaining agreements can influence the outcome of a conflict between management and staff in a health-care organization.

A collective bargaining contract is a legal document that governs the relationship between management and staff, which is represented by the union (for nurses, it may be the nurses' association or another health-care workers' union). The contract may cover some or all of the following:

- **Economic issues:** Salaries, shift differentials, length of the workday, overtime, holidays, sick leave, breaks, health insurance, pensions, severance pay
- **Management issues:** Promotions, layoffs, transfers, reprimands, grievance procedures, hiring and firing procedures
- **Practice issues:** Adequate staffing, standards of care, code of ethics, safe working environment, other quality-of-care issues, staff development opportunities

Better patient-nurse staffing ratios, more reasonable workloads, opportunities for professional development, and better relationships with management are among the most important issues (Budd, Warino, & Patton, 2004).

The Pros and Cons of Collective Bargaining

Some nurses believe it is unprofessional to belong to a union. Others point out that physicians and teachers are union members and that the protections offered by a union outweigh the downside. There is no easy answer to this question.

Probably the greatest advantages of collective bargaining are protection of the right to fair treatment

Case 3

Collective Bargaining

The chief executive officer (CEO) of a large home health agency in a southwestern resort area called a general staff meeting. She reported that the agency had grown rapidly and was now the largest in the area. "Much of our success is due to the professionalism and commitment of our staff members," she said. "With growth come some problems, however. The most serious problem is the fluctuation in patient census. Our census peaks in the winter months when seasonal residents are here and troughs in the summer. In the past, when we were a small agency, we all took our vacations during the slow season. This made it possible to continue to pay everyone his or her full salary all year. However, given pressures to reduce costs and the large number of staff members we now have, we cannot continue to do this. We are very concerned about maintaining the high quality of patient care currently provided, but we have calculated that we need to reduce staff by 30 percent over the summer in order to survive financially."

The CEO then invited comments from the staff members. The majority of the nurses said they wanted and needed to work full-time all year. Most supported families and had to have a steady income all year. "My rent does not go down in the summer," said one. "Neither does my mortgage payment or the grocery bill," said another. A small number said that they would be happy to work part-time in the summer if they could be guaranteed full-time employment from October through May. "We have friends who would love this work schedule," they added.

"That's not fair," protested the nurses who needed to work full-time all year. "You can't replace us with part-time staff." The discussion grew louder and the participants more agitated. The meeting ended without a solution to the problem. Although the CEO promised to consider all points of view before making a decision, the nurses left the meeting feeling very confused and concerned about the security of their future income. Some grumbled that they probably should begin looking for new positions "before the ax falls."

The next day the CEO received a telephone call from the nurses' union representative. "If what I heard about the meeting yesterday is correct," said the representative, "your plan is in violation of our collective bargaining contract." The CEO reviewed the contract and found that the representative was correct. A new solution to the financial problems caused by the seasonal fluctuations in patient census would have to be found.

and the availability of a written grievance procedure that specifies both the employee's and the employer's rights and responsibilities if an issue arises that cannot be settled informally (Forman & Merrick, 2003). Having a say in practice and work-related issues empowers nurses (Budd, Warino, & Patton, 2004; Crochette, 2008). Another advantage is salary: nurses working under a collective bargaining agreement can earn as much as 28% more than those who do not (Pittman, 2007).

The greatest disadvantage of using collective bargaining as a way to deal with conflict is that it clearly separates management-level people from staff-level people, often creating an adversarial relationship. Any nurses who make staffing decisions may be classified as supervisors and, therefore, may be ineligible to join the union, separating them from the rest of their colleagues (Martin, 2001). The result is that management and staff are treated as opposing parties rather than as people who are trying to work together to provide essential services to their clients. The collective bargaining contract also adds another layer of rules and regulations between staff members and their supervisors. Because management of such employee-related rules and regulations can take almost a quarter of a manager's time (Drucker, 2002), this can become a drain on a nurse manager's time and energy.

Conclusion

Conflict is inevitable within any large, diverse group of people who are trying to work together over an extended period. However, conflict does not have to be destructive, nor does it have to be a negative experience. If it is handled skillfully by everyone involved, conflict can stimulate people to learn more about each other and how to work together in more effective ways. Resolving a conflict, when done well, can lead to improved working relationships, more creative methods of operation, and higher productivity.

Study Questions

1. Debate the question of whether conflict is constructive or destructive. How can good leadership affect the outcome of a conflict?

2. Give an example of how each of the seven sources of conflict listed in this chapter can lead to a serious problem. Then discuss ways to prevent the occurrence of conflict from each of the eight sources.

3. What is the difference between problem resolution and negotiation? Under what circumstances would you use one or the other?

4. Identify a conflict (actual or potential) in your clinical area, and explain how either problem resolution or negotiation could be used to resolve it.

Case Study to Promote Critical Reasoning

A not-for-profit hospice center in a small community received a generous gift from the grateful family of a patient who had died recently. The family asked only that the money be "put to the best use possible."

Everyone in this small facility had an opinion about the "best" use for the money. The administrator wanted to renovate the old, run-down headquarters. The financial officer wanted to put the money in the bank "for a rainy day." The chaplain wanted to add a small chapel to the building. The nurses wanted to create a food bank to help the poorest of their clients. The social workers wanted to buy a van to transport clients to health-care providers. The staff agreed that all the ideas had merit, that all of the needs identified were important ones. Unfortunately, there was enough money to meet only one of them.

The more the staff members discussed how to use this gift, the more insistent each group became that their idea was best. At their last meeting, it was evident that some were becoming frustrated and that others were becoming angry. It was rumored that a shouting match between the administrator and the financial officer had occurred.

1. In your analysis of this situation, identify the sources of the conflict that are developing in this facility.

2. What kind of leadership actions are needed to prevent the escalation of this conflict?

3. If the conflict does escalate, how could it be resolved?

4. Which idea do you think has the most merit? Why did you select the one you did?

5. Try role-playing a negotiation among the administrator, the financial officer, the chaplain, a representative of the nursing staff, and a representative of the social work staff. Can you suggest a creative solution?

References

Block, P. (2004). A time to heal. *Reflections.* Fourth Quarter, 20, 22.

Browne, M.M., & Kelley, S.M. (1994). *Asking the Right Questions: A Guide to Critical Thinking.* Englewood Cliffs, N.J.: Prentice-Hall.

Budd, K.W., Warino, L.S., & Patton, M.E. (2004, January). Traditional and non-traditional collective bargaining strategies to improve the patient care environment. *The Online Journal of Issues in Nursing,* 9(1). Retrieved September 8, 2008, from http://cms.nursingworld.org/MainMenuCategories/ANAMarketplace/ANAPeriodicals/OJIN/TableofContents/Volume92004/No1Jan04/CollectiveBargainingStrategies.aspx

Crochette, C.A. (2008). Employment low, negotiation, and the business environment. *Journal of Legal Studies,* 25(1), 127–182.

Drucker, P.F. (2002). They're not employees, they're people. *Harvard Business Review,* 80(2), 70–77, 128.

Ehrlich, H.J. (1995). Prejudice and ethnoviolence on campus. *Higher Education Extension Service Review,* 6(2), 1–3.

Fiumano, J. (2005). Navigate through conflict, not around it. *Nursing Management,* 36(8), 14, 18.

Forman, H., & Merrick, F. (2003). Grievances and complaints: Valuable tools for management and for staff. *Journal of Nursing Administration,* 33(3), 136–138.

Hart, L.B., & Waisman, C.S. (2005). *The Leadership Training Activity Book.* N.Y.: AMACOM.

Haslan, S.A. (2001). *Psychology in Organizations.* Thousand Oaks, Calif.: Sage.

Horton-Deutsch, S.L., & Wellman, D.S. (2002). Christman's principles for effective management. *Journal of Nursing Administration,* 32, 596–601.

Jordan, P., & Troth, A.C. (2004). Managing emotions during team problem solving: Emotional intelligence and conflict resolution. *Human Performance,* 17(2), 195–218.

Ketter, J. (1994). Protecting RNs with the Fair Labor Standards Act. *American Nurse,* 26(9), 1–2.

Lazoritz, S., & Carlson, P.J. (2008). Descriptive physician behavior. *American Nurse Today,* 3(3), 20–22.

Martin, R.H. (June 2001). Ruling may limit ability to unionize. *Advance for Nurses,* 9.

McDonald, D. (2008). Revisiting a theory of negotiation: The utility of Markiewicz (2005) proposed six principles. *Evaluation and Program Planning,* 31(3), 259–265.

McElhaney, R. (1996). Conflict management in nursing administration. *Nursing Management,* 27(3), 49–50.

McVicar, A. (2003). Workplace stress in nursing: A literature review. *Journal of Advanced Nursing,* 44(6), 633–642.

Patterson, K., Grenny, J., McMillan, R., & Surtzler, A. (18 March 2003). Crucial conversations: Making a difference between being healed and being seriously hurt. *Vital Signs,* 13(5), 14–15.

Pittman, J. (2007). Registered nurse job satisfaction and collective bargaining unit membership status. *Journal of Nursing Administration,* 37(10), 471–476.

Qureshi, P. (1996). The effects of threat appraisal. *Nursing Management,* 27(3), 31–32.

Ramos, M.C. (2006). Eliminate destructive behaviors through example and evidence. *Nursing Management,* 34–41.

Rees, F. (2005). *25 Activities for Developing Team Leaders.* San Francisco: Pfeiffer.

Rondeau, K.V., & Wagar, T.H. (2002). Reducing the hospital workforce: What is the role of human resource management practices? *Hospital Topics,* 89(1), 12–18.

Sanon-Rollins, G. (2000). Surviving conflict on the job. *Nursing Spectrum Career Fitness Guide,* 6767–6868. Barrington, Ill.: Gannett.

Schwartz, R.W., & Pogge, C. (2000). Physician leadership: Essential skills in a changing environment. *American Journal of Surgery,* 180(3), 187–192.

Shapiro, R.M., & Jankowski, M.A. (1998). *The Power of Nice.* N.Y.: John Wiley & Sons.

Siu, H., Laschinger, H.R.S., & Finegan, J. (2008). Nursing professional practice environments: Setting the stage for constructive conflict resolution and work effectiveness. *Journal of Nursing Administration,* 38(5), 250–257.

Smialek, M.A. (2001). *Team Strategies for Success.* Lanham, Md.: Scarecrow Press.

Sportsman, S. (2005). Build a framework for conflict assessment. *Nursing Management,* 36(4), 32–40.

Tappen, R.M. (2001). *Nursing Leadership and Management: Concept and Practice.* Philadelphia: FA Davis.

Thompson, L., & Fox, C.R. (2001). Negotiation within and between groups in organizations: Levels of analysis. In Turner, M.E. (ed.). *Groups at Work,* 221–266. Mahwah, N.J.: Laurence Erlbaum.

Tjosvold, D., & Tjosvold, M.M. (1995). *Psychology for Leaders: Using Motivation, Conflict, and Power to Manage More Effectively.* N.Y.: John Wiley & Sons.

Van de Vliert, E., & Janssen, O. (2001). Description, explanation, and prescription of intragroup conflict behaviors. In Turner, M.E. (ed.). *Groups at Work,* 267–297. Mahwah, N.J.: Laurence Erlbaum.

Vivar, C.G. (2006). Putting conflict management into practice: A nursing case study. *Journal of Nursing Management,* 14, 201–206.

Walker, M.A., & Harris, G.L. (1995). *Negotiations: Six Steps to Success.* Upper Saddle River, N.J.: Prentice Hall.

Walsh, B. (3 June 1996). When past perfect isn't. *Forbes ASAP,* 18.

Wenckus, E. (21 February 1995). Working with an interdisciplinary team. *Nursing Spectrum,* 5, 12–14.

Willis, E., Taffoli, L., Henderson, J., & Walter, B. (2008). Enterprise bargaining: A case study in the de-intensification of nursing work in Australia. *Nursing Inquiry,* 15(2), 148–157.

chapter 8

People and the Process of Change

OBJECTIVES

After reading this chapter, the student should be able to:

- Describe the process of change.
- Recognize resistance to change and identify its sources.
- Suggest strategies to reduce resistance to change.
- Assume a leadership role in implementing change.

When asked the theme of a nursing management conference, a top nursing executive replied, "Change, change, and more change." Whether it is called innovation, turbulence, or change, this theme seems to be a constant in the workplace today. Mismanaging change is common. In fact, as many as three out of four major change efforts fail (Cameron & Quinn, 2006; Hempel, 2005). This chapter discusses how people respond to change, how you can influence change, and how you can help people cope with it when it becomes difficult.

Change

A Natural Phenomenon

Change is a part of everyone's lives. Every day, people have new experiences, meet new people, and learn something new. People grow up, leave home, graduate from college, begin a career, and perhaps start a family. Some of these changes are milestones, ones for which people have prepared and have anticipated for some time. Many are exciting, leading to new opportunities and challenges. Some are entirely unexpected, sometimes welcome and sometimes not. When change occurs too rapidly or demands too much, it can make people uncomfortable (Bilchik, 2002), even anxious or stressed.

Macro and Micro Change

The "ever-whirling wheel of change" (Dent, 1995, p. 287) in health care seems to spin faster every year. By itself, managed care profoundly changed the way health care is provided in the United States (Trinh & O'Connor, 2002). Medicare and Medicaid cuts, increasing numbers of people who are uninsured or underinsured, restructuring, downsizing, and staff shortages are major concerns. Such changes sweep through the health-care system, affecting patients and caregivers alike. They are the *macro-level* (large-scale) changes that affect virtually every health-care facility.

Change anywhere in a system creates "ripples throughout the system" (Parker & Gadbois, 2000, p. 472). Every change that occurs at this macro level filters down to the *micro level* (small-scale change), to teams and to individuals. Nurses, colleagues in other disciplines, and patients are participants in these changes. This micro level of change is the primary focus of this chapter.

Change and the Comfort Zone

The basic stages of the change process described by Kurt Lewin in 1951 are *unfreezing, change,* and *refreezing* (Lewin, 1951; Schein, 2004). Imagine a work situation that is basically stable. People are generally accustomed to each other, have a routine for doing their work, and believe they know what to expect and how to deal with whatever problems come up. They are operating within their "comfort zone" (Farrell & Broude, 1987; Lapp, 2002). A change of any magnitude is likely to move people out of this comfort zone into discomfort. This move out of the comfort zone is called *unfreezing* (Fig. 8.1). For example:

Many health-care institutions offer nurses the choice of weekday or weekend work. Given these choices, nurses with school-age children are likely to find their comfort zone on weekday shifts. Imagine the discomfort they would experience if they were transferred to weekends. Such a change would rapidly unfreeze their usual routine and move them into the discomfort zone. They might have to find a new babysitter or begin a search for a new child-care center that is open on weekends. Another alternative would be to establish a child-care center where they work. Yet another alternative would be to find a position that offers better working hours.

Figure 8.1 The change process. (Based on Farrell, K., & Broude, C. [1987]. *Winning the Change Game: How to Implement Information Systems With Fewer Headaches and Bigger Paybacks.* Los Angeles: Breakthrough Enterprises; and Lewin, K. [1951]. *Field Theory in Social Science: Selected Theoretical Papers.* N.Y.: Harper & Row.)

Whatever alternative they chose, the nurses were being challenged to find a solution that enabled them to move into a new comfort zone. To accomplish this, they would have to find a consistent, dependable source of child care suited to their new schedule and to the needs of their children and then refreeze their situation. If they did not find a satisfactory alternative, they could remain in an unsettled state, in a discomfort zone, caught in a conflict between their personal and professional responsibilities.

As this example illustrates, even what seems to be a small change can greatly disturb the people involved in it. The next section considers the many reasons why change provokes resistance and how change can be unsettling.

Resistance to Change

People resist change for a variety of reasons that vary from person to person and situation to situation. You might find that one patient-care technician is delighted with an increase in responsibility, whereas another is upset about it. Some people are eager to risk change; others prefer the status quo (Hansten & Washburn, 1999). Managers may find that one change in routine provokes a storm of protest and that another is hardly noticed Why does this happen?

Receptivity to Change

Recognizing Different Information Processing Styles

An interesting research study suggests that nurse managers are more receptive to change than their staff members (Kalisch, 2007). Nurse managers were found to be more innovative and decisive, whereas staff nurses preferred proven approaches, thus being resistant to change. Nursing assistants, unit secretaries, and licensed practical nurses were also unreceptive to change, adding layers of people who formed a "solid wall of resistance" to change. Kalisch suggests that helping teams recognize their preference for certainty (as opposed to change) will increase their receptivity to necessary changes in the workplace.

Speaking to People's Feelings

Although both thinking and feeling responses to change are important, Kotter (1999) says that the heart of change lies in the emotions surrounding it.

He suggests that a *compelling story* will increase receptivity to a change more than a carefully crafted analysis of the need for change. How is this done? The following are some examples of appeals to feelings.

- Instead of presenting statistics about the number of people who are re-admitted due to poor discharge preparation, providing a story is more persuasive: an older man collapsed at home the evening after discharge because he had not been able to control his diabetes post surgery. Trying to break his fall, he fractured both wrists and is now unable to return home or take care of himself.
- Even better, videotape an interview with this man, letting him tell his story and describe the repercussions of poor preparation for discharge.
- Drama may also be achieved through visual display. A culture plate of pathogens grown from swabs of ventilator equipment and patient room furniture is more attention-getting than an infection control report. A display of disposables with price tags attached used for just one surgical patient is more memorable than an accounting sheet listing the costs.

The purpose of these activities is to present a compelling image that will affect people emotionally, increasing their receptivity to change and moving them into a state of readiness to change (Kotter, 1999).

Sources of Resistance

Resistance to change comes from three major sources: technical concerns, psychosocial needs, and threats to a person's position and power (Araujo Group).

Technical Concerns

Some resistance to change is based on concerns about whether the proposed change is a good idea. The change itself may have *design flaws.*

The Professional Practice Committee of a small hospital, in order to save money, suggested replacing a commercial mouthwash with a mixture of hydrogen peroxide and water. A staff nurse objected to this proposed change, saying that she had read a research study several years ago that found peroxide solutions to be an irritant to the oral mucosa (Tombes & Gallucci, 1993). Fortunately, the chairperson of the committee recognized that this objection was based on technical concerns and requested a study of the evidence before instituting the change. "It's important to investigate the evidence supporting a proposed change thoroughly before recommending it," she said.

A change may provide resistance for *practical* reasons. For example, if the bar codes on patients' armbands are difficult to scan, nurses may develop a way to work around this safety feature by taping a duplicate armband to the bed or to a clipboard (Englebright & Franklin, 2005), defeating the purpose of instituting electronically monitored medication administration.

Psychosocial Needs

Change often creates anxiety, much of it related to what people fear they might lose (Berman-Rubera, 2008; Johnston, 2008). According to Maslow (1970), human beings have a hierarchy of needs, from the basic physiological needs for oxygen, fluids, and nutrients to the higher-order needs for belonging, self-esteem, and self-actualization (Fig. 8.2). Maslow observed that the more basic needs (those lower on the hierarchy) must be at least partially met before a person is motivated to seek fulfillment of the higher-order needs.

Change may make it more difficult for a person to meet any or all of his or her needs. It may threaten the powerful safety and security needs that Maslow discussed (Hunter, 2004). For example, if a massive downsizing occurs and a person's job is eliminated, fulfillment of all of these levels of needs may be threatened, from having enough money to pay for food and shelter to opportunities to fulfill one's career potential.

In other cases, the threat is subtler and may be harder to anticipate. For example, an institution-wide reevaluation of the effectiveness of the advanced practice role would be a great concern to a staff nurse who is working toward accomplishing a lifelong dream of becoming an advanced practice nurse in oncology. In contrast, it would have little effect on unlicensed assistive personnel (UAPs), but a staff reorganization that moves UAP to different units could threaten the belonging needs of those who have close friends on the unit but few friends outside.

Position and Power

Once gained within an organization, status, power, and influence are hard to give up. This applies to people anywhere in the organization, not just those at the top. For example:

A clerk in the surgical suite had been preparing the operating room schedule for many years. Although his supervisor was expected to review the schedule before it was posted, she rarely did so because the clerk was skillful in balancing the needs of various parties, including some very demanding surgeons. When the supervisor was transferred to another facility, her replacement decided that she had to review the schedules before they were posted because they were ultimately her responsibility. The clerk became defensive. He tried to avoid the new supervisor and posted the schedules without her approval. This surprised her. She knew the clerk was skilled and did not think that her review of them would be threatening.

Why did this happen? The supervisor had not realized the importance of this task to the clerk. The opportunity to tell others when and where they could perform surgery gave the clerk a feeling of power and importance. The supervisor's insistence on reviewing his work reduced the importance of his position. What seemed to the new supervisor to

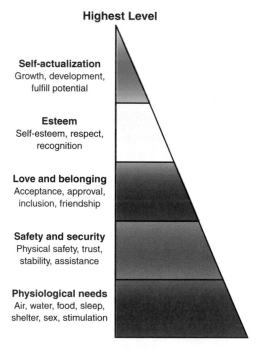

Figure 8.2 Maslow's hierarchy of needs. (Based on Maslow, A.H. [1970]. *Motivation and Personality.* N.Y.: Harper & Row.)

be a very small change in routine had provoked surprisingly strong resistance because it threatened the clerk's sense of importance and power.

Recognizing Resistance

Resistance may be *active* or *passive* (Heller, 1998). It is easy to recognize resistance to a change when it is expressed directly. When a person says to you, "That's not a very good idea," "I'll quit if you schedule me for the night shift," or "There's no way I'm going to do that," there is no doubt you are encountering resistance. Active resistance can take the form of outright refusal to comply, such as these statements, writing memos that destroy the idea, quoting existing rules that make the change difficult to implement, or encouraging others to resist.

When resistance is less direct, however, it can be difficult to recognize unless you know what to look for. Passive approaches usually involve avoidance: canceling appointments to discuss implementation of the change, being too busy to make the change, refusing to commit to changing, agreeing to it but doing nothing to change, and simply ignoring the entire process as much as possible (Table 8-1). Once resistance has been recognized, action can be taken to lower or even eliminate it.

Lowering Resistance

A great deal can be done to lower people's resistance to change. Strategies fall into four categories: sharing information, disconfirming currently held beliefs, providing psychological safety, and dictating (forcing) change (Tappen, 2001).

Sharing Information

Much resistance is simply the result of misunderstanding a proposed change. Sharing information about the proposed change can be done on a one-to-one basis, in group meetings, or through written materials distributed to everyone involved via print or electronic means.

Disconfirming Currently Held Beliefs

Disconfirming current beliefs is a primary force for change (Schein, 2004). Providing evidence that what people are currently doing is inadequate, incorrect, or inefficient can increase people's willingness to change. The dramatic presentations described in the section on receptivity disconfirm current beliefs and practices. The following is a less dramatic example but still persuasive:

Jolene was a little nervous when her turn came to present information to the Safe Clinical Practice Committee on a new enteral feeding procedure. Committee members were very demanding: they wanted clear, research-based information presented in a concise manner. Opinions and generalities were not acceptable. Jolene had prepared thoroughly and had practiced her presentation at home until she could speak without referring to her notes. The presentation went well. Committee members commented on how thorough she was and on the quality of the information presented. To her disappointment, however, no action was taken on her proposal.

Returning to her unit, she shared her disappointment with the nurse manager. Together, they used the unfreezing-change-refreezing process as a guide to review the presentation. The nurse manager agreed that Jolene had thoroughly reviewed the information on enteral feeding. The problem, she explained, was that Jolene had not attended to the need to unfreeze the situation. Jolene realized that she had not put any emphasis on the high risk of contamination and resulting gastrointestinal disturbances of the procedure currently in use. She had left members of the committee feeling comfortable with current practice because she had not emphasized the risk involved in failing to change it.

At the next meeting, Jolene presented additional information on the risks associated with the current enteral feeding procedures. This disconfirming evidence was persuasive. The committee accepted her proposal to adopt the new, lower-risk procedure.

Without the addition of the disconfirming evidence, it is likely that Jolene's proposed change would never have been implemented. The *inertia* (tendency to remain in the same state rather than to move toward change) exhibited by the Safe Clinical Practice Committee is not unusual (Pearcey & Draper, 1996).

table 8-1	
Resistance to Change	
Active	**Passive**
Attacking the idea	Avoiding discussion
Refusing to change	Ignoring the change
Arguing against the change	Refusing to commit to the change
Organizing resistance of other people	Agreeing but not acting

Providing Psychological Safety

As indicated earlier, a proposed change can threaten people's basic needs. Resistance can be lowered by reducing that threat, leaving people feeling more comfortable with the change. Each situation poses different kinds of threats and, therefore, requires different actions to reduce the levels of threat; the following is a list of useful strategies to increase psychological safety:

- Express approval of people's interest in providing the best care possible.
- Recognize the competence and skill of the people involved.
- Provide assurance (if possible) that no one will lose his or her position because of the change.
- Suggest ways in which the change can provide new opportunities and challenges (new ways to increase self-esteem and self-actualization).
- Involve as many people as possible in the design or plan to implement change.
- Provide opportunities for people to express their feelings and ask questions about the proposed change.
- Allow time for practice and learning of any new procedures before a change is implemented.

Dictating Change

This is an entirely different approach to change. People in authority in an organization can simply require people to make a change in what they are doing or can reassign people to new positions (Porter-O'Grady, 1996). This may not work well if there are ways for people to resist; for example:

- When passive resistance can undermine the change
- When high motivational levels are necessary to make the change successful
- When people can refuse to obey the order without negative consequences

The following is an example of an unsuccessful attempt to dictate change:

A new and insecure nurse manager believed that her staff members were taking advantage of her inexperience by taking more than the two 15-minute coffee breaks allowed during an 8-hour shift. She decided that staff members would have to sign in and out for their coffee breaks and their 30-minute meal break. Staff members were outraged. Most had been taking fewer than 15 minutes for coffee breaks or 30 minutes for lunch because of the heavy care demands of the unit. They refused to sign the coffee break sheet. When asked why they had not signed it, they replied "I forgot," "I couldn't find it," or "I was called away before I had a chance." This organized passive resistance was sufficient to overcome the nurse manager's authority. The nurse manager decided that the coffee break sheet had been a mistake, removed it from the bulletin board, and never mentioned it again.

For people in authority, dictating a change often seems to be the easiest way to institute change: just tell people what to do, and do not listen to any arguments. There is risk in this approach, however. Even when staff members do not resist authority-based change, overuse of dictates can lead to a passive, dependent, unmotivated, and unempowered staff. Providing high-quality patient care requires staff members who are active, motivated, and highly committed to their work.

Leading the Implementation of Change

New graduates may find themselves given responsibility for bringing about change. Following are examples of the kinds of changes they might be asked to help implement:

- Introduce a new technical procedure
- Implement evidence-based practice guidelines
- Develop new policies for staff evaluation and promotion
- Participate in quality-improvement and patient-safety projects
- Prepare for accreditation reviews and safety inspections

Now that you understand how change can affect people and have learned some ways to lower their resistance to change, taking a leadership role in successful implementation of change is presented.

The entire process of bringing about change can be divided into four phases: designing the change, deciding how to implement the change, carrying out the actual implementation, and following through to ensure the change has been integrated into the regular operation of the facility (Fig. 8.3).

Designing the Change

This is the starting point. The first step in bringing about change is to craft the change carefully. Not every change is for the better: some changes fail

Figure 8.3 Four phases of planned change.

because they are poorly conceived in the first place. Ask yourself:

- What are we trying to accomplish?
- Is the change necessary?
- Is the change technically correct?
- Will it work?
- Is this change a better way to do things?

This is a good time to use creativity and innovation (Handy, 2002). Encourage people to talk about the changes planned, to express their doubts, and to provide their input (Fullan, 2001). Those who do are usually enthusiastic supporters later in the process.

Planning

Now is the time to build a "road map" to guide you on the journey from status quo to completed change (McCarthy, 2005). All the information presented previously about sources of resistance and ways to overcome that resistance should be taken into consideration when deciding how to implement a change.

Remember that some research has found nursing staff to be resistant to change. You are likely to find supporters, "fence-sitters," and resisters within your group (McCarthy, 2005). The supporters will help you lead people on the path to change, but be sure to include those who are neutral (the fence-sitters) and opposed (the resisters) in the process and to analyze why they might be resistant. Ask yourself:

- Why might people resist this change?
- Is their resistance justified?

- What can be done to prevent or overcome this resistance?

The context in which the change will take place is another factor to consider when assessing resistance to change (Lichiello & Madden, 1996). This includes the amount of change occurring at the same time, the organizational climate, the environment surrounding the organization, and past history of change in the organization. Is there goodwill toward change because it has gone well in the past? Or have the changes gone badly, generating ill will and resistance to additional change (Maurer, 2008)? There may be external pressure to change because of the competitive nature of the healthcare market in the community. In other situations, government regulations may make it difficult to bring about a desired change.

Almost everything you have learned about effective leadership is useful in planning the implementation of change: communicating the vision, motivating people, involving people in decisions that affect them, dealing with conflict, eliciting cooperation, providing coordination, and fostering teamwork. People have to be moved out of their comfort zone to unfreeze the situation and get them ready to change (Flower & Guillaume, 2002). Consider all these things when formulating a plan to implement a proposed change, then act on them in the next step: implementing the change.

Implementing the Change

You are finally ready to embark on the journey that has been carefully planned. Consider the following factors:

- **Magnitude:** Is it a major change that affects almost everything people do, or is it a minor one?
- **Complexity:** Is this a difficult change to make? Does it require much new knowledge and skill? How much time will it take to acquire them?
- **Pace:** How urgent is this change? Can it be done gradually, or must it be implemented all at once?
- **Stress:** Is this the only change that is taking place, or is it just one of many taking place? How stressful are these changes? How can you help people keep their stress at tolerable levels?

A simple change, such as introducing a new thermometer, may be planned, implemented, and integrated easily into everyone's work routine. A complex change, such as introducing a medication error reduction system, may require experimentation with the new system, feedback on what works and what does not, and revising the plan several times before the system really works.

Some discomfort is likely to occur with almost any change, but it is important to keep it within tolerable limits. Exert pressure to make people pay attention to the change process, but do not exert so much pressure that they are overstressed by it. In other words, you want to raise the heat enough to get them moving but not so much that they boil over (Heifetz & Linsky, 2002).

Integrating the Change

Finally, after the change has been made, make sure that everyone has moved into a new comfort zone. Ask yourself:

■ Is the change well integrated into everyday operations?
■ Are people comfortable with it?
■ Is it well accepted? Is there any residual resistance that could still undermine full integration of the change?

It usually takes some time before a change is fully integrated into everyday routines (Hunter, 2004). As Kotter noted, change "sticks" when, instead of being the new way to do something, it has become "the way we always do things around here" (1999, p. 18).

Personal Change

The focus of this chapter is on leading others through the process of change. However, choosing to change is also an important part of your own development as a leader. Hart and Waisman (2005) compare personal change with the story of the caterpillar and the butterfly:

Caterpillars cannot fly. They have to crawl or climb to find their food. Butterflies, on the other hand, can soar above an obstacle. They also have a different perspective on their world because they can fly. It is not easy to change from a caterpillar to a butterfly. Indeed, the transition (metamorphosis) may be quite uncomfortable and involves some risk. Are you ready to become a butterfly?

The process of personal change is similar to the process described throughout this chapter: first recognize the need for change, then learn how to do things differently, and then become comfortable

with the "new you" (Guthrie & King, 2004). A more detailed step-by-step process is given in Table 8-2. You might, for example, decide that you need to stop interrupting people when they speak with you. Or you might want to change your leadership style from laissez-faire to participative.

Would a small change be easier to accomplish than the radical change in your leadership style? Perhaps not. Deutschman (2005) reports research that indicates radical change might be easier to accomplish because the benefits are evident much more quickly. An extreme example: many people could avoid a second coronary bypass or angioplasty by changing their lifestyle, yet 90% do not do so. Deutschman compares the typical advice (exercise, stop smoking, eat healthier meals) with Dean Ornish's radical vegetarian diet (only 10% of calories from fat). After 3 years, 77% of the patients who went through this extreme change had continued these lifestyle changes. Why? Ornish suggests several reasons: (1) after several weeks, people felt a change—they could walk or have sex without pain; (2) information alone is not enough—the emotional aspect is dealt with in support groups and through meditation, relaxation, yoga, and aerobic exercise; and (3) the motivation to pursue this change is redefined—instead of focusing on fear of death, which many find too frightening, Ornish focuses on the joy of living, feeling better, and being active without pain.

The traditional approach to change is turned on its head in this approach: radical change appears easier to accomplish than a minor change, and people are not stressed but feel better making the change. Deutschman's five commonly accepted myths about change that have been refuted by new insights from research summarize this approach (Table 8-3).

It remains to be seen whether these new insights on changing behavior will be useful in the workplace as well.

Conclusion

Change is an inevitable part of living and working. How people respond to change, the amount of stress it causes, and the amount of resistance it provokes can be influenced by leadership. Handled well, most changes can become opportunities for professional growth and development rather than just additional stressors with which nurses and their clients have to cope.

table 8-2

Which Stage of Change Are You In?

While studying how smokers quit the habit, Dr. James Prochaska, a psychologist at the University of Rhode Island, developed a widely influential model of the "stages of change." What stage are you in? See if any of the following statements sound familiar.

Typical Statement	Stage	Risks
"As far as I'm concerned, I don't have any problems that need changing." "I guess I have faults, but there's nothing that I really need to change."	1 Precontemplation ("Never")	You are in denial. You probably feel coerced by other people who are trying to make you change. But they are not going to shame you into it—their meddling will backfire.
"I've been thinking that I wanted to change something about myself." "I wish I had more ideas on how to solve my problems."	2 Contemplation ("Someday")	Feeling righteous because of your good intentions, you could stay in this stage for years. But you might respond to the emotional persuasion of a compelling leader.
"I have decided to make changes in the next 2 weeks." "I am committed to join a fitness club by the end of the month."	3 Preparation ("Soon")	This "rehearsal" can become your reality. Some 85% of people who need to change their behavior for health reasons never get to this stage or progress beyond it.
"Anyone can talk about changing. I'm actually doing something about it." "I am doing okay, but I wish I was more consistent."	4 Action ("Now")	It is an emotional struggle. It is important to change quickly enough to feel the short-term benefits that give a psychic lift and make it easier to stick with the change.
"I may need a boost right now to help me maintain the changes I've already made." "This has become part of my day, and I feel it when I don't follow through."	5 Maintenance ("Forever")	Relapse. Even though you have created a new mental pathway, the old pathway is still there in your brain, and when you are under a lot of stress, you might fall back on it.

Adapted from Deutschman's Which Stage of Change Are You In? *"Typical statements" adapted from* Stages of Change: Theory and Practice *by Michael Samuelson, executive director of the National Center for Health Promotion.*

table 8-3

Five Myths About Changing Behavior

Myth	Reality
1. Crisis is a powerful impetus for change.	Ninety percent of patients who have had coronary bypasses do not sustain changes in the unhealthy lifestyles, which worsens their severe heart disease and greatly threatens their lives.
2. Change is motivated by fear.	It is too easy for people to go into denial of the bad things that might happen to them. Compelling positive visions of the future are a much stronger inspiration for change.
3. The facts will set us free.	Our thinking is guided by narratives, not facts. When a fact does not fit people's conceptual "frames"—the metaphors used to make sense of the world—people reject the fact. Also, change is best inspired by emotional appeals rather than factual statements.
4. Small, gradual changes are always easier to make and sustain.	Radical, sweeping changes are often easier because they yield benefits quickly.
5. People cannot change because the brain becomes "hardwired" early in life.	Brains have extraordinary "plasticity," meaning that people can continue learning complex new things throughout life—assuming they remain truly active and engaged.

Adapted from Deutschman's Fact Take: Five Myths About Changing Behavior. *Deutschman, A. (2005/May).* Change or die. Fast Company, 94, *52–62.*

Study Questions

1. Why is change inevitable? What would happen if no change at all occurred in health care?

2. Why do people resist change? Why do nursing staff members seem particularly resistant to change?

3. How can leaders overcome resistance to change?

4. Describe the process of implementing a change from beginning to end. Use an example from your clinical experience to illustrate this process.

Case Study to Promote Critical Reasoning

A large health-care corporation recently purchased a small, 50-bed rural nursing home. A new director of nursing was brought in to replace the former one, who had retired after 30 years. The new director addressed the staff members at the reception held to welcome him. "My philosophy is that you cannot manage anything that you haven't measured. Everyone tells me that you have all been doing an excellent job here. With my measurement approach, we will be able to analyze everything you do and become more efficient than ever." The nursing staff members soon found out what the new director meant by his measurement approach. Every bath, episode of incontinence care, feeding of a resident, or trip off the unit had to be counted, and the amount of time each activity required had to be recorded. Nurse managers were required to review these data with staff members every week, questioning any time that was not accounted for. Time spent talking with families or consulting with other staff members was considered time wasted unless the staff member could justify the "interruption" in his or her work. No one complained openly about the change, but absenteeism rates increased rapidly. Personal day and vacation time requests soared. Staff members nearing retirement crowded the tiny personnel office, overwhelming the single staff member with their requests to "tell me how soon I can retire with full benefits." The director of nursing found that shortage of staff was becoming a serious problem and that no new applications were coming in, despite the fact that this rural area offered few good job opportunities.

1. What evidence of resistance to change can you find in this case study?

2. What kind of resistance to change did the staff members exhibit?

3. If you were a staff nurse at this facility, how do you think you would have reacted to this change in administration?

4. Why did staff members resist this change?

5. What could the director of nursing do to increase acceptance of this change? What could the nurse managers and staff nurses do?

References

Araujo Group. A compilation of opinions of experts in the field of the management of change. Unpublished report.

Berman-Rubera, S. (2008, August 10). Leading and embracing change. *Business/Change-Management*. Retrieved August 20, 2008, from http://ezinearticles.com/?Leading-And-Embracing-Change&id=1180585

Bilchik, G.S. (May 2002). Are you the problem? *Hospitals and Health Networks Magazine,* 38–42.

Cameron, K.S. & Quinn, Q.E. (2006). *Diagnosing and Changing Organizational Culture.* N.Y.: Jossey-Bass.

Dent, H.S. (1995). *Job Shock: Four New Principles Transforming Our Work and Business.* N.Y.: St. Martin's Press.

Deutschman, A. (2005). Change or die. *Fast Company,* 94, 52–62.

Englebright, J.D., & Franklin, M. (2005). Managing a new medication administrative process. *Journal of Nursing Administration,* 35(9), 410–413.

Farrell, K., & Broude, C. (1987). *Winning the Change Game: How to Implement Information Systems With Fewer Headaches and Bigger Paybacks.* Los Angeles: Breakthrough Enterprises.

Flower, J., & Guillaume, P. (March/April 2002). Surfing the edge of chaos. *Health Forum Journal,* 17–20.

Fullan, M. (2001). *Leading in a Culture of Change.* San Francisco: Jossey-Bass.

Guthrie, V.A., & King, S.N. (2004). Feedback-intensive programs. In McCauley, C.D., & Van Velson, E. (eds.). *The Center for Creative Leadership Handbook of Leadership Development.* San Francisco: Jossey-Bass.

Handy, C. (June 2002). The elephant and the flea: Looking backward to the future. *Times Literary Supplement,* 5157, 30.

Hansten, R.I., & Washburn, M.J. (1999). Individual and organizational accountability for development of critical thinking. *Journal of Nursing Administration,* 29(11), 39–45.

Hart, L.B., & Waisman, C.S. (2005). *The Leadership Training Activity Book.* N.Y.: AMACOM.

Heifetz, R.A., & Linsky, M. (June 2002). A survival guide for leaders. *Harvard Business Review,* 65–74.

Heller, R. (1998). *Managing Change.* N.Y.: DK Publishing.

Hempel, J. (2005). Why the boss really had to say goodbye. *Business Week,* July 4, p. 10.

Hunter, J.C. (2004). *The World's Most Powerful Leadership Principle: How to Become a Servant Leader.* N.Y.: Crown Business.

Johnston, G. (2008, March 8). Change management—Why the high failure rate. *Business/Change-Management.* Retrieved August 20, 2008, from http://ezinearticles.com/?Change-Management—Why-the-High-Failure-Rate?&id=1028294

Kalisch, B.J. (2007). Don't like change? Blame it on your strategic style. *Reflections on Nursing Leadership,* 33(3). Retrieved August 20, 2008, from http://nursingsociety.org/RNL/3Q_2007/features/feature5.html

Kotter, J.P. (1999). Leading change: The eight steps to transformation. In Conger, J.A., Spreitzer, G.M., & Lawler, E.E. (eds.). *The Leader's Change Handbook: An Essential Guide to Setting Direction and Taking Action.* San Francisco: Jossey-Bass.

Lapp, J. (May 2002). Thriving on change. *Caring Magazine,* 40–43.

Lewin, K. (1951). *Field Theory in Social Science: Selected Theoretical Papers.* N.Y.: Harper & Row.

Lichiello, P., & Madden, C.W. (1996). Context and catalysts for change in health care markets. *Health Affairs,* 15(2), 121–129.

Maslow, A.H. (1970). *Motivation and Personality.* N.Y.: Harper & Row.

Maurer, R. (2008, August 13). The 4 reasons why people resist change. *Business/Change-Management.* Retrieved August 20, 2008, from http://ezinearticles.com/?The-7-Reasons-Why-People-Resist-Change&id=1053595

McCarthy, J.E. (2005). Five concepts for creating change. *Nursing Management,* 36(5), 20–22.

Parker, M., & Gadbois, S. (2000). Building community in healthcare workplace. Part 3: Belonging and satisfaction at work. *Journal of Nursing Administration,* 30, 466–473.

Pearcey, P., & Draper, P. (1996). Using the diffusion of innovation model to influence practice: A case study. *Journal of Advanced Nursing,* 23, 724–726.

Porter-O'Grady, T. (1996). The seven basic rules for successful redesign. *Journal of Nursing Administration,* 26(1), 46–53.

Schein, E.H. (2004, August 1). Kurt Lewin's change theory in the field and in the classroom: Notes toward a model of managed learning. Retrieved August 20, 2008, from http://www.a2zpsychology.com/articles/kurt_lewin's_change_theory.htm

Tappen, R.M. (2001). *Nursing Leadership and Management: Concepts and Practice.* Philadelphia: F.A. Davis.

Tombes, M.B., & Gallucci, B. (1993). The effects of hydrogen peroxide rinses on the normal oral mucosa. *Nursing Research,* 42, 332–337.

Trinh, H.Q., & O'Connor, S.J. (2002). Helpful or harmful? The impact of strategic change on the performance of U.S. urban hospitals. *Health Services Research,* 37(1), 145–171.

chapter 9

Delegation of Client Care

⊙ ○ ○ ○ ○ ○ ○ ○ ○ ○

OBJECTIVES

After reading this chapter, the student should be able to:

- Define the term delegation.
- Define the term unlicensed assistive personnel.
- Understand the legal implications of making assignments to other health-care personnel.
- Recognize barriers to successful delegation.
- Make appropriate assignments to team members.
- Explain the various nursing care delivery models.

Linda is a new graduate and has just finished her orientation. She works from 7 p.m. to 7 a.m. on a busy, monitored neuroscience unit. The client census is 48, making this a full unit. Although there is an associate nurse manager for the shift, Linda is the charge nurse. Her responsibilities include receiving and transcribing orders, contacting physicians with any information or requests, accessing laboratory reports from the computer, reviewing them and giving them to the appropriate staff members, checking any new medication orders and placing them in the appropriate medication administration records, relieving the monitor technician for dinner and breaks, and assigning staff to dinner and breaks. When Linda comes to work, she discovers that one registered nurse (RN) called in sick. She has two RNs and three unlicensed assistive personnel (UAP) for staff. She panics and wants to refuse to take report. After a discussion with the charge nurse from the previous shift, she realizes that not taking report is not an option. She sits down to evaluate the acuity of the clients and the capabilities of her staff.

Introduction to Delegation

Delegation is not a new concept. In her *Notes on Nursing,* Florence Nightingale (1859) clearly stated: "Don't imagine that if you, who are in charge, don't look to all these things yourself, those under you will be more careful than you are...." She continued by directing, "But then again to look to all these things yourself does not mean to do them yourself. If you do it, it is by so much the better certainly than if it were not done at all. But can you not insure that it is done when not done by yourself? Can you insure that it is not undone when your back is turned? This is what being in charge means. And a very important meaning it is, too. The former only implies that just what you can do with your own hands is done. The latter that what ought to be done is always done. Head in charge must see to house hygiene, not do it herself" (p. 17).

Definition of Delegation

By definition, delegation is the reassigning of responsibility for the performance of a job from one person to another (American Nurses Association [ANA], 1996). RNs maintain accountability for supervising those to whom tasks are delegated (ANA, 2005). Although the responsibility for the task is transferred, the accountability for the

process or outcome of the task remains with the delegator, or the person delegating the activity. Nightingale referred to this delegation responsibility when she inferred that the "head in charge" does not necessarily carry out the task but still sees that it is completed.

An assignment is not the same as delegation. In an assignment, power is not transferred. Assignments refer to practical or routine functions that are part of a job description or client needs. For example, the team leader assigns three clients to the licensed practical nurse (LPN). That is part of the job description for the LPN. However, giving medications to all the clients on the team is a delegated responsibility.

According to the ANA, specific overlying principles remain firm regarding delegation. These include the following:

- The nursing profession delineates the scope of nursing practice.
- The nursing profession identifies and supervises the necessary education, training, and use of ancillary roles concerned with the delivery of direct client care.
- The RN assumes responsibility and accountability for the provision of nursing practice.
- The RN directs care and determines the appropriate utilization of any ancillary personnel involved in providing direct client care.
- The RN accepts assistance from ancillary nursing personnel in delivering nursing care for the client (ANA, 2005, p. 6).

Nurse-related principles are also designated by the ANA. These are important when considering what tasks may be delegated and to whom. These principles are:

- The RN has the duty to be accountable for personal actions related to the nursing process.
- The RN considers the knowledge and skills of any ancillary personnel to whom aspects of care are delegated.
- The decision to delegate or assign is based on the RN's judgment regarding the following: the condition of the client; the competence of the members of the nursing team; the amount of supervision that will be required of the RN if a task is delegated.
- The RN uses critical thinking and professional judgment when following the Five Rights of

Delegation delineated by the National Council of State Boards of Nursing (NCSBN) (Box 9-1).

- The RN recognizes that a relational aspect exists between delegation and communication. Communication needs to be culturally appropriate, and the individual receiving the communication should be treated with respect.
- Chief nursing officers are responsible for creating systems to assess, monitor, verify, and communicate continuous competence requirements in areas related to delegation.
- RNs monitor organizational policies, procedures, and job descriptions to ensure they are in compliance with the nurse practice act, consulting with the state board of nursing as needed (ANA, 2005, p. 6).

Delegation may be direct or indirect. *Direct delegation* is usually "verbal direction by the RN delegator regarding an activity or task in a specific nursing care situation" (ANA, 1996, p. 15). In this case, the RN decides which staff member is capable of performing the specific task or activity. *Indirect delegation is* "an approved listing of activities or tasks that have been established in policies and procedures of the health care institution or facility" (ANA, 1996, p. 15). The ANA also differentiated the delegation of a task from the assignment of a task. Although the terms are often used interchangeably, according to the ANA (1996), assignment is the "downward or lateral transfer of both the responsibility and the accountability of an activity from one person to another." When one RN "delegates" to another RN, that RN, based on knowledge and skill, may be responsible and accountable. UAP may also be assigned, rather than "delegated," a task. For example, UAP have the knowledge and skills required for some routine tasks (Ellis & Hartley, 2004).

The recent changes occurring in the health-care environment continue to modify the scope of nursing practice and the activities delegated to UAP. A main concern in almost all health-care settings is

that UAP are performing inappropriate functions that belong within the legal realm of nursing (ANA, 2002).

Permitted tasks vary from institution to institution. For example, a certified nursing assistant (CNA) performs specific activities designated by the job description approved by the particular healthcare institution. Although the institution delineates tasks and activities, this does not mean that the RN cannot decide to assign other personnel in specific situations. Take the following example:

Ms. Ross was admitted to the neurological unit from the neuroscience intensive care unit. She suffered a grade II subarachnoid hemorrhage 2 weeks ago and has a left hemiparesis. She has difficulty with swallowing and receives tube feedings through a percutaneous endoscopic gastrostomy (PEG) tube; however, she has been advanced to a pureed diet. She needs assistance with personal care, toileting, and feeding. A physical therapist comes twice a day to get her up for gait training; otherwise, the physician wants her in a chair as much as possible.

Assessing this situation, the RN might consider assigning an LPN to this client. The swallowing problems place the client at risk for aspiration, which means that feeding may present a problem. There is a potential for injury. The LPN is capable of managing the PEG tube feeding. While assisting with bathing, the LPN can perform range-of-motion exercises to all the client's extremities and assess her skin for breakdown. The LPN also knows the appropriate way to assist the client in transferring from the bed to the chair. The RN may not assign an individual to perform a task or activity not specified in that person's job description or within the scope of practice, such as allowing a nursing assistant to administer medications or perform certain types of dressing changes.

Supervision

Do not confuse delegation with supervision. Supervision is more direct and requires directly overseeing the work or performance of others. Supervision includes checking with individuals throughout the day to see what activities have been completed and what may still need to be finished. For example, a nursing assistant has been assigned to take all the vital signs on the unit and give the morning baths to eight clients. Three hours into the morning, she is far behind. At this point, it is

---

box 9-1
The Five Rights of Delegation
1. Right task
2. Right circumstances
3. Right person
4. Right direction/communication
5. Right supervision/evaluation

important that the RN discover why. Perhaps one of the clients required more care than expected, or the nursing assistant needed to do an errand off the floor. Reevaluation of the assignment may be necessary. When one RN works with another, then supervision is not needed. This is a collaborative relationship and includes consulting and giving advice when needed.

Individuals who supervise others also delegate tasks and activities. Chief nursing officers often delegate tasks to associate directors. This may include record reviews, unit reports, or client acuities. Certain administrative tasks, such as staff scheduling, may be delegated to another staff member, such as an associate manager. The chief nursing officer remains accountable for ensuring the activities are completed.

Supervision sometimes entails more direct evaluation of performance, such as performance evaluations and discussions regarding individual interactions with clients and other staff members.

Regardless of where you work, you cannot assume that only those in the higher levels of the organization delegate work to other people. You, too, will be responsible at times for delegating some of your work to other nurses, to technical personnel, or to another department. Decisions associated with this responsibility often cause some difficulty for new nurses. Knowing each person's capabilities and job description can help you decide which personnel can assist with a task.

The Nursing Process and Delegation

Before deciding who should care for a particular client, the nurse must assess each client's particular needs, set client-specific goals, and match the skills of the person assigned with the tasks that need to be accomplished *(assessment)*. Thinking this through before delegating helps prevent problems later *(plan)*. Next, the nurse assigns the tasks to the appropriate person *(implementation)*. The nurse must then oversee the care and determine whether client care needs have been met *(evaluation)*. It is also important for the nurse to allow time for feedback during the day. This enables all personnel to see where they are and where they want to go.

Often, the nurse must first coordinate care for groups of clients before being able to delegate tasks to other personnel. The nurse also needs to consider his or her own responsibilities. This includes assisting other staff members with setting priorities, communicating clearly, clarifying instructions, and reassessing the situation.

In 1995 the NCSBN published a paper addressing the issue of delegation. The NCSBN developed a concept called the Five Rights of Delegation (see Box 9-1), similar to the five rights regarding medication administration. In 2006 the NCSBN, along with the ANA, prepared a joint statement on delegation that clarified the profession's practice guidelines and the legal requisites for delegation. Before being able to delegate tasks and activities to other individuals, however, the nurse must understand the needs of each client.

Coordinating Assignments

One of the most difficult tasks for new nurses to master is coordinating daily activities. Often, you have clients for whom you provide direct care, and you must supervise the work of others, such as non-nurse caregivers, LPNs, or vocational nurses. Although care plans, critical (or clinical) pathways, concept maps, and computer information sheets are available to help identify client needs, these items do not provide a mechanism for coordinating the delivery of care. To do this, personalized worksheets can be developed that prioritize tasks to perform for each client. Using the worksheets helps the nurse identify tasks that require the knowledge and skill of an RN and those that can be carried out by UAP.

On the worksheet, tasks are prioritized on the basis of client need, not nursing convenience. For example, an order states that a client is to receive continuous tube feedings. Although it may be convenient for the nurse to fill the feeding container with enough supplement to last 6 hours, it is not good practice and not safe for the client. Instead, the nurse should plan to check the tube feeding every 2 hours.

As for Linda at the beginning of the chapter, a worksheet can help her determine who can do what. First, she needs to decide what particular tasks she must do. These include receiving and transcribing orders; contacting physicians with information or requests; accessing laboratory reports from the computer, reviewing them, and giving them to the appropriate staff members; and checking any new medication orders and placing them in the medication administration records. Another RN may be able to relieve the monitor technician for dinner and breaks, and a second RN may be able to assign staff to dinner and breaks. Next, Linda needs to look at the needs of each client on the unit and prioritize them. She is now ready to delegate to her staff effectively.

Some activities must be done at a certain time, and their timing may be out of one's control. Examples include medication administration and clients who need special preparation for a scheduled procedure. The following are some tips for organizing work on personalized worksheets to help establish client priorities (Tappen, Weiss, & Whitehead, 2004):

- Plan your time around these activities.
- Do high-priority activities first.
- Determine which activities are best done in a cluster.
- Remember that you are responsible for activities delegated to others.
- Consider your peak energy time when scheduling optional activities.

This list acts as a guideline for coordinating client care. The nurse needs to use critical thinking skills in the decision-making process. Remember that this is one of the ANA nurse-related principles of delegation (ANA, 2005). For example, activities that are usually clustered include bathing, changing linen, and parts of the physical assessment. Some clients may not be able to tolerate too much activity at one time. Take special situations into consideration when coordinating client care and deciding who should carry out some of the activities. Remember, however, that even when you delegate, you remain accountable.

Figure 9.1 is an example of a personalized worksheet. (See Chapter 11, Time Management, for a complete discussion.)

The Need for Delegation

The 1990s brought rapid change to the health-care environment. Several forces came together at one time, including the nursing shortage, health-care reform, an increased need for nursing services, and demographic trends. These changes continue to have an impact on the delivery of nursing care, requiring institutions to hire other personnel to assist nurses with client care (Zimmerman, 1996).

Health-care institutions often use UAP to perform certain client care tasks (Habel, 2001;

Hansten & Jackson, 2004; Huber, Blegan, & McCloskey, 1994). As the nursing shortage becomes more critical, there is a greater need for institutions to recruit the services of UAPs (ANA, 2002). A survey conducted by the American Hospital Association revealed that 97% of hospitals currently employ some type of UAP. Because a high percentage of institutions employ these personnel, many nurses believe they know how to work with and safely delegate tasks to them. This is not the case. Therefore, many nursing organizations have developed definitions for UAP and criteria regarding their responsibilities. The ANA defines UAP as follows:

Unlicensed assistive personnel are individuals who are trained to function in an assistive role to the registered nurse in the provision of patient/client care activities as delegated by and under the supervision of the registered professional nurse. Although some of these people may be certified (e.g., certified nursing assistant [CNA]), it is important to remember that certification differs from licensure. When a task is delegated to an unlicensed person, the professional nurse remains personally responsible for the outcomes of these activities (ANA, 2005).

As work on the UAP issue is ongoing, the ANA has recently updated its position statements to define direct and indirect patient care activities that may be performed by UAP. Included in these updates are specific definitions regarding UAP and technicians and acceptable tasks.

Use of the RN to provide all the care a client needs may not be the most efficient or cost-effective use of professional time. More hospitals are moving away from hiring LPNs and utilizing all RN staffing with UAP. For this reason, the nursing focus is directed at diagnosing client care needs and carrying out complex interventions.

The ANA cautions against delegating nursing activities that include the foundation of the nursing process and that require specialized knowledge, judgment, or skill (ANA, 1996, 2002, 2005). Non-nursing functions, such as performing clerical or receptionist duties, taking trips or doing errands off the unit, cleaning floors, making beds, collecting trays, and ordering supplies, should not be carried out by the highest paid and most educated member of the team. These tasks are easily delegated to other personnel.

Nurse/Team _____DNR 8607/Code 99

Patient Room # _____ Name _____ Age _____

Allergies_____

Diagnosis_____

Diet _____Fluids: PO _____IV_____ Type _____

Restrictions: BR _____ BRP _____OOB/Chair_____ Ambulate with assist_____

Activity _____

Assessment_____

Treatments

1. _____

2. _____

3. _____

4. _____

5. _____

Monitor

1. Vital signs: Temp _____ Pulse _____AHR_____ BP _____Parameters _____

2. Cardiac Monitor: Rhythm_____ Rate _____

3. Neurologic Status _____

4. CMS: _____ Traction:_____

Figure 9.1 Personalized patient worksheet.

Safe Delegation

In 1990 the NCSBN adopted a definition of delegation, stating that delegation is "transferring to a competent individual the authority to perform a selected nursing task in a selected situation" (p. 1). In its publication *Issues* (1995), the NCSBN again presented this definition. Likewise, the ANA Code for Nurses (1985) stated, "The nurse exercises informed judgment and uses individual competence and qualifications as criteria in seeking consultation, accepting responsibilities, and delegating nursing activities to others" (p. 1). In 2005, the ANA defined delegation as "the transfer of responsibility for the performance of an activity from one individual to another while retaining accountability for the outcome" (p. 4). To delegate tasks safely, nurses must delegate appropriately and supervise adequately.

In 1997 the NCSBN developed a Delegation Decision-Making Grid. This grid is a tool to help nurses delegate appropriately. It provides a scoring instrument for seven categories that the nurse should consider when making delegation decisions. The categories for the grid are listed in Box 9-2.

Scoring the components helps the nurse evaluate the situations, the client needs, and the healthcare personnel available to meet the needs. A low score on the grid indicates that the activity may be safely delegated to personnel other than the RN, and a high score indicates that delegation may not be advisable. Figure 9.2 shows the Delegation Decision-Making Grid. The grid is also available on the NCSBN Web site at ncsbn.com

Nurses who delegate tasks to UAP should evaluate the activities being considered for delegation (Keeney, Hasson, & McKenna, 2005). The American Association of Critical Care Nurses (AACN) (1990) recommended considering five factors, which are listed in Box 9-3, in making a decision to delegate.

It is the responsibility of the RN to be well acquainted with the state's nurse practice act and regulations issued by the state board of nursing regarding UAP (ANA, 2005). State laws and regulations supersede any publications or opinions set forth by professional organizations. As stated earlier, the NCSBN provides criteria to assist nurses with delegation.

LPNs are trained to perform specific tasks, such as basic medication administration, dressing changes, and personal hygiene tasks. In some states, the LPN, with additional training, may start and monitor intravenous (IV) infusions and administer certain medications.

Criteria for Delegation

The purpose of delegation is not to assign tasks to others that you do not want to do yourself. When you delegate to others effectively, the result is you have more time to perform the tasks that only a professional nurse is permitted to do.

In delegating, the nurse must consider both the *ability* of the person to whom the task is delegated and the *fairness* of the task to the individual and the team (Tappen, Weiss, & Whitehead, 2004). In other words, both the *task aspects* of delegation (Is this a complex task? Is it a professional responsibility? Can this person do it safely?) and the *interpersonal aspects* (Does the person have time to do this? Is the work evenly distributed?) must be considered.

The ANA (2005) has specified tasks that RNs may not delegate because they are specific to the discipline of professional nursing. These activities include (Boysen & Fischer, 2000):

- Initial nursing and follow-up assessments if nursing judgment is indicated
- Decisions and judgments about client outcomes
- Determination and approval of a client plan of care
- Interventions that require professional nursing knowledge, decisions, or skills
- Decisions and judgments necessary for the evaluation of client care

Task-Related Concerns

The primary task-related concern in delegating work is whether the person assigned to do the task has the ability to complete it. Team priorities and efficiency are also important considerations.

Abilities

To make appropriate assignments, the nurse needs to know the knowledge and skill level, legal definitions, role expectations, and job description for each member of the team. It is equally important to be aware of the different skill levels of

---

box 9-2

Seven Components of the Delegation Decision-Making Grid

- Level of client acuity
- Level of unlicensed assistive personnel capability
- Level of licensed nurse capability
- Possibility for injury
- Number of times the skill has been performed by the unlicensed assistive personnel
- Level of decision making needed for the activity
- Client's ability for self-care

Adapted from the National Council of State Boards of Nursing. Delegation Decision-Making Grid. National State Boards of Nursing, Inc., 1997 (ncsbn.org).

Elements for Review		Client A	Client B	Client C	Client D
Activity/task	**Describe activity/task:**				
Level of Client Stability	**Score the client's level of stability:** 0. Client condition is chronic/stable/predictable 1. Client condition has minimal potential for change 2. Client condition has moderate potential for change 3. Client condition is unstable/acute/strong potential for change				
Level of UAP Competence	**Score the UAP competence in completing delegated nursing care activities in the defined client population:** 0. UAP - expert in activities to be delegated, in defined population 1. UAP - experienced in activities to be delegated, in defined population 2. UAP - experienced in activities, but not in defined population 3. UAP - novice in performing activities and in defined population				
Level of Licensed Nurse Competence	**Score the licensed nurse's competence in relation to both knowledge of providing nursing care to a defined population and competence in implementation of the delegation process:** 0. Expert in the knowledge of nursing needs/activities of defined client population and expert in the delegation process 1. Either expert in knowledge of needs/activities of defined client population and competent in delegation or experienced in the needs/activities of defined client population and expert in the delegation process 2. Experienced in the knowledge of needs/activities of defined client population and competent in the delegation process 3. Either experienced in the knowledge of needs/activities of defined client population or competent in the delegation process 4. Novice in knowledge of defined population and novice in delegation				
Potential for Harm	**Score the potential level of risk the nursing care activity has for the client (risk is probability of suffering harm):** 0. None 1. Low 2. Medium 3. High				
Frequency	**Score based on how often the UAP has performed the specific nursing care activity:** 0. Performed at least daily 1. Performed at least weekly 2. Performed at least monthly 3. Performed less than monthly 4. Never performed				
Level of Decision Making	**Score the decision making needed, related to the specific nursing care activity, client (both cognitive and physical status), and client situation:** 0. Does not require decision making 1. Minimal level of decision making 2. Moderate level of decision making 3. High level of decision making				
Ability for Self-Care	**Score the client's level of assistance needed for self-care activities:** 0. No assistance 1. Limited assistance 2. Extensive assistance 3. Total care or constant attendance				
	Total Score				

Figure 9.2 Delegation decision-making grid.

box 9-3

Five Factors for Determining if Client Care Activity Should Be Delegated

- Potential for harm to the patient
- Complexity of the nursing activity
- Extent of problem solving and innovation required
- Predictability of outcome
- Extent of interaction

Adapted from American Association of Critical Care Nurses (AACN). (1990). Delegation of Nursing and Non-Nursing Activities in Critical Care: A Framework for Decision-Making. Irvine, CA: AACN.

caregivers within each discipline because ability differs with each level of education. Additionally, individuals within each level of skill possess their own strengths and weaknesses. Prior assessment of the strengths of each member of the team will assist in providing safe and efficient care to clients. Figure 9.3 outlines the skills of various health-care personnel.

People should not be assigned a task that they are not skilled in or knowledgeable to perform, regardless of their professional level. People are often reluctant to admit they cannot do something. Instead of seeking help or saying they are not comfortable with a task, they may avoid doing it, delay starting it, do only part of it, or even bluff their way through it, a risky choice in health care.

Regardless of the length of time individuals have been in a position, employees need orientation when assigned a new task. Those who seek assistance and advice are showing concern for the team and the welfare of their clients. Requests for assistance or additional explanations should not be ignored, and the person should be praised, not criticized, for seeking guidance (Tappen, Weiss, & Whitehead, 2004).

Priorities

The work of a busy unit rarely ends up going as expected. Dealing with sick people, their families, physicians, and other team members all at the same time is a difficult task. Setting priorities for the day should be based on client needs, team needs, and organizational and community demands. The values of each may be very different, even opposed. These differences should be discussed with team members so that decisions can be made based on team priorities.

One way to determine patient priorities is to base decisions on Maslow's hierarchy of needs. Maslow's hierarchy is frequently used in nursing to provide a framework for prioritizing care to meet client needs. The basic physiological needs come first because they are necessary for survival. For example, oxygen and medication administration, IV fluids, and enteral feedings are included in this group.

Identifying priorities and deciding the needs to be met first help in organizing care and in deciding which other team members can meet client needs. For example, nursing assistants can meet many hygiene needs, allowing licensed personnel to administer medications and enteral feedings in a timely manner.

Efficiency

Efficiency means that all members of the team know their jobs and responsibilities and work together like gears in a well-built clock. They mesh together and keep perfect time.

Figure 9.3 Diagram of delegation decision-making grid.

The current health-care delivery environment demands efficient, cost-effective care. Delegating appropriately can increase efficiency and save money. Likewise, incorrect delegation can decrease efficiency and cost money. When delegating tasks to individuals who cannot perform the job, the RN must often go back to perform the task.

Although institutions often need to "float" staff to other units, maintaining continuity, if at all possible, is important. Keeping the same staff members on the unit all the time, for example, allows them to develop familiarity with the physical setting and routines of the unit as well as the types of clients the unit services. Time is lost when staff members are reassigned frequently to different units. Although physical layouts may be the same, client needs, unit routines, use of space, and availability of supplies are often different. Time spent to orient reassigned staff members takes time away from delivery of client care. However, when staff members are reassigned, it is important for them to indicate their skill level and comfort in the new setting. It is just as important for the staff members who are familiar with the setting to identify the strengths of the reassigned person and build on them.

Appropriateness

Appropriateness is another task-related concern. Nothing can be more counterproductive than, for example, floating a coronary care nurse to labor and delivery. More time will be spent teaching the necessary skills than on safe mother-baby care. Assigning an educated, licensed staff member to perform non-nursing functions to protect safety is also poor use of personnel.

Relationship-Oriented Concerns

Relationship-oriented concerns include fairness, learning opportunities, health concerns, compatibility, and staff preferences.

Fairness

Fairness means distributing the workload evenly in terms of both the physical requirements and the emotional investment in providing health care. The nurse who is caring for a dying client may have less physical work to do than another team member, but in terms of emotional care to the client and family, he or she may be doing double the work of another staff member.

Fairness also means considering equally all requests for special consideration. The quickest way to alienate members of a team is to be unfair. It is important to discuss with team members any decisions that have been made that may appear unfair to any one of them. Allow the team members to participate in making decisions regarding assignments. Their participation will decrease resentment and increase cooperation. In some health-care institutions, team members make such decisions as a group.

Learning Opportunities

Including assignments that stimulate motivation, learning, and assisting team members to learn new tasks and take on new challenges is part of the role of the RN.

Health

Some aspects of caregiving jobs are more stressful than others. Rotating team members through the more difficult jobs may decrease stress and allow empathy to increase among the members. Special health needs, such as family emergencies or special physical problems of team members, also need to be addressed. If some team members have difficulty accepting the needs of others, the situation should be discussed with the team, bearing in mind the employee's right to privacy when discussing sensitive issues.

Compatibility

No matter how hard you may strive to get your team to work together, it just may not happen. Some people work together better than others. Helping people develop better working relationships is part of team building. Creating opportunities for people to share and learn from each other increases the overall effectiveness of the team.

As the leader, you may be forced to intervene in team member disputes. Many individuals find it difficult to work with others they do not like personally. It sometimes becomes necessary to explain that liking another person is a plus but not a necessity in the work setting and that personal problems have no place in the work environment. For example:

Laura had been a labor and delivery room supervisor in a large metropolitan hospital for 5 years before she moved to another city. Because a position similar to the one she left was not available, she became a staff nurse at a small local hospital. The hospital had just opened its new birthing center. The first day on the job went well. The other staff members seemed cordial. As the weeks went by, however, Laura began to have problems getting other staff to help her. No one would offer to relieve her for meals or a break. She noticed that certain groups of staff members always went to lunch together but that she was never invited to join them. She attempted to speak to some of the more approachable coworkers, but she did not get much information. Disturbed by the situation, Laura went to the nurse manager. The nurse manager listened quietly while Laura related her experiences. She then asked Laura to think about the last staff meeting. Laura realized that she had alienated the staff during the meeting because she had said repeatedly that in "her hospital" things were done in a particular way. Laura also realized that, instead of asking for help, she was in the habit of demanding it. Laura and the nurse manager discussed the difficulties of her changing positions, moving to a new place, and trying to develop both professional and social ties. Together, they came up with several solutions to Laura's problem.

Staff Preferences

Considering the preferences of individual team members is important but should not supersede other criteria for delegating responsibly. Allowing team members to always select what they want to do may cause the less assertive members' needs to be unmet.

It is important to explain the rationale for decisions made regarding delegation so that all team members may understand the needs of the unit or organization. Box 9-4 outlines basic rights for professional health-care team members. Although written originally for women, the concepts are applicable to all professional health-care providers.

Barriers to Delegation

Many nurses, particularly new ones, have difficulty delegating. The reasons for this include experience issues, licensure issues, and quality-of-care issues.

Experience Issues

Many nurses received their education during the 1980s, when primary care was the major delivery system. These nurses lacked the education and skill needed for delegation (Mahlmeister, 1999). Nurses

---

box 9-4

Basic Entitlements of Individuals in the Workplace

Professionals in the workplace are entitled to:
- Respect from others in the work setting
- A reasonable and equitable workload
- Wages commensurate with the job
- Determine his or her own priorities
- Ask for what he or she wants
- Refuse without guilt
- Make mistakes and be accountable for them
- Give and receive information as a professional nurse
- Act in the best interest of the client
- Be human

Adapted from Chevernet, M. (1988). STAT: Special Techniques in Assertiveness Training for Women in Healthcare Professions, 2nd ed. St. Louis, Mo.: Mosby.

---

educated before the 1970s worked in settings with LPNs and nursing assistants, where they routinely delegated tasks. However, client acuity was lower and the care less complex. Older nurses have considerable delegation experience and can be a resource for younger nurses.

The added responsibility of delegation creates some discomfort for nurses. Many believe they are unprepared to assume this responsibility, especially in deciding the competency of another person. To decrease this discomfort, nurses need to participate in establishing guidelines for UAP within their institution. The ANA Position Statements on Unlicensed Assistive Personnel address this. Table 9-1 lists the direct and indirect client care activities that may be performed by UAP.

Licensure Issues

The current health-care environment requires nurses to delegate. Many nurses voice concerns about the personal risk regarding their licensure if they delegate inappropriately. The courts have usually ruled that nurses are not liable for the negligence of other individuals, provided that the nurse delegated appropriately. Delegation is within the scope of nursing practice. The art and skill of delegation are acquired with practice.

Legal Issues and Delegation

State nurse practice acts establish the legal boundaries for nursing practice. Professional nursing organizations define practice standards, and the policies of the health-care institution create job descriptions and establish policies that guide appropriate delegation decisions for the organization.

table 9-1	

Direct and Indirect Client Care Activities

Direct Client Care Activities	Indirect Client Care Activities
Assisting with feeding and drinking	Providing a clean environment
Assisting with ambulation	Providing a safe environment
Assisting with grooming	Providing companion care
Assisting with toileting	Providing transportation for noncritical clients
Assisting with dressing	Assisting with stocking nursing units
Assisting with socializing	Providing messenger and delivery services

Adapted from American Nurses Association. (2002). Position Statement on Utilization of Unlicensed Assistive Personnel. Washington, DC: American Nurses Association.

Inherent in today's health-care environment is the safety of the client. The quality of client care and the delievery of safe and effective care are central to the concept of delegation. RNs are held accountable when delegating care activities to others. This means that they have an obligation to intervene whenever they deem the care provided is unsafe or unethical. It is also important to realize that a delegated task may not be "sub-delegated." In other words, if the RN delegated a task to the LPN, the LPN cannot then delegate the task to the UAP, even if the LPN has decided that it is within the abilities of that particular UAP. There may be legal implications if a client is injured as a result of inappropriate delegation. Take the following case:

In Hicks v. New York State Department of Health, a nurse was found guilty of patient neglect because of her failure to appropriately train and supervise the UAP working under her. In this particular situation, a security guard discovered an elderly nursing home client in a totally dark room undressed and covered with urine and fecal material. The client was partially in his bed and partially restrained in an overturned wheelchair. The court found the nurse guilty on the following: the nurse failed to assess whether the UAP had delivered proper care to the client, and this subsequently led to the inadequate delivery of care (1991).

Quality-of-Care Issues

Nurses have expressed concern over the quality of client care when tasks and activities are delegated to others. Remember Nightingale's words earlier in the chapter, "Don't imagine that if you, who are in charge, don't look to all these things yourself, those under you will be more careful than you are." She added that you do not need to do everything yourself to see that it is done correctly. When you delegate, you control the delegation. You decide to whom you will delegate the task. Remember that there are levels of acceptable performance and that not every task needs to be done perfectly.

Assigning Work to Others

Assigning work can be difficult for several reasons:

1. Some nurses think they must do everything themselves.
2. Some nurses distrust subordinates to do things correctly.
3. Some nurses think that if they delegate all the technical tasks, they will not reinforce their own learning.
4. Some nurses are more comfortable with the technical aspects of client care than with the more complex issues of client teaching and discharge planning.

Families and clients do not always see professional activities. Rather, they see direct client care (Keeney, Hasson, McKenna, & Gillen, 2005). Nurses believe that when they do not participate directly in client care, they do not accomplish anything for the client. The professional aspects of nursing, such as planning care, teaching, and discharge planning, help to promote positive outcomes for clients and their families. When working with LPNs, knowing their scope of practice helps in making delegation decisions.

Models of Care Delivery

Functional nursing, team nursing, total client care, and primary nursing are models of care delivery that developed in an attempt to balance the needs of the client with the availablity and skills of nurses. Both delegation and communication skills are essential to successfully follow through with any given model of care delivery.

Functional Nursing

Functional nursing or task nursing evolved during the mid-1940s due to the loss of RNs who left home to serve in the armed forces during the Second World War. Prior to the war, RNs comprised the majority of hospital staffing. Because of the lack of nurses to provide care at home, hospitals used more LPNs or licensed vocational nurses and UAP to care for clients.

When implementing functional nursing, the focus is on the task and not necessarily holistic client care. The needs of the clients are categorized by task, and then the tasks are assigned to the "best person for the job." This method takes into consideration the skill set and licensure scope of practice of each caregiver. For example, the RN would perform and document all assessments and administer all IV medications; the LPN or LVN would adminster treatments and perform dressing changes. UAP would be responsible for meeting hygiene needs of clients, obtaining and recording vital signs, and assisting in feeding clients. This method is efficient and effective; however, when implemented, continuity in client care is lost. Many times, re evaluation of client status and follow-up does not occur, and a breakdown in communication among staff occurs.

Team Nursing

Team nursing grew out of functional nursing; nursing units often resort to this model when appropriate staffing is unavailable. A group of nursing personnel or a team provides care for a cluster of clients. The manner in which clients are divided varies and depends on several issues: the layout of the unit, the types of clients on the unit, and the number of clients on the unit. The organization of the team is based on the number of available staff and the skill mix within the group.

An RN assumes the role of the team leader. The team may consist of another RN, an LPN, and UAP. The team leader directs and supervises the team, which provides client care. The team knows the condition and needs of all the clients on the team.

The team leader acts as a liaison between the clients and the health-care provider/physician. Responsibilities include formulating a client plan of care, transcribing and communicating orders and treatment changes to team members, and solving problems of clients and/or team members. The nurse manager confers with the team leaders, supervises the client care teams and, in some institutions, conducts rounds with the health-care providers.

For this method to be effective, the team leader needs strong delegation and communication skills. Communication among team members and the nurse manager avoids duplication of efforts and decreases competition for control of assignments that may not be equal based on client acuity and the skills sets of team members.

Total Client Care

During the 1920s total client care was the original model of nursing care delivery. Much nursing was in the form of private duty nursing, in which nurses cared for clients in homes and in hospitals. Schools of nursing located in hospitals provided students who staffed the nursing units and delivered care under the watchful eyes of nursing supervisors and directors. In this model, one RN assumes the responsibility of caring for one client. This includes acting as a direct liason among the client, family, health-care provider, and other members of the health-care team. Today, this model is seen in high acuity areas such as critical care units, postanesthesia recovery units, and in labor and delivery units. This model requires RNs to engage in non-nursing tasks that might be assumed by individuals without the educational level of an RN.

Primary Nursing

In the 1960s nursing care delivery models started to move away from team nursing and placed the RN in the role of giving direct client care. The central principle of this model is to distribute nursing decision making to the nurses caring for the client. As the primary nurse, the RN devises, implements, and is responsible for the nursing care of the client during the time the client remains on the nursing unit. The primary nurse along with associate nurses gives direct care to the client.

In its ideal form, primary nursing requires an all-RN staff. Although this model provides continuity of care and nursing accountability, staffing is difficult and expensive. Some view it as ineffective as many tasks that consume the time of the RN could be carried out by other personnel.

Conclusion

The concept of delegation is not new. The delegation role is essential to the RN-LPN and RN-UAP relationship. Personal organizational skills are a prerequisite to delegation. Before the nurse can delegate tasks to others, he or she needs to understand individual client needs. Using worksheets and Maslow's hierarchy helps the nurse understand these individual client needs, set priorities, and identify which tasks can be delegated to others. Using the Delegation Decision-Making Grid helps the nurse delegate safely and appropriately.

It is also important the nurse be aware of the capabilities of each staff member, the tasks that may be delegated, and the tasks that the RN needs to perform. When delegating, the RN uses professional judgment in making decisions. Professional judgment is directed by the state nurse practice act and national standards of nursing. Institutions develop their own job descriptions for UAP and other health-care professionals, but institutional policies cannot contradict the state nurse practice act. Although the nurse delegates the task or activity, he or she remains accountable for the delegated decision.

Understanding the concept of delegation helps the new nurse organize and prioritize client care. Knowing the staff and their capabilities simplifies delegation. Utilizing staff members' capabilities creates a pleasant and productive working environment for everyone involved. Understanding delegation and proper application of delegation principles is needed in the implementation of the various nursing practice models.

Study Questions

1. What are the responsibilities of the professional nurse when delegating tasks to an LPN or UAP?

2. What factors need to be considered when delegating tasks?

3. What is the difference between the delegation and the assignment of a task?

4. What are the nurse manager's legal responsibilities in supervising UAP?

5. If you were the nurse manager, how would you have handled Laura's situation?

6. How would you have handled the situation if you were Linda?

7. Bring the client census from your assigned clinical unit to class. Using the Delegation Decision-Making Grid, decide which clients you would assign to the personnel on the unit. Give reasons for your decision.

8. What type of nursing delivery model is implemented on your assigned clinical unit? Give examples of the roles of the personnel engaged in client care to support your answer.

Case Study to Promote Critical Reasoning

Julio works at a large teaching hospital in a major metropolitan area. This institution services the entire geographical region, including indigent clients, and, because of its reputation, administers care to international clients and individuals who reside in other states. Like all health-care institutions, this one has been attempting to cut costs by using more UAP. Nurses are often floated to other units. Lately, the number of indigent and foreign clients on Julio's unit has increased. The acuity of these clients has been quite high, requiring a great deal of time from the nursing staff.

Julio arrived at work at 6:30 a.m., his usual time. He looked at the census board and discovered that the unit was filled, and Bed Control was calling all night to have clients discharged or transferred to make room for several clients who had been in the emergency department since the previous evening. He also discovered that the other RN assigned to his team called in sick. His team consists of himself, two UAP, and an LPN who is shared by two teams. He has eight clients on his team: two need to be readied for surgery, including preoperative and postoperative teaching, one of whom is a 35-year-old woman scheduled for a modified radical mastectomy for the treatment of breast cancer; three are second-day postoperative clients, two of whom require extensive dressing changes, are receiving IV antibiotics, and need to be ambulated; one postoperative client who is required to remain on total bedrest, has a nasogastric tube to suction as well as a chest tube, is on total parenteral nutrition and lipids, needs a central venous catheter line dressing change, has an IV, is taking multiple IV medications, and has a Foley catheter; one client who is ready for discharge and needs discharge instruction; and one client who needs to be transferred to a subacute unit, and a report must be given to the RN of that unit. Once the latter client is transferred and the other one is discharged, the emergency department will be sending two clients to the unit for admission.

1. How should Julio organize his day? Set up an hourly schedule.

2. What type of client management approach should Julio consider in assigning staff appropriately?

3. If you were Julio, which clients and/or tasks would you assign to your staff? List all of them, and explain your rationale.

4. Using the Delegation Decision-Making Grid, make staff and client assignments.

References

American Association of Critical Care Nurses (AACN). (1990). *Delegation of Nursing and Non-Nursing Activities in Critical Care: A Framework for Decision Making.* Irvine, Calif.: AACN.

American Nurses Association (ANA). (1985). *Code for Nurses.* Washington, DC: ANA.

American Nurses Association (ANA). (1996). *Registered Professional Nurses and Unlicensed Assistive Personnel.* Washington, DC: ANA.

American Nurses Association (ANA). (2002). *Position Statements on Registered Nurse Utilization of Unlicensed Assistive Personnel.* Washington, DC: ANA.

American Nurses Association (ANA). (2005). *Principles for Delegation.* Washington, DC: ANA.

Boysen, R., & Fischer, C. (2000). Delegation/practice boundaries. South Dakota State University College of Nursing. Retrieved July 29, 2002, from learn.sdstate. edu/nursing/ DelegationModule2

Chevernet, M. (1988). *STAT: Special Techniques in Assertiveness Training for Women in Healthcare Professions,* 2nd ed. St. Louis, Mo.: Mosby.

Ellis, J.R., & Hartley, C.L. (2004). *Nursing in Today's World.* Philadelphia: Lippincott, Williams & Wilkins.

Habel, M. (Winter 2001). Delegating nursing care to unlicensed assistive personnel. *Continuing Education for Florida Nurses,* 39–54.

Hansten, R.I, & Jackson, M. (2004). *Clinical Delegation Skills: A Handbook for Professional Practice.* Sudbury, Mass.: Jones & Bartlett.

Hicks v. New York State Department of Health. (1991). 570 N.Y.S. 2d 395 (A.D. 3 Dept).

Huber, D., Blegan, M., & McCloskey, J. (1994). Use of nursing assistants: Staff nurse opinions. *Nursing Management,* 25(5), 64–68.

Keeney, S., Hasson, F., McKenna, H., & Gillen, P. (2005). Health care assistants: The view of managers of health care agencies on training and employment. *Journal of Nursing Management,* 13(1), 83–92.

Keeney, S., Hasson, F., & McKenna, H. (2005). Nurses', midwives', and patients' perceptions of trained health care assistants. *Journal of Advanced Nursing,* 50(4), 345–355.

Mahlmeister, L. (1999). Professional accountability and legal liability for the team leader and charge nurse. *Journal of Obstetric, Gynecologic, and Neonatal Nursing,* 28, 300–309.

National Council of State Boards of Nursing. (1990). *Concept Paper on Delegation.* Chicago: NCSBN.

National Council of State Boards of Nursing. (1995). Delegation: Concepts and decision-making process. *Issues* (December), 1–2.

National Council of State Boards of Nursing. (1997). *Delegation Decision-Making Grid.* Chicago: NCSBN.

National Council of State Boards of Nursing. (2007). The five rights of delegation. Retrieved November 30, 2008, from www.ncsbn.org/Joint_statement.pdf

Nightingale, F. (1859). *Notes on Nursing: What It Is and What It Is Not.* London: Harrison and Sons. (Reprint 1992. Philadelphia: JB Lippincott.)

Tappen, R., Weiss, S.A., & Whitehead, D.K. (2004). *Essentials of Leadership and Management.* Philadelphia: FA Davis.

Zimmerman, P.G. (1996). Delegating to assistive personnel. *Journal of Emergency Nursing,* 22, 206–212.

⦿ ○ ○ ○ ○ ○ ○ ○ ○ ○ ○

OBJECTIVES

After reading this chapter, the student should be able to:

- Discuss the history of quality and safety within the U.S. health-care system.
- Analyze historical, social, political, and economic trends affecting the nursing profession and the health-care delivery system.
- Explain the importance of quality improvement (QI) for the nurse, patient, organization, and health-care delivery system.
- Discuss the role of the nurse in continuous quality improvement (CQI) and risk management.
- Examine factors contributing to medical errors and evidence-based methods for the prevention of medical errors.
- Explain the use of technology to enhance and promote safe patient care, educate patients and consumers, evaluate health-care delivery, and enhance the nurse's knowledge base.
- Describe the effects of communication on patient-centered care, interdisciplinary collaboration, and safety.
- Promote the role of the nurse in the contemporary health-care environment.

History and Overview

You are entering professional nursing at a time when issues pertaining to quality and safety of the U.S. health-care system have come to the forefront in the delivery of health care. Considering the complexity of the decisions you make every day in managing patient care at the bedside, it may be easy to dismiss the theory that you must also consider quality and safety within the health-care system. However, each day as a professional registered nurse (RN), you will participate in activities to support quality and safety initiatives at the bedside, within your organization, and as part of the health-care system. First, this chapter identifies trends and issues that have brought quality and safety to the forefront.

Historical Trends and Issues

The rapidly changing health-care delivery system is driven by many forces (Baldwin, Conger, Maycock, & Ableggen, 2002; Davis, 2001; Elwood, 2007; Ervin, Bickes, & Schim, 2006; Menix, 2000) that are influencing the current movement toward improved quality and safety. Some of these forces include economics, societal demographics and diversity, regulation and legislation, technology, health-care delivery and practice, and environment and globalization.

Economics. U.S health-care delivery has been affected by many economic trends and issues. Businesses, government, and the media decry the cost of health care within the United States when compared with that of other developed nations (Jackson, 2006; Kersbergen, 2000). The cost of research and the cost to develop new treatments and technology are rising. Nurses need to be prepared to support consumers with a thorough knowledge of quality, accountability, and cost-effectiveness (AACN, 1997). Educated consumers will expect safe, quality care with associated satisfaction and health outcomes. Improvements in quality and safety will reduce costs (Cronenwett et al., 2007; Institute of Medicine [IOM], 2003a).

Societal demographics and diversity. Increased numbers of racial and ethnic groups /will influence health-care delivery (Billings & Halsted, 2005; Elwood 2007; Heller, Oros, & Durney-Crowley, 2000). Increased numbers of elderly people, increased lifespan, and improvements in technology mean an emphasis on specialized geriatric care.

Both the elderly and ethnic minorities are at-risk populations who suffer disadvantages in access, payment, and quality of care (U.S. Department of Health & Human Services, 2001).

Regulation and legislation. The diverse interests of consumers, insurance companies, government, and regulation affect health-care legislation. For health-care leaders and providers of care, unprecedented challenges will continue despite the attention that quality and safety has received during the evolution of the existing health-care system.

Technology. The use of technology will improve cost, clinical outcomes, quality, and safety (IOM, 2003a). Nursing practice must accommodate this health-care delivery trend with the inclusion of concepts in interdisciplinary collaboration, patient-focused systems, and information literacy (Booth, 2006). Additionally, nurses must utilize technology and informatics to incorporate evidenced-based practices for improved quality and safety in the health-care delivery system.

Technology also produces advancements in disease treatments, especially in the areas of genetics and genomics, and all professionals must integrate these areas into practice (Jenkins & Calzone, 2007). Advances in genetics and genomics lead to breakthroughs in the treatments of a variety of genetic disorders, QI, and outcomes in clinical practice often related to pharmacotherapeutics (Trossman, 2006).

Health-care delivery and practice. Health-care professionals should be prepared to provide safe, quality care in all settings, including acute care and community settings. Nurses and other health-care professionals need the knowledge, skills, attitudes, and competencies to function in a variety of settings and the ability to support the needs of the elderly (Ervin, Bickes, & Schim, 2006; Heller, Oros, Durney-Crowley, 2000).

The integration of evidenced-based practice will serve to improve quality and safety for patients, as it will improve collaboration and interdisciplinary teamwork (Brady et al., 2001; IOM, 2003a; O'Neill, 1998). Both the IOM (2003a) and the Pew Health Professions Commission (O'Neill, 1998) identified the need for the health-care delivery system and its professionals to improve collaboration and to work in an interdisciplinary team to improve quality and safety.

Environment and globalization. The emergence of a global economy, the ease of travel, and advances in communication technology affect the movement of people, money, and disease (Heller, Oros, & Durney-Crowley, 2000; Kirk, 2002). Global warming and climate change have been linked to the emergence of new drug-resistant organisms, an increase in vector-borne and water-borne disease, and migration of affected populations. Safe, quality health care will need to confront the challenges of increasing multiculturalism,

potential for pandemic, and the effect of climate change and pollution on health.

In addition, many health-care professionals, government agencies, and supporting organizations have contributed to the evolution of quality and safety within the health-care system. The Historical Timeline (Table 10-1) highlights significant organizations and initiatives of importance to quality and safety.

table 10-1

Historical Timeline

1896	Nurses Associated Alumnae of the United States and Canada formed, later called the American Nurses Association (ANA)
1906	Food and Drug Act signed, which began the regulation of food and drugs to protect consumers
1918	American College of Surgeons founded, which initiated minimum standards for hospitals and on-site hospital inspections for adherence to standards
1930s	Employers began offering *health benefits*, and the first commercial insurance companies arose
1945	Quality management principles developed by Edward Deming were applied successfully to industries such as manufacturing, government, and health care
1951	Joint Commission on Accreditation of Healthcare Organizations (JCAHO) founded; currently referred to as the Joint Commission (JC)
1955	Social Security Act passed; hospitals that had volunteered for accreditation by JCAHO were approved for participation in Medicare and Medicaid
1966	*Quality of health-care services* defined in the literature
1970	IOM established as a nonprofit adviser to the nation to improve health in the national academies
1979	National Committee on Quality Assurance (NCQA) established
1986	National Center of Nursing Research founded at the National Institutes of Health (NIH)
1989	Agency for Healthcare Research and Quality (AHRQ) established
1990	NCQA began accrediting managed care organizations by using data from Health Plan Employer Data and Information Set (HEDIS)
1990	Institute of Healthcare Improvement (IHI) founded
1991	Nursing's Agenda for Health Care Reform published by the ANA
1996	National Patient Safety Foundation (NPSF) founded; JC established Sentinel Event Policies
1996	IOM launched three-part initiative to study health-care system quality
1998	IOM National Roundtable on Health Care Quality released *Consensus Statement*
1999	IOM published *To Err is Human: Building a Safer Health System*
2001	IOM published *Crossing the Quality Chasm: A New Health System for the 21st Century*
2001	IOM published *Envisioning the National Health Care Quality Report*
2001	ANA's National Database for Nursing Quality Indicators (NDNQI) demonstrated the positive impact of the appropriate mix of nursing staff on patient outcomes
2001	JC mandated hospital-wide patient safety standards
2003	IOM published *Priority Areas for National Action: Transforming Health Care Quality*, which established priority areas for national action to improve quality of care and outcomes (Box 10-1)
2003	JC established first set of National Patient Safety Goals (NPSG)
2003	IOM published *Health Professions Education: A Bridge to Quality*
2004	IOM published *Keeping Patients Safe: Transforming the Work Environment of Nurses*
2004	IOM published *Patient Safety: Achieving a New Standard of Care*
2005	ANA updated its Health Care Agenda, urging system reform
2006	IOM published *Preventing Medication Errors: Quality Chasm Series*

box 10-1

Institute of Medicine Priority Areas (IOM, 2003b).

• Asthma	• Ischemic heart disease
• Cancer screening	• Major depression
• Care coordination	• Nosocomial infections
• Children with special care needs	• Obesity
• Diabetes	• Pain control in advanced cancer
• End-of-life issues	• Pregnancy and childbirth
• Frail elderly	• Self-management
• Health literacy	• Severe, persistent mental illness
• Hypertension	• Stroke
• Immunizations	• Tobacco dependence in adults

The IOM and the Committee on the Quality of Health Care in America

The IOM is a private, nonprofit organization chartered in 1970 by the U.S government. The IOM's role is to provide unbiased, expert health and scientific advice for the purpose of improving health. The result of the IOM's work supports government policy making, the health-care system, health-care professionals, and consumers.

In 1998 the IOM National Roundtable on Health Care Quality released *Statement on Quality of Care* (Donaldson, 1998), which urged health-care leaders to make urgent changes in the U.S. health-care system. The Roundtable reached consensus in four areas regarding the U.S. health-care system:

1. Quality can be defined and measured;
2. Quality problems are serious and extensive;
3. Current approaches to QI are inadequate; and
4. There is an urgent need for rapid change.

This IOM statement launched today's movement to improve quality and safety for the 21st century U.S. health-care system.

In 1998 the IOM charged the Committee on the Quality of Health Care in America to develop a strategy to improve health-care quality in the coming decade (IOM, 2000). The Committee completed a systematic review and critique of literature that highlighted and quantified severe shortcomings in the heath-care system. Its work led to the series of reports that serves as the foundation and strategy for health system reform (Box 10-2). Two in particular, *To Err is Human: Building a Safer Health System* (IOM, 2000) and *Crossing the Quality Chasm: A New Health System for the 21st Century* (IOM, 2001), provide a framework

upon which the 21st-century health-care system is being built.

To Err is Human—discussed later in this chapter—quantified unnecessary death in the U.S. health-care system and placed emphasis on system failures as the foundation for errors and mistakes. According the report, it is the flawed systems in patient care that often leave the door open for human error. The report made a series of eight recommendations in four areas (Box 10-3) that aimed to decreased errors by at least 50% over 5 years. The goal of the recommendations was "for the external environment to create sufficient pressure to make errors costly to health-care organizations and providers, so they are compelled to take action to improve safety" (IOM, 2000, p. 4). The recommendations sparked pubic interest in health-care quality and safety and caused prompt responses by the government and national quality organizations.

Crossing the Quality Chasm addressed broad quality issues in the U.S. health-care system. The report indicated that the health-care system is fundamentally flawed with "gaps," and it proposed a system-wide

box 10-2

IOM Quality Reports (IOM, 2006)

- *Crossing the Quality Chasm: The IOM Quality Health Care Initiative* (1996)
- *To Err Is Human: Building a Safer Health System* (2000)
- *Crossing the Quality Chasm: A New Health System for the 21st Century* (2001)
- *Envisioning the National Health Care Quality Report* (2001)
- *Priority Areas for National Action: Transforming Health Care Quality* (2003b)
- *Leadership by Example: Governmental Roles* (2003)
- *Health Professions Education: A Bridge to Quality* (2003a)
- *Patient Safety: Achieving a New Standard of Care* (2003)
- *Keeping Patients Safe: Transforming the Work Environment for Nurses* (2004)
- *Academic Health Centers: Leading Change in the 21st Century* (2004)
- *Preventing Medication Errors: Quality Chasm Series* (2006)

box 10-3

Focus Areas of *To Err is Human* Recommendations (IOM, 2000)

- Enhance knowledge and leadership regarding safety.
- Identify and learn from errors.
- Set performance standards and expectations for safety.
- Implement safety systems within health-care organizations.

strategy and action plans to redesign the health-care system. The report stated that the gaps between actual care and high-quality care could be attributed to four key inter-related areas in the health-care system: the growing complexity of science and technology, an increase in chronic conditions, a poorly organized delivery system of care, and constraints on exploiting the revolution in information technology. With the overarching goal of improving the health-care system by closing identifiable gaps, the report made 13 recommendations, some of which are in Box 10-4. Additionally, the report addressed the importance of aligning and designing health-care payer systems, professional education, and the health-care environment for quality enhancements, improved outcomes in care, and use of best practices.

As a professional nurse, you have a responsibility to acknowledge the complexity and deficits of the health-care system. In managing patient care, you must continually consider the impact of the system on the care you provide and participate in the quality and safety initiatives at the bedside, in your unit, and within your organization to promote quality and safety within the system.

Quality in the Health-Care System

The IOM defines **quality** as "the degree to which health services for individuals and populations increase the likelihood of desired health outcomes and are consistent with current and professional knowledge" (IOM, 2001, p. 232). This definition is used by U.S. organizations and many international health-care organizations, and it is the basis for nursing management of patient care. Box 10-5 elaborates on this definition by outlining six primary aims of health care.

---

box 10-4

Ten Rules to Govern Health-Care Reform for the 21st Century (IOM, 2001, p. 61)

- Care is based on a continuous healing relationship
- Care is provided based on patient needs and values
- Patient is source of control of care
- Knowledge is shared and free-flowing
- Decisions are evidence-based
- Safety as a system property
- Transparency is necessary; secrecy is harmful
- Anticipate patient needs
- Waste is continually decreased
- Cooperation between health-care providers

---

box 10-5

Six Aims for Improving Quality in Health-Care (IOM, 2001, p. 39).

Health care should be:

1. **Safe:** Avoiding injuries to patients from the care that is intended to help them
2. **Effective:** Providing services based on scientific knowledge to all who could benefit and refraining from providing services to those not likely to benefit (avoiding underuse and overuse)
3. **Patient-centered:** Providing care that is respectful of and responsive to individual patient preferences, needs, and values and ensuring that patient values guide all clinical decisions
4. **Timely:** Reducing waits and sometimes harmful delays for those who receive and those who give care
5. **Efficient:** Avoiding waste, in particular that of equipment, supplies, ideas, and energy
6. **Equitable:** Providing care that does not vary in quality because of characteristics such as gender, ethnicity, geographic location, and socioeconomic status

---

QI

QI activities have been part of nursing care since Florence Nightingale evaluated the care of soldiers during the Crimean War (Nightingale & Barnum, 1992). To achieve quality health care, QI activities use evidence-based methods for gathering data and achieving desired results.

QI usually involves common characteristics (McLaughlin & Caluzny, 2006, p 3):

- A link to key elements of the organization's strategic plan
- A quality council consisting of the institution's top leadership
- Training programs for all levels of personnel
- Mechanisms for selecting improvement opportunities
- Formation of process improvement teams
- Staff support for process analysis and redesign
- Personnel policies that motivate and support staff participation in process improvement

QI is called by many names: quality assurance, FADE, PDSA, total quality management (TQM), Six Sigma, and CQI. Regardless of the term used, QI is a structured organizational process for involving personnel in planning and executing a continuous flow of improvements to provide quality health care that meets or exceeds expectations (McLaughlin & Kaluzny, 2006, p. 3). The following sections focus on CQI.

Using CQI to Monitor and Evaluate Quality of Care

Continuous quality improvement (CQI) is a process of identifying areas of concern (indicators), continuously collecting data on these indicators, analyzing and evaluating the data, and implementing needed changes. When one indicator is no longer a concern, another indicator is selected. Common indicators include, for example, number of falls, medication errors, and infection rates. Indicators can be identified by the accrediting agency or by the facility itself. The purpose of CQI is to improve the capability continuously of everyone involved in providing care, including the organization itself. CQI aims to avoid a blaming environment and attempts to provide a means to improve the entire system.

CQI relies on collecting information and analyzing it. The time frame used in a CQI program can be retrospective (evaluating past performance, often called *quality assurance*), concurrent (evaluating current performance), or prospective (future-oriented, collecting data as they come in). The procedures used to collect data depend on the purpose of the program. Data may be obtained by observation, performance appraisals, patient satisfaction surveys, statistical analyses of length-of-stay and costs, surveys, peer reviews, and chart audits (Huber, 2000).

In the CQI framework, data collection is everyone's responsibility. Collecting comprehensive, accurate, and representative data is the first step in the CQI process. You may be asked to brainstorm your ideas with other nurses or members of the interdisciplinary team, complete surveys or checklists, or keep a log of your daily activities. How do you administer medications to groups of patients? What steps are involved? Are the medications always available at the right time and in the right dose, or do you have to wait for the pharmacy to bring them to the floor? Is the pharmacy technician delayed by emergency orders that must be processed? Looking at the entire process and mapping it out on paper in the form of a flowchart may be part of the CQI process for your organization (Fig. 10.1).

QI at the Organizational and Unit Levels

Strategic Planning

Leaders and managers are so often preoccupied with immediate issues that they lose sight of their ultimate objectives. Quality cannot be found at the

Figure 10.1 Unit level QI process. (Adapted from Hunt, D.V. [1992]. *Quality in America: How to Implement a Competitive Quality Program.* Homewood, IL: Business One Irwin; and Duquette, A.M. [1991]. Approaches to monitoring practice: Getting started. In Schroeder, P. [ed.]. *Monitoring and Evaluation in Nursing.* Gaithersburg, MD: Aspen.)

unit level if the organization is not focusing on quality issues. To stay on track, an organization needs a strategic plan. A **strategic plan** is a short, visionary, conceptual document that:

- Serves as a framework for decisions or for securing support/approval
- Provides a basis for more detailed planning
- Explains the business to others in order to inform, motivate, and involve

■ Assists benchmarking and performance monitoring

■ Stimulates change and becomes the building block for the next plan (planware.org/strategy.htm)

During the strategic planning process, the organization develops or reviews its vision, mission statement, and corporate values. A group develops business objectives and key strategies to meet these objectives. In order to do this, a SWOT analysis is done—a review of the organization's Strengths, Weaknesses, Opportunities, and Threats. Key strategies are identified, and action plans are developed. The organization's mission, goals, and strategic plan ultimately drive the outcomes and QI plan for that organization. Be proactive, and participate in the process. Ask your nurse manager if there are opportunities for the staff to participate in the planning process.

Issues related to QI may also come out of the strategic planning process. Quality issues are not often apparent to senior managers. Staff members at the unit level can often identify quality issues because they are the ones who can feel the impact when quality is lacking. Once a process that needs improvement is identified, an interdisciplinary team is organized whose members have knowledge of the identified process. The team members meet to identify and analyze problems, discuss solutions, and evaluate changes. The team clarifies the current knowledge of the process; it identifies causes for variations in the process and works to unify the process. Box 10-6 identifies questions that team members might ask as they work on the QI plan.

---

box 10-6

Questions the Team Needs to Ask

1. Who are our customers, stakeholders, markets?
2. What do they expect from us?
3. What are we trying to accomplish?
4. What changes do we think will make an improvement?
5. How and when will we pilot-test our predicted improvement?
6. What do we expect to learn from the pilot test?
7. What will we do with negative results? positive results?
8. How will we implement the change?
9. How will we measure success?
10. What did we learn as a team from this experience?
11. What changes would we make for the future?

Adapted from McLaughlin, C., & Kaluzny, A. (2006). Continuous Quality Improvement in Health Care: Theory, Implementations, and Applications. 3rd ed. Massachusetts: Jones & Bartlett.

Structured Care Methodologies

Most agencies have tools for tracking outcomes. These tools are called *structured care methodologies* (SCMs). SCMs are interdisciplinary tools to "identify best practices, facilitate standardization of care, and provide a mechanism for variance tracking, quality enhancement, outcomes measurement, and outcomes research" (Cole & Houston, 1999, p. 53). SCMs include guidelines, protocols, algorithms, standards of care, critical pathways, and order sets.

■ **Guidelines.** Guidelines first appeared in the 1980s as statements to assist health-care providers and patients in making appropriate health-care decisions. Guidelines are based on current research strategies and are often developed by experts in the field. The use of guidelines is seen as a way to decrease variations in practice.

■ **Protocols.** Protocols are specific, formal documents that outline how a procedure or intervention should be conducted. Protocols have been used for many years in research and specialty areas but have been introduced into general health care as a way to standardize approaches to achieve desired outcomes. An example in many facilities is a chest pain protocol.

■ **Algorithms.** Algorithms are systematic procedures that follow a logical progression based on additional information or patient responses to treatment. They were originally developed in mathematics and are frequently seen in emergency medical services. Advanced cardiac life support algorithms are now widely used in health-care agencies.

■ **Standards of care.** Standards of care are often discipline-related and help to operationalize patient care processes and provide a baseline for quality care. Lawyers often refer to a discipline's standards of care in evaluating whether a patient has received appropriate services.

■ **Critical (or clinical) pathways.** A critical pathway outlines the expected course of treatment for patients with similar diagnoses. The critical pathway should orient the nurse easily to the patient outcomes for the day. In some institutions, nursing diagnoses with specific time frames are incorporated into the critical pathway, which describes the course of events that lead to successful patient outcome within the diagnosis-related group (DRG)–defined time frame. For the patient with an uncomplicated myocardial infarction (MI), a proposed course of events leading to a successful patient outcome within the 4-day DRG-defined time frame might be as follows (Doenges, Moorhouse, & Geissler, 1997): (1) Patient states that chest pain is relieved; (2) ST- and T-wave changes resolve and pulse oximeter reading is greater than 90%; patient has clear breath sounds; (3) Patient ambulates in hall without experiencing extreme fatigue or chest pain; (4) Patient verbalizes feelings about having an MI and future fears; (5) Patient identifies effective coping strategies; (6) Ventricular dysfunction, dysrhythmia, or crackles resolved

SCMs may be used alone or together. A patient who is admitted for an MI may have care planned using a critical pathway for an acute MI, a heparin protocol, and a dysrhythmia algorithm. In addition, the nurses may refer to the standards of care in developing a traditional nursing care plan.

SCMs can improve physiological, psychological, and financial outcomes. Services and interventions are sequenced to provide safe and effective outcomes in a designated time and with most effective use of resources. They also give an interdisciplinary perspective that is not found in the traditional nursing care plan. Computer programs allow health-care personnel to track variances (differences from the identified standard) and use these variances in planning QI activities.

The use of SCMs does not take the place of the expert nursing judgment. The fundamental purpose of the SCM is to assist health-care providers in implementing practices identified with good clinical judgment, research-based interventions, and improved patient outcomes. Data from SCMs allow comparisons of outcomes, development of research-based decisions, identification of high-risk patients, and identification of issues and problems before they escalate into disasters. Do not be afraid to learn and understand the different SCMs.

Critical Pathways

Critical pathways are clinical protocols involving all disciplines. They are designed for tracking a planned clinical course for patients based on average and expected lengths of stay. Financial outcomes can be evaluated from critical pathways by assessing any variances from the proposed length of stay. The health-care agency can then focus on problems within the system that extend the length of stay or drive up costs because of overutilization or repetition of services. For example:

Mr. J. was admitted to the telemetry unit with a diagnosis of MI. He had no previous history of heart disease and no other complicating factors such as diabetes, hypertension, or elevated cholesterol levels. His DRG-prescribed length of stay was 4 days. He had an uneventful hospitalization for the first 2 days. On the third day, he complained of pain in the left calf. The calf was slightly reddened and warm to the touch. This condition was diagnosed as thrombophlebitis, which increased his length of hospitalization. The case manager's review of the events leading up to the complaints of calf pain indicated that, although the physician had ordered compression stockings for Mr. J., the stockings never arrived, and no one followed through on the order. The variances related to his proposed length of stay were discussed with the team providing care, and measures were instituted to make sure that this oversight would not occur again.

Critical pathways provide a framework for communication and documentation of care. They are also excellent teaching tools for staff members from various disciplines. Institutions can use critical pathways to evaluate the cost of care for different patient populations (Capuano, 1995; Crummer & Carter, 1993; Flarey, 1995; Lynam, 1994).

Most institutions have adopted a chronological, diagrammatic format for presenting a critical pathway. Time frames may range from daily (day 1, day 2, day 3) to hourly, depending on patient needs. Key elements of the critical pathway include discharge planning, patient education, consultations, activities, nutrition, medications, diagnostic tests, and treatment (Crummer & Carter, 1993). Table 10-2 is an example of a critical pathway. Although originally developed for use in acute care institutions, critical pathways can be developed for home care and long-term care. The patient's nurse is usually responsible for monitoring and recording any deviations from the critical pathway. When deviations occur, the reasons are discussed with all members of the health-care team, and the appropriate changes in care are made. The nurse must identify general trends in patient outcomes and develop plans to improve the quality of care to reduce the number of deviations. Through this close monitoring, the health-care team can avoid last-minute surprises that may delay patient discharge and can predict lengths of stay more effectively.

Aspects of Health Care to Evaluate

A CQI program can evaluate three aspects of health care: the structure within which the care is given, the process of giving care, and the outcome of that care. A comprehensive evaluation should include all three aspects (Brook, Davis, & Kamberg, 1980; Donabedian, 1969, 1977, 1987). When evaluation focuses on nursing care, the independent, dependent, and interdependent functions of nurses may be added to the model (Irvine, 1998). Each of these dimensions is described here, and their interrelationship is illustrated in Table 10-3.

Structure

Structure refers to the setting in which the care is given and to the resources (human, financial, and material) that are available. The following structural aspects of a health-care organization can be evaluated:

- *Facilities*. Comfort, convenience of layout, accessibility of support services, and safety
- *Equipment*. Adequate supplies, state-of-the-art equipment, and staff ability to use equipment
- *Staff*. Credentials, experience, absenteeism, turnover rate, staff-patient ratios
- *Finances*. Salaries, adequacy, sources

Although none of these structural factors alone can guarantee quality care, they make good care more likely. A higher level of nurses each shift and a higher proportion of RNs are associated with shorter lengths of stay; higher proportions of RNs are also related to fewer adverse patient outcomes (Lichtig, Knauf, & Milholland, 1999; Rogers et al., 2004).

Process

Process refers to the activities carried out by the health-care providers and all the decisions made while a patient is interacting with the organization (Irvine, 1998). Examples include:

- Setting an appointment
- Conducting a physical assessment
- Ordering a radiograph and magnetic resonance imaging scan
- Administering a blood transfusion
- Completing a home environment assessment

- Preparing the patient for discharge
- Telephoning the patient post discharge

Each of these processes can be evaluated in terms of timeliness, appropriateness, accuracy, and completeness (Irvine, 1998). Process variables include psychosocial interventions, such as teaching and counseling, and physical care measures. Process also includes leadership activities, such as interdisciplinary team conferences. When process data are collected, a set of objectives, procedures, or guidelines is needed to serve as a standard or gauge against which to compare the activities. This set can be highly specific, such as listing all the steps in a catheterization procedure, or it can be a list of objectives, such as offering information on breastfeeding to all expectant parents or conducting weekly staff meetings.

The American Nurses Association (ANA) Standards of Care are process standards that answer the question: What should the nurse be doing, and what process should the nurse follow to ensure quality care?

Outcome

An *outcome* is the result of all the health-care providers' activities. Outcome measures evaluate the effectiveness of nursing activities by answering such questions as: Did the patient recover? Is the family more independent now? Has team functioning improved? Outcome standards address indicators such as physical and mental health; social and physical function; health attitudes, knowledge, and behavior; utilization of services; and customer satisfaction (Huber, 2000).

The outcome questions asked during an evaluation should measure observable behavior, such as the following:

- Patient: Wound healed; blood pressure within normal limits; infection absent
- Family: Increased time between visits to the emergency department; applied for food stamps
- Team: Decisions reached by consensus; attendance at meetings by all team members

Some of these outcomes, such as blood pressure or time between emergency department visits, are easier to measure than other, equally important outcomes, such as increased satisfaction or changes in attitude. Although the latter cannot be measured as precisely, it is important to include the full spectrum

table 10-2

Sample Critical Pathway: Heart Failure, Hospital; ELOS 4 Days Cardiology or Medical Unit

ND and Categories of Care	Day 1 _____	Day 2 _____	Day 3 _____	Day 4 _____
Decreased cardiac output R/T: Decreased myocardial contractility, altered electrical conduction, structural changes	Goals: Participate in actions to reduce cardiac workload	Display VS within acceptable limits; dysrhythmias controlled; pulse oximetry within acceptable range	→ Dysrhythmias controlled or absent Free of signs of respiratory distress	→ → →
		Meet own self-care needs with assistance as necessary	Demonstrate measurable increase in activity tolerance	
Fluid volume excess R/T compromised regulatory mechanisms: hypertension, sodium/water retention	Verbalize understanding of fluid/food restrictions	Verbalize understanding of general condition and health-care needs	Plan for lifestyle/ behavior changes	Plan in place to meet postdischarge needs
		Breathing sounds clearing	Breath sounds clear	
		Urinary output adequate	Balanced I&O	
		Weight loss (reflecting fluid loss)	Edema resolving	Weight stable or continued loss if edema present
Referrals	Cardiology Dietitian	Cardiac rehabilitation Occupational therapist (for ADLs) Social services Home care	Community resources	
Diagnostic studies	ECG, echo, Doppler ultrasound, stress test, cardiac scan	Echo-Doppler (if not done day 1) or other cardiac scans		
	CXR		CXR	
	ABGs/pulse oximeter			
	Cardiac enzymes	Cardiac enzymes (if ↑)		
	ANP, BNP			
	BUN/Cr	BUN/Cr	BUN/Cr	
	CBC/electrolytes, MG++	Electrolytes	Electrolytes	
	PT/aPTT	PT/aPTT (if taking anti-coagulants)	PT/aPTT (as indicated)	
	Liver function studies			
	Serum glucose			
	Albumin/total protein			
	Thyroid studies			
	Digoxin level (as indicated)		Repeat digoxin level (if indicated)	
	UA			

table 10-2

Sample Critical Pathway: Heart Failure, Hospital; ELOS 4 Days Cardiology or Medical Unit—cont'd

ND and Categories of Care	Day 1 _____	Day 2 _____	Day 3 _____	Day 4 _____
Additional assessments	Apical pulse, heart/breath sounds q8h	→	→ bid	→
	Cardiac rhythm (telemetry) q4h	→	→ D/C	
	BP, P, R q2h until stable, q4h	→ q8h	→	→
	Temp q8h	→	→	→
	I&O q8h	→	→	→ D/C
	Weight qAM	→	→	→
	Peripheral edema q8h	→	→ bid	→ qd
	Peripheral pulses q8h	→	→ bid	→ D/C
	Sensorium q8h	→	→ bid	→ D/C
	DVT check qd	→	→	→
	Response to activity	→	→	→
	Response to therapeutic interventions	→	→	→
Medication allergies:	IV diuretic	→ PO	→	→
	ACEI, ARB, vasodialtors, beta blocker	→	→	→
	IV/PO potassium	⟩	→ D/C	
	Digoxin	→	→	→
	PO/cutaneous nitrates	→	→	→
	Morphine sulfate	→	→ D/C	
	Daytime/hs sedation	→	→	→ D/C
	PO/low-dose anticoagulant	→	→ PO or D/C	→
	Stool softener/laxative	→	→	→
Patient education	Orient to unit/room	Cardiac education per protocol	Signs/symptoms to report to health-care provider	Provide written instructions for home care
	Review advance directives	Review medications: Dose, times, route, purpose, side effects	Plan for home-care needs	Schedule for follow-up appointments
	Discuss expected outcomes, diagnostic tests/results	Progressive activity program		
	Fluid/nutritional restrictions/needs	Skin care		
Additional nursing actions	Bed/chair rest	→ BPR/ambulate as tolerated, cardiac program	→ Up ad lib/graded program	→
	Assist with physical care	→	→	→
	Pressure-relieving mattress	→	→	→ (send home)
	Dysrhythmia/angina care per protocol	→	→	→
	Supplemental O$_2$	→	→ D/C if able	→
	Cardiac diet	→	→	

CP = critical path; ELOS = estimated length of stay; ND = nursing diagnosis.

Doenges, M.E., Moorhouse, M.F., and Geissler, A.C. (2010). *Nursing Care Plans: Guidelines for Individualizing Patient Care*, ed. 8. Philadelphia: FA Davis, with permission.

table 10-3

Dimensions of QI in Nursing: Examples

	Independent Function	Dependent Function	Interdependent Function
Structure	Pressure ulcer risk assessment form available	High-speed automatic dial-up system puts nurses in touch with physicians rapidly	Nursing case management model of care adopted on rehabilitation unit
Process	Assesses risk for development of pressure ulcer and implements preventive measures	Order to increase dosage of pain medication obtained and processedwithin 1 hour	Communicates with therapists about need for customized wheelchair
Outcome	Skin intact at discharge	Relief from pain	Able to enter narrow doorway to bathroom unassisted

Adapted from Irvine, D. (1998). Finding value in nursing care: A framework for quality improvement and clinical evaluation. Nursing Economics, 16(3), 110–118.

of biological, psychological, and social aspects (Strickland, 1997). For this reason, considerable effort has been put into identifying the patient outcomes that are affected by the quality of nursing care. For example, the ANA identified 10 quality indicators in acute care that are likely to relate to the availability and quality of professional nursing services in hospitals. Across the United States, data are being collected from nursing units using these quality indicators.

A major problem in using and interpreting outcome measures is that outcomes are influenced by many factors. For example, the outcome of patient teaching done by a nurse on a home visit is affected by the patient's interest and ability to learn, the quality of the teaching materials, the presence or absence of family support, information (which may conflict) from other caregivers, and the environment in which the teaching is done. If the teaching is successful, can the nurse be given full credit for the success? If it is not successful, who has failed?

It is necessary to evaluate the process as well as the outcome to determine why an intervention such as patient teaching succeeds or fails. A comprehensive evaluation includes all three aspects: structure, process, and outcome. However, it is much more difficult to gather and monitor outcome data than to measure structure or process.

Risk Management

An important part of CQI is **risk management,** a process of identifying, analyzing, treating, and evaluating real and potential hazards. The Joint Commission (JC) recommends the integration of a quality control/risk management program to maintain continuous feedback and communication. To plan proactively, an organization must identify real or potential exposures that might threaten it. As a nurse, it is your responsibility to report adverse incidents to the risk manager, according to your organization's policies and procedures. In many states, this is a legal requirement.

Risk events are categorized according to severity. Although all untoward events are important, not all carry the same severity of outcomes (Benson-Flynn, 2001).

1. **Service occurrence.** A service occurrence is an unexpected occurrence that does not result in a clinically significant interruption of services and that is without apparent patient or employee injury. Examples include minor property or equipment damage, unsatisfactory provision of service at any level, or inconsequential interruption of service. Most occurrences in this category are addressed within the patient complaint process.
2. **Serious incident.** A serious incident results in a clinically significant interruption of therapy or service, minor injury to a patient or employee, or significant loss or damage of equipment or property. Minor injuries are usually defined as needing medical intervention outside of hospital admission or physical or psychological damage.
3. **Sentinel events.** A sentinel event is an unexpected occurrence involving death or serious/permanent physical or psychological injury, or the risk thereof. The phrase, "or the risk thereof" includes any process variation for which a recurrence would carry a significant chance of a serious adverse outcome. Such events are called sentinel because they signal the need for immediate investigation and response. When a sentinel event occurs, appropriate individuals

within the organization must be made aware of the event; they must investigate and understand the causes of the event; and they must make changes in the organization's systems and processes to reduce the probability of such an event in the future (jcaho.org/ptsafety_frm.html).

The subset of sentinel events that is subject to review by JC includes any occurrence that meets any of the following criteria:

■ The event has resulted in an unanticipated death or major permanent loss of function, not related to the natural course of the patient's illness or underlying condition.
■ The event is one of the following (even if the outcome was not death or major permanent loss of function): suicide of a patient in a setting where the patient receives around-the-clock care (e.g., hospital, residential treatment center, crisis stabilization center), infant abduction or discharge to the wrong family, rape, hemolytic transfusion reaction involving administration of blood or blood products having major blood group incompatibilities, surgery on the wrong patient or wrong body part (jcaho.org/ptsafety_frm.html)

Adhering to nursing standards of care as well as the policies and procedures of the institution greatly decreases the nurse's risk. Common areas of risk for nursing include:

■ Medication errors
■ Documentation errors and/or omissions
■ Failure to perform nursing care or treatments correctly
■ Errors in patient safety that result in falls
■ Failure to communicate significant data to patients and other providers (Swansburg & Swansburg, 2002)

Risk management programs also include attention to areas of employee wellness and prevention of injury. Latex allergies, repetitive stress injuries, carpal tunnel syndrome, barrier protection for tuberculosis, back injuries, and the rise of antibiotic-resistant organisms all fall under the area of risk management (Huber, 2000).

Adhering to standards of care and exercising the amount of care that a reasonable nurse would demonstrate under the same or similar circumstances can protect the nurse from litigation. Understanding what actions to take when something goes wrong is

imperative. The main goal is patient safety. Reporting and remediation must occur quickly (Huber, 2000).

Once an incident has occurred, you must complete an incident report immediately. The incident report is used to collect and analyze data for future determination of risk. The report should be accurate, objective, complete, and factual. If there is future litigation, the plaintiff's attorney can subpoena the report. The report should be prepared in only a single copy and never placed in the medical record (Swansburg & Swansburg, 2002). It is kept with internal hospital correspondence.

Nurses have a responsibility to remain educated and informed and to become active participants in understanding and identifying potential risks to their patients and to themselves. Ignorance of the law is no excuse. Maintaining a knowledgeable, professional, and caring nurse-patient relationship is the first step in decreasing your own risk.

The Economic Climate in the Health-Care System

For many years, decisions about care were based primarily on providing the best quality care, whatever the cost. As the economic support for health care is challenged, however, health-care providers are pressured to seek methods of care delivery that achieve quality outcomes at lower cost.

Economic Perspective

The economic perspective is rooted in three fundamental observations:

1. **Resources are scarce.** Due to scarce resources, three choices result:

■ The amount to be spent on health-care services and the composition of those services
■ The methods for producing those services
■ The method of distribution of health care, which influences the equity with which these services are distributed

2. **Resources have alternative uses.** As a result of this scarcity, the choice to expend resources in one area eliminates the use of those same resources in another area. If more nursing homes are going to be built, for example, then there will be fewer hospitals, less housing, less education, or other uses of those same resources.

3. **Individuals want different services or have different preferences.** Some people choose alternative treatment modalities such as acupuncture, herbal therapy, or massage therapy rather than traditional health care. Health-care services are marketed extensively.

Regulation and Competition

During the past three decades, federal and state governments have attempted to restrain the cost of health care by focusing. *Regulation* attempts to control cost through government actions; *competition* uses market forces. Competition can drive aspects of health care through consumers, providers, and suppliers. Among the attempts to control cost were:

1. **Medicare Prospective Payment System (PPS).** In 1983 the federal government changed its method of paying hospitals for treating Medicare patients. Instead of paying for actual costs, the PPS pays hospitals a fixed, predetermined sum for a particular admission. If a hospital can provide the service at a cost below the fixed amount, it pockets the difference. If more resources and money are used than the predetermined amount, the hospital incurs a loss.

2. **DRGs.** Tied to the PPS, DRGs are the patient classification systems by which the Medicare PPS determines payment. Each of the 495 DRGs represents a particular case type.

3. **Managed care.** Managed care is a system of health care that combines the financing and delivery of health services into a single entity. Currently, more than 75% of people with private health insurance are enrolled in managed care plans. Managed care plans are seen as cost-saving alternatives to traditional fee-for-service delivery systems. Through provider networks and selective provider contracting, they attempt to control resource use and health-care costs (Chang, Price, & Pfoutz, 2001). Figure 10.2 depicts the current factors increasing and containing health-care costs.

4. **Cost sharing.** With rising health-care costs, employers purchasing health plans have begun to shift some of the increase cost in premiums, prescriptions, and specialty services to employees. Higher cost for consumers and shifting financial burdens have left more Americans without health-care coverage.

Factors Increasing Costs

- Expansion of national economy
- General inflation
- Aging population
- Growth of third-party payments
- Employer-provided health insurance
- Tax deduction for medical expenses
- Increased costs of labor and equipment
- Expansion of medical technology and products
- Malpractice insurance and litigation

Factors Containing Costs

- Federal economic stabilization program
- Voluntary effort hospital regulation program
- State-level health-care payment programs
- Medicare prospective payment system (PPS) with payments of fixed amount per admission
- Diagnostic-related groups (DRGs) for hospital payments
- Resource-based relative value scale (RBRVS) for physician payments
- Managed care plans

Figure 10.2 Factors affecting the cost of health care. (From Chang, C.F., Price, S.A., & Pfoutz, S.K. [2001]. *Economics and Nursing: Critical Professional Issues.* Philadelphia: FA Davis, p. 79.)

5. **Medical savings accounts (MSA).** As a regulatory tool, MSAs are a cost-sharing method for incentivizing consumers to plan and share in the cost of their own health-care expenditures. Money that would normally be spent on health-care premiums by the employer-consumer is deposited into an MSA. Accounts created under the Medicare Modernization Act of 2003 are the property of the employee-consumer, giving more choice into how and where the money is spent. The account is tax-deferred until it is used for allowable health-related spending as in high-deductible health plans and tax-deferred plans. Other types of consumer-directed plans exist, such as the flexible spending account, health reimbursement account, and medical saving accounts, all of which have stipulations for use.

6. Single-Payer/National Health Coverage.
A single-payer system aims to decrease the cost of care by eliminating third-party insurers, costly overhead, and bureaucracy while providing coverage for all. Plans may offer choices to consumers regarding providers, hospitals, and specialty services, and physicians and hospitals are paid through negotiates, fee-for-service, or salary. Costs are controlled through budgeting, bulk purchasing, and negotiation (Physicians for a National Health Plan, 2008).

Proponents of a single-payer system cite lower costs per capita while ensuring access to care for all Americans. Opponents cite that the possible trade-off for decreased cost and improved access leads to increased mortality, poorer outcomes of care, limited to no-cost savings, and loss of control by consumers (National Center for Policy Analysis, 2008).

The intended effects of regulation and competition are to decrease cost. Despite the variety of attempts over the years to drive down costs, they continue to go up, imposing a heavy burden on consumers or employers (Center for Studying Health System Change, 2008). However, improved quality and safety prevent unnecessary deaths and errors that contribute to the high cost of care (IOM, 2000; IOM 2003a). The U.S. government, consumers, providers, and organizations have a vested interest in controlling health-care expenditures and in preventing waste while maintaining quality care.

Nursing Labor Market

RNs comprise 77% of the nurse workforce, and almost 60% of RNs are employed by hospitals. The nationwide unemployment rate for RNs is only 1%. Vacancy rates nationwide are reported at anywhere from 13% to 20% and are rising. A serious nursing shortage is here, and it will continue until at least 2020. The demand for nurses is expected to increase even more dramatically as the baby boomers reach their 60s, 70s, and beyond. From now until 2030, the population age 65 years and older will double.

Defining and Identifying the Nursing Shortage

The nursing shortage is defined simply as a supply-demand issue. Unfortunately, the current nursing shortage is more complex and severe than previous shortages in terms of the available supply, the

demand from employers, and the new graduate pipeline for RNs.

- **Supply of existing RNs.** The total supply of U.S. RNs is estimated at 2.9 million and is projected to remain the same though 2020. The supply of active RNs, including those who are licensed, working, or seeking employment as an RN, is projected be 2.1–2.3 million from 2000 to 2020 (U.S. Department of Health and Human Services [HRSA], 2006).
- **New graduate supply pipeline.** Nursing program graduation and NCLEX-RN pass rates affect supply. The American Association of Colleges of Nursing (AACN) reported an increase in baccalaureate level–entry enrollments, up by 5.4% in 2006 (AACN, 2008). According to the National Council of State Boards of Nursing (2008), first-time candidates for nursing licensure in 2007 numbered 200,209, with a pass rate of 69.4%. However, HRSA (2006) projected that U.S. nursing programs must graduate 90% more nurses to meet the U.S. demands for nurses (p. 2).
- **Demand from employers.** The Bureau of Labor Statistics predicts the RN job to be among the top 10 in growth rate (U.S. Department of Labor, 2008). Total job openings for RNs will exceed 1.1 million, including new job growth and replacement of retiring nurses.

In a survey of over 5000 community hospitals, the American Hospital Association (2007) reported 116,000 RN vacancies as of December 2006. The effects of these vacancies contribute to decreased employee and patient satisfaction and increased hiring of foreign-educated nurses. The majority of urban hospital emergency departments reported capacity issues and spend time on by-pass or diversion due to a lack of properly staffed critical care beds.

In 2002 more than 100,000 new RNs were hired; the majority were foreign-born nurses and nurses over age 50 returning to the workforce in tough economic times. Although the new hires and a sharp increase in RN salaries are positive, the current nursing shortage is far from over.

Factors Contributing to the Nursing Shortage

Many complex factors have led to and continue to contribute to the current critical nursing shortage:

- **High acuity, increasing age of patients in hospitals.** Medically complex patients require skilled nursing care. The number of aging baby boomers will significantly increase the demands on the health-care systems and increase the needs for RNs.

■ **Increased demand for nurses.** As health care moves to a variety of community settings, only the most acute patients remain in the hospital. The transfer of less acute patients to nursing homes and community settings creates additional job opportunities. Research supporting improved patient outcomes when patient care is provided by RNs as opposed to unlicensed personnel will also increase demand for RNs.

■ **Aging nursing workforce.** In 2000, fewer than one in three RNs was younger than 40 years of age. The percentage of nurses age 40–49 years is currently more than 35%.

In March 2004 the average age of the RN population was 46.8 years of age, up from 45.2 in 2000. The RN population under the age of 30 dropped from 9% of the nursing population in 2000 to 8% in 2004 (AACN, 2008).

■ *Job dissatisfaction.* Staffing levels, heavy workloads, increased use of overtime, lack of sufficient support staff, and salary discrepancies between nurses and other health-care professionals have contributed to growing dissatisfaction and lower retention of nurses. Many facilities are now using workplace issues and incentives as a retention strategy.

■ *Reduction in and shortage of nursing faculty.* As retirements for faculty continue, the shortage of faculty continues to affect the number of students admitted to nursing programs. In 2007 nursing programs reported more than 750 open nursing faculty positions (AACN, 2008). In addition, nursing programs turned away over 40,000 qualified nursing applicants, in part, due to the shortage of nursing faculty (AACN, 2008).

■ The need to control spiraling health-care costs, along with the issues of supply and demand for nursing services will continue. According to the ANA, more than 40% of nurses graduate initially from associate-degree nursing programs. You, personally, will be affected by trends in health-care delivery, but you can also be a major voice in decision making (Nelson, 2002). As in the past, cost control and demand for nursing services will most likely involve changing nurse

staffing, the model of care, and professional nursing practice (Ritter-Teitel, 2002).

Safety in the U.S. Health-Care System

Patient safety is the prevention of harm caused by errors. The IOM defines errors as "the failure of a planned action to be completed as intended (e.g., error of execution) or the use of a wrong plan to achieve an aim (e.g., error of planning) (IOM, 2000, p. 57). It is important to note that errors are unintentional and that not all errors lead to an adverse event causing harm or death.

Types of Errors

To Err is Human (2000) relied on the work of Leape et al. (1993) to categorize types of errors (Box 10-7). After categorizing types of errors, Leape and colleagues found that 70% of all errors were preventable.

Human errors can occur for many reasons. *Skill-based errors* can be slips or lapses when the actions taken by the provider were not what was intended (Duke University Medical Center, 2005). An example of rule-based error is an experienced nurse administering the wrong medication by picking up the wrong syringe.

---

box 10-7

Types of Errors (IOM, 2000, p. 36)

Diagnostic
Error or delay in diagnosis
Failure to employ indicated tests
Use of outmoded tests or therapy
Failure to act on results of monitoring or testing

Treatment
Error in the performance of an operation, procedure, or test
Error in administering the treatment
Error in the dose or method of using a drug
Avoidable delay in treatment or in responding to an abnormal test
Inappropriate (not indicated) care

Preventive
Failure to provide prophylactic treatment
Inadequate monitoring or follow-up of treatment

Other
Failure of communication
Equipment failure
Other system failure

Leape, Lucian; Lawthers, Ann G.; Brennan, Troyen A., et al. Preventing medical injury. Qual Rev Bull. 19(5):144–149, 1993.

Not all errors lead to patient harm or to an adverse event. Each type of event can be studied to glean data used to improve safety.

- *Near miss.* A near miss is an error that results in no harm or very minimal patient harm (IOM, 2000, p. 87). Near misses are useful in identifying and remedying vulnerabilities in a system before harm can occur.
- *Adverse event.* An adverse event is injury to a patient caused by medical management rather than an underlying condition of the patient (IOM, 2000). The IOM reports have highlighted the prevalence of errors, especially preventable adverse events. Adverse events have been classified into four types (see Box 10-7).
- *Accident.* An accident is an event that involves damage to a defined system that disrupts the ongoing or future output of that system. Accidents occur when multiple systems fail and tend to be unplanned or unforeseen. Accidents provide information about systems.

Error Identification and Reporting

Nurses are on the front line in identifying and reporting errors. However, many errors are not reported or go undetected. Providers and organizations may fear blame or punishment for mistakes or errors.

Developing a Culture of Safety

To achieve safe patient care, a *culture of safety* must exist. Organizations and senior leadership must drive change to develop a culture of safety—a blame-free environment in which reporting of errors is promoted and rewarded. A culture of safety promotes trust, honesty, openness, and transparency. Teamwork and involvement of the patient contribute to promoting a culture of safety. When a culture of safety exists, individual providers do not fear reprisal and are not blamed for identifying or reporting errors. Reported errors provide data and information necessary to understand why or how the error occurred, thus improving care and preventing harm.

Event-reporting systems hold organizations accountable and lead to improved safety. Mandatory reporting systems are operated by regulatory agencies and have a strong focus on errors associated with serious harm or death. As of 2005, 24 states had either mandatory or voluntary reporting

systems (Rosenthal & Booth, 2005). In addition, the Food and Drug Administration (FDA) mandates reporting of serious harm or death (adverse events) related to drugs and medical devices. Failure to report mandatory requirements may lead to fines, withdrawal of participation in clinical trials, or loss of licensure to operate.

The Joint Commission relied on *root cause analysis* from each sentinel event. Root cause analysis is the process of learning from consequences. The consequences can be desirable, but most root cause analysis deals with adverse consequences. An example of a root cause analysis is a review of a medication error, especially one resulting in a death or severe complications. Principles of root cause analysis include:

1. Determine what influenced the consequences, i.e., determine the necessary and sufficient influences that explain the nature and the magnitude of the consequences.
2. Establish tightly linked chains of influence.
3. At every level of analysis, determine the necessary and sufficient influences.
4. Whenever feasible, drill down to root causes.
5. Know that there are always multiple root causes.

The Joint Commission also developed the International Center for Patient Safety, which establishes National Patient Safety Goals each year and publishes Sentinel Event Strategies. Box 10-8

---

box 10-8

Joint Commission International Center for Patient Safety

1. Sets patient safety standards
2. Implements and oversees sentinel event policy and advisory group
3. Publishes *Sentinel Event Alert* newsletter and quality check reports
4. Sets yearly national patient safety goals
5. Developed the universal protocol related to surgical procedures
6. Evaluates organizations' monitoring of quality of care issues
7. Conducts patient safety research
8. Provides patient safety resources
9. Supports the Speak Up program
10. Involved with patient safety coalitions and legislative efforts

Adapted from Joint Commission on Accreditation of Healthcare Organizations (JCAHO), accessed November 26, 2005, from jcpatientsafety.org describes the work of the International Center for Patient Safety. These tools developed by the Joint Commission offer health-care organizations goals and strategies to prevent harm and death based on what has been learned from sentinel events.

Organizations, Agencies, and Initiatives Supporting Quality and Safety in the Health-Care System

The ongoing movement to improve quality and safety has led to the development of governmental and private organizations (see Box 10-9) in addition to those mentioned in the historical perspective at the beginning of this chapter. These organizations and agencies currently monitor, evaluate, accredit, influence, research, finance, and advocate for quality within the health delivery system. Each organization works inside and outside the system to drive change leading to improved health outcomes and improved system quality. Each organization works within its mission to address various characteristics of the health-care system or to address patient needs. Some organizations serve multiple roles beyond their primary mission.

Government Agencies

Federal and state-level government agencies provide tools and resources for improving quality and safety within the U.S. health-care system. Government agencies also oversee regulation, licensure, and mandatory and voluntary reporting programs.

Within the U.S. Department of Health and Human Services (HHS) reside multiple agencies that support quality and safety. HHS is the U. S. government's principal agency for protecting the health of all Americans and providing essential human services, including health care (HHS, 2008). HHS works closely with state and local governments to meet the nation's health and human needs.

In addition to administering Medicare and Medicaid, the Center for Medicare and Medicaid (CMS) administers quality initiatives intended "to assure quality health care for all Americans through accountability and public exposure" (CMS, 2008). Initiatives include:

■ MedQIC. This initiative aims to ensure each Medicare recipient receives the appropriate level of care. MedQIC is a community-based QI program that provides tools and resources to

---

box 10-9

Organizations and Agencies Supporting Quality and Safety

Government Agencies
- U.S. Department of Health and Human Services http://www.hhs.gov/
- Food and Drug Administratoin (FDA) http://www.fda.gov/
- Initiatives: Medwatch and Sentinel Initiative
- Health Resources and Services Administration (HRSA) http://www.hrsa.gov/
- Initiatives: Health Information Technology and National Practitioner Database
- Center for Medicare and Medicaid Services (CMS) http://www.cms.hhs.gov/
- Initiatives: Hospital Quality Initiative, MedQIC, American Health Quality Association (AHQA),
- Agency for Healthcare Research and Quality (AHRQ) http://www.ahrq.gov/
- Initiatives: Health IT, Improving Health Care Quality, Medical Errors and Patient Safety, Measuring Quality
- VA National Center for Patient Safety http://www.va.gov/ncps/

Health-Care Provider Professional Organizations
- American Nurses Association http://nursingworld.org/
- Initiative: National Database of Nursing Quality Indicators (NDNQI)
- Association of Perioperative Registered Nurses (AORN) https://www.aorn.org/
- Initiative: Patient Safety First and AORN Toolkits
- American Hospital Association (AHA) http://www.aha.org/
- Initiative: AHA Quality Center
- Association of Academic Health Centers http://www.aahcdc.org/index.php
- Priorities: Health Profession Workforce and Health Care Reform

Non-Profit Organizations, Foundations, and Research
- The Leapfrog Group http://www.leapfroggroup.org/
- Kaiser Family Foundation http://www.kff.org/
- Markel Foundation-Connecting for Health http://www.connectingforhealth.org/aboutus/index.html#
- Robert Wood Johnson Foundation-Quality Equality in Healthcare http://www.rwjf.org/qualityequality/index.jsp
- National Patient Safety Foundation http://www.npsf.org/
- The Commonwealth Fund http://www.commonwealthfund.org/aboutus/

Quality Organizations
- Institute for Healthcare Improvement (IHI) http://www.ihi.org/ihi
- The Joint Commission http://www.jointcommission.org/
- National Committee for Quality Assurance (NCQA) http://web.ncqa.org/
- National Quality Forum http://www.qualityforum.org/

encourage changes in processes, structures, and behaviors within the health-care community.

■ **Post–Acute Care Reform Plan.** CMS is examining post-acute transfers with the aim of reducing care fragmentation and unsafe transitions.

■ **Hospital Quality Initiative.** This is a major initiative aimed at improving quality of care at the provider and organization level. Organizations provide data through public reporting of quality measures that translate information to assist consumers in health decisions. This initiative creates a uniform set of quality measurement by which consumers can compare organizations and by which organizations can benchmark progress toward achieving goals in specified areas of care, such as acute myocardial infarct, congestive heart failure, pneumonia, and postsurgical infections. These data feed the *Hospital Compare* Web site (www.hospitalcompare.hhs.gov). Organizations are incentivized to participate with an offering of increased reimbursement.

Also under the HHS is the Agency for Healthcare Research and Quality (AHRQ), which is the lead federal agency charged with improving the quality, safety, efficiency, and effectiveness of health care for all Americans (HHS, 2008). Through multiple initiatives, the support of research, and evidence-based decision-making, the AHRQ aims to fulfill its mission:

■ **Health IT.** A multifaceted initiative that includes (a) research support of $260 million in grants and contracts to support and stimulate investment in health information technology (IT); (b) the newly created AHRQ National Resource Center, which provides technical assistance and research funding to aid technology implementation within communities; and (c) learning laboratories at more than 100 hospitals nationwide to develop and test health IT applications

■ **National Quality Measures Clearinghouse (NQMC).** Web-accessible database provides access to evidence-based quality measures and measure sets; NQMC provides access for obtaining detailed information on quality measures and to further their dissemination, implementation, and use in order to inform health-care decisions

■ **Medical Errors and Patient Safety.** Web site providing access to evidence-based tools and resources for consumers and providers

■ **AHRQ Quality Indicators.** Set of quality indicators used by organizations to highlight potential quality concerns, identify areas that need further study and investigation, and track changes over time

The U. S. Department of Defense (DoD) and the Veterans Health Administration (VHA) have taken leadership positions in developing tools, resources, and programs aimed at improving safety, promoting change, and promoting a culture of safety within the DoD and VHA. The VHA National Center for Patient Safety developed a toolkit for fall prevention and management, tools for escape and elopement management, and cognitive aids for root cause analysis and health failure mode and effect analysis.

Health-Care Provider Professional Organizations

Professional organizations directly address the missions and concerns regarding quality and safety of the professionals they represent. Each organization offers programs, access to evidence-based practices, toolkits, and newsletters to aid their members in driving quality within their own practice and organization.

The vital quality and safety initiative of the ANA is the National Database of Nursing Quality Indicators (NDNQI), a database of unit-specific nurse-sensitive information collected at hospitals. Data are collected and evaluated to improve quality. The indicators reflect the structure, process, and outcomes of nursing care and lead to improved quality and safety at the bedside. The ANA also has a strong focus on safe nurse staffing levels to promote safe, quality patient care.

Nonprofit Organizations and Foundations

With few exceptions, nonprofit organizations and foundations are generally focused on consumer education, policy development, and research to improve quality and safety within the health-care system. Many organizations serve multiple missions. The Kaiser Family Foundation (2005) has a strong emphasis on U.S. and international nonpartisan health policy and health policy research. Self-funded research and public opinion polling on topics related to quality and safety in the health-care system contribute to policy and legislation development.

Also having a multifaceted mission, the renowned Robert Wood Johnson Foundation (RWJF) serves multiple missions and seeks to improve health and health care for all Americans. RWJF's success comes from leveraging partnerships and its endowment to "building evidence and producing, synthesizing and distributing knowledge, new ideas and expertise" (RWJF, 2008) in eight program areas. RWJF is responsible for sucessfully funded projects and research that improve quality and safety for all Americans.

The Leapfrog Group is a nonprofit organization interested in improving safety, quality, and affordability of health care through incentives and rewards to those who use and pay for health care (Leapfrog Group, 2007). With a focus on reducing preventable medical mistakes, the Leapfrog Group touted their benefits to improve safety and quality to consumers and business owners with three *leaps:* (a) improve transparency by reporting hospital survey results addressing quality and safety indicators; (b) incentivize better quality and safety performance; and (c) collaborate with other organizations to improve quality and safety. To date, there is limited evidence that the Leapfrog Group has effectively improved quality or safety. Limitations to success may be in part because too few hospitals have participated in the surveys and too few consumers have used the available information to make health decisions; however, there is an indication that, with time, participation could improve with adjustments in strategy by the Leapfrog Group (Galvin, Delbanco, Milstein, & Belden, 2005).

Quality Organizations

Each of the quality organizations strives to improve system-wide quality for Americans through a variety of programs and methods.

The National Committee for Quality Assurance (NCQA) was established in 1990 to accredit health plans and certify organizations. Its success in supporting quality and safety resides in its Health Effectiveness Data and Information Set (HEDIS). Over 90% of U.S. health plans use HEDIS to measure performance. HEDIS allows for consumers and employers to evaluate health plans using data from HEDIS as a report card of the plan's success.

JC was established in 1951 with a focus on structural measures of quality, assessment of the physical plant, number of patient beds per nurse, credentialing of service providers, and other standards for each department. This system of evaluation has given way to a more process- and outcome-focused model: CQI. Today, the JC accredits more than 19,000 health-care organizations. Evaluation of nursing services is an important part of the accreditation. JC–accredited agencies are measured against national standards set by health-care professionals. Hospitals, health-care networks, long-term care facilities, ambulatory care centers, home health agencies, behavioral health-care facilities, and clinical laboratories are among the organizations seeking JC accreditation. Although accreditation by the JC is voluntary, Medicare and Medicaid reimbursement cannot be sought by organizations not accredited by JCAHO.

Integrating Initiatives and Evidenced-Based Practices Into Patient Care

As you familiarize yourself with each of these organizations and their respective initiatives, consider how they will affect the management of patient care. Your responsibility as a professional RN is to acknowledge their presence, understand and value their importance, and participate in your facility-adopted initiatives and evidence-based practices. Additionally, as a leader and manager, you will be expected to drive changes based upon endeavors of many of these organizations, agencies, and initiatives ensuring that quality and safety continue to improve.

Health-Care System Reform

Eighty-two percent of Americans believe the U.S. health-care system is in need of either fundamental change or complete rebuilding (How, Shih, Lau, & Shoen, 2008). Americans want leadership to address quality, cost, coverage, and access. The debate rests on *how* best to achieve necessary reform.

The IOM report proposed five core competencies (Box 10-10) in which all health-care professionals will need to be effective as providers and leaders in the 21st-century health-care system.

By integrating these competencies into 21st-century health profession education, you can begin to support health-care reform while managing

---

box 10-10

Core Competencies for Health Professionals (IOM, 2003a, p. 4)

Provide patient-centered care. Identify, respect, and care about patients; differences, values, preferences, and expressed needs; relieve pain and suffering; coordinate continuous care; listen to, clearly inform, communicate with, and educate patients; share decision making and management; and continuously advocate disease prevention, wellness, and promotion of healthy lifestyles, including a focus on population health.

Work in interdisciplinary teams. Cooperate, collaborate, communicate, and integrate care in teams to ensure that care is continuous and reliable.

Employ evidence-based practice. Integrate best research with clinical expertise and patient values for optimum care, and participate in learning and research activities to the extent feasible.

Apply quality improvement. Identify errors and hazards in care; understand and implement basic safety design principles, such as standardization and simplification; continually understand and measure quality of care in terms of structure, process, and outcomes in relation to patient and community needs; and design and test interventions to change processes and systems of care with the objective of improving quality.

Utilize informatics. Communicate, manage knowledge, mitigate error, and support decision making using information technology.

---

patient care. As a practicing professional, you can use the competencies to guide future professional development and ensure positive impact on health-care reform while improving quality and safety.

Role of Nursing in System Reform

The ANA's Agenda

In 1989, taking a leadership position regarding health-care reform, the ANA began to address concerns regarding quality, safety, and cost of care as well as the potential health-care reform within the United States Working with more than 60 nursing and health-care organizations, the ANA published *Nursing's Agenda for Health Care Reform* (ANA, 1991). This document was positioned as its blueprint for reform.

Building on the ANA's report from 1991, the ANA's *Health Care Agenda* (ANA, 2005) describes the organization's policy on health system reform. This policy includes four basic principles:

1. Health care is a basic human right. A restructured health-care system should include universal access to essential services.
2. The development of health policies that incorporate the IOM's six aims of health care will save money.
3. The health-care system must be reshaped and redirected away from the overuse of expensive, technology-driven, acute, hospital-based services in the model we now have to one in which a balance is struck between high-technology treatment and community-based and preventive services, with emphasis on the latter.

4. The ANA supports a single-payer health-care system (ANA, 2005, p. 2).

Although updated in 2008, the ANA's policy still maintains the same four principles.

Influence of Nursing

Nurses are empowered through self-determination, meaning, competence, and impact (Whitehead, Weiss, & Tappen, 2007, p. 71). Additionally, nurses play vital roles in collective bargaining and decision making within their organizations, empowered through professional organization such as the ANA (see Chapter 5).

Nurses are respected and trusted health-care professionals. To influence change in the health-care system, professional nurses must first acknowledge power within the profession and recognize their central role in health care. To be effective, nurses must leverage their professional expertise and the trust and respect they have garnered. It is critical that nurses speak up and seek an active role in shaping health-care reform:

- **Become informed.** Research topics of interest to *you* and your practice. Rely on the Internet and your professional organizations as resources for current policy and legislative topics.
- **Plan.** After selecting a topic, prepare your plan: gather facts and figures that will support your ideas and position. Outline them, and address your audience in person, on paper, or via the Web. The most influential people are prepared and believe in their topic.
- **Take action.** Shape public opinion by the method of your choice. Start small, and build

your impact. (1) Write a letter to your representative (local, state, federal), ANA leadership or state-level delegate, the editor of your local newspaper, or to the editor of your favorite nursing journal/magazine. (2) Attend a meeting where your topic will be addressed in a public forum or at a professional gathering. Meet the people who are influential, and share your ideas or learn from others. (3) Vote for candidates and officers in your professional organizations and within the government. (4) Visit your representative (local, state, federal) or ANA leadership or state-level delegate to share your ideas. (5) Volunteer. Ask what you can do to help. (6) Testify before decision-making bodies.

Conclusion

Pressure from quality organizations, consumers, payers, and providers has caused the focus in the health-care system to shift from patient care to issues of cost and quality. Experts indicate that quality promotes decreased costs and increased satisfaction. This is an opportunity for nurses to become more professional and empowered to organize and manage patient care so that it is safe, efficient, and of the highest quality. Begin early in your career to participate actively in QI initiatives. Regardless of the care model used or the indicators

selected, focus attention on the following in patient care delivery (Hansten & Washburn, 2001, p. 24D):

1. **Think critically.** Use your creative, intuitive, logical, and analytical processes continually in working with patients.
2. **Plan and report outcomes.** Emphasizing results is a necessary part of managing resources in today's cost-conscious environment. Focusing on the outcomes moves the nurse out of the mindset of focusing just on tasks.
3. **Make introductory rounds.** Begin each shift with the health-care team members introducing themselves, describing their roles, and providing patients updates.
4. **Plan in partnership with the patient.** In conjunction with the introductory rounds, spend a few minutes early in the shift with each patient, discussing shift objectives and long-term goals. This event becomes the center of the nursing process for the shift and ensures that the patient and nurse are working toward the same outcomes.
5. **Communicate the plan.** Avoid confusion among members of the team by communicating the intended outcomes and the important role that each member plays in the plan.
6. **Evaluate progress.** Schedule time during the shift quickly to evaluate outcomes and the progress of the plan and to make revisions as necessary.

Study Questions

1. How have historical, social, political, and economic trends affected your practice? Give specific examples and their implications.

2. What problems have you identified during your clinical experiences that could be considered issues to be addressed using CQI?

3. What SCMs have you seen implemented in practice? Which ones might you use to assist you in planning care? If you have not seen any, ask the nurse manager what is used on the unit.

4. Review the section in this chapter on risk management. In what areas of risk do you feel you are the most vulnerable? How will you work on correcting your risk?

5. Discuss the role of the nurse in CQI and risk management.

6. Based on patient safety goals for the current year, what will you do to ensure adherence to these goals?

7. What are evidence-based practices that promote quality and safety within the health-care system?

8. Describe how regulatory agencies and accrediting agencies affect patient care and outcomes at the bedside.

9. Review the nonprofit organizations and government agencies that influence and advocate for quality and safety in the health-care system. What do the organizations or agencies do that supports the hallmarks of quality? What have been the results of their efforts for patients, facilities, the health-care delivery system, and the nursing profession? How have the organizations or agencies affected your facility and professional practice?

10. Explain how technology enhances and promotes safe patient care, educates patients and consumers, evaluates health-care delivery, and enhances the nurse's knowledge base in your practice and at your organization.

11. How would you begin discussion on quality and safety issues with the nurse manager or colleague?

12. What issues may arise when the care delivery system is changed? What does the RN need to consider when implementing these changes?

Case Study to Promote Critical Reasoning

The director of CQI has called a meeting of all the staff members on your floor. Based on last quarter's statistics, the length of stay of patients with uncontrolled diabetes is 2.6 days longer than that of patients for the first half of the year. She has requested that the staff identify members who wish to be CQI team members looking at this problem. You, the staff nurse, have volunteered to be a member of the team. The team will consist of the diabetes educator, a patient-focused care assistant, a pharmacist, and you.

1. Why were these people selected for the team?

2. What data need to be collected to evaluate this situation?

3. What are the potential outcomes for patients with uncontrolled diabetes?

4. Develop a flowchart of a typical hospital stay for a patient with uncontrolled diabetes.

References

American Association of Colleges of Nursing. (October 1997). A vision of baccalaureate and graduate nursing education: The next decade. Retrieved July 17, 2007, from http://www.aacn.nche.edu/Publications/positions/vision.htm

American Association of Colleges of Nursing. (2008). Nursing shortage fact sheet. Retrieved September 15, 2008, from http://www.aacn.nche.edu/media/FactSheets/NursingShortage.htm

American Hospital Association. (2007). The 2007 state of American hospitals. Retrieved September 16, 2008, from http://www.aha.org

American Nurses Association. (1991). Nursing's agenda for health care reform (1991). Retrieved August 23, 2008, from http://www.nursingworld.org/

American Nurses Association. (2005). ANA's health care agenda. Retrieved August 24, 2008, from http://www.nursingworld.org/

Baldwin, J. H., Conger, C. O., Maycock, C., & Abegglen, J. C. (2002). Health care delivery system influences changes in nursing educational materials. *Public Health Nursing,* 19(4), 246–254.

Benson-Flynn, J. (2001). Incident reporting: Clarifying occurrences, incidents, and sentinel events. *Home Healthcare Nurse,* 19, 701–706.

Billings, D. M., & Halstead, J. A. (2005). *Teaching in Nursing: A Guide for Faculty,* 2nd ed. St. Louis: Elsevier Saunders.

Booth, R.G. (2006). Educating the future health professional nurse. *International Journal of Nursing Education Scholarship,* 3(1), 1–10.

Brady, M., Leuner, J. D., Bellack, J. P., Loquist, R. S., et al. (2001). A proposed framework for differentiating the 21 Pew competencies by level of nursing education. *Nursing & Health Care Perspectives,* 22(1), 30–35.

Brook, R.H., Davis, A.R., & Kamberg, C. (1980). Selected reflections on quality of medical care evaluations in the 1980s. *Nursing Research,* 29(2), 127.

Capuano, T.A. (1995). Clinical pathways. *Nursing Management,* 26(1), 34–37.

Center for Studying Health System Change. (2008). Health care cost and access challenges persist. Retrieved August 2, 2008, from http://www.hschange.org/CONTENT/947/

Centers for Medicare and Medicaid. (2008). About CMS. Retrieved August 20, 2008, from http://www.cms.hhs.gov/

Chang, C., Price, S., & Pfoutz, S. (2001). *Economics and Nursing.* Philadelphia: FA Davis.

Cole, L., & Houston, S. (1999). Structured care methodologies: Evolution and use in patient care delivery. *Outcomes Management for Nursing Practice,* 3(2), 53–60.

Cronenwett, L., Sherwood, G., Barnsteiner, J., Disch, J., et al. (2007). Quality and safety education for nurses. *Nursing Outlook,* 55(3), 122–131.

Crummer, M.B., & Carter, V (1993). Critical pathways: The pivotal tool. *Cardiovascular Nursing,* 7(4), 30–37.

Davis, K. (2001). Preparing for the future: A 2020 vision for American health care. *Academic Medicine,* 76(4), 304–306.

Doenges, M.E., Moorhouse, M.F., & Geissler, A.C. (1997). *Nursing Care Plans: Guidelines for Individualizing Patient Care,* 4th ed. Philadelphia: FA Davis.

Donabedian, A. (1969). A guide to medical care administration. In *Medical care appraisal: Quality and Utilization,* vol. II. New York: American Public Health Association.

Donabedian, A. (1977). Evaluating the quality of medical care. *Milbank Memorial Fund Quarterly,* 44 (part 2), 166.

Donabedian, A. (1987). Some basic issues in evaluating the quality of health care. In Rinke, L.T. (ed.). *Outcome measures in home care.* N.Y.: National League of Nursing.

Donaldson, M.S. (ed.). (1998). Statement on quality of care. Washington, D.C.: National Academy Press. Retrieved August 1, 2008, from http://www.nap.edu/

Duke University Medical Center. (2005). Anatomy of an error: Basic tenet of human error. Retrieved August 7, 2008, from http://patientsafetyed.duhs.duke.edu/index.html

Elwood, T. W. (2007). The future of health care in the United States. *Journal of Allied Health,* 36(1), 3–10.

Ervin, N. E., Bickes, J. T., & Schim, S. M. (2006). Environments of care: A curriculum model for preparing a new generation of nurses. *Journal of Nursing Education,* 45(2), 75–80.

Flarey, D.L. (1995). *Redesigning Nursing Care Delivery.* Philadelphia: JB Lippincott.

Galvin, R. S., Delbanco, S., Milstein, A., & Belden, G. (2005, Jan/Feb). Has the Leapfrog Group had an impact on the health care market? *Health Affairs,* 24(1), 228–233.

Hansten, R., & Washburn, M. (2001). Outcomes-based care delivery. *American Journal of Nursing,* 101(2), 24A–D.

Heller, B. R., Oros, M. T., & Durney-Crowley, J. (2000). The future of nursing education: 10 trends to watch. *Nursing and Health Care Perspectives,* 21(1), 9.

How, S. K. H., Shih, A., Lau, J., Schoen, C. (Aug 2008). Public views on U.S. health system organization: A call for new directions. The Commonwealth Fund. Retrieved August 25, 2008, from http://www.commonwealthfund.org/usr_doc/ How_Public_Views_8-4-08.pdf?section=4039

Huber, D. (2000). *Leadership and Nursing Care Management,* 2nd ed. Philadelphia: WB Saunders.

Hunt, D.V. (1992). *Quality in America: How to Implement a Competitive Quality Program.* Homewood, Ill.: Business One Irwin.

Institute of Medicine. (2000). To err is human: Building a safer health system. Kohn, L. T., Corrigan, J. M., & Donaldson, M. S. (eds.). Washington, D.C.: National Academy Press.

Institute of Medicine. (2001). Crossing the quality chasm: A new health system for the 21st century. Washington, D.C.: National Academy Press.

Institute of Medicine. (2003a). Health professions education: A bridge to quality. Washington, D.C.: National Academy Press.

Institute of Medicine. (2003b). Priority areas for national actions: Transforming health care quality. *Quality Chasm Series.* Washington, D.C.: National Academies Press.

Institute of Medicine. (2004). Keeping patients safe: Transforming the work environment for nurses. Washington, D.C.: National Academy Press.

Institute of Medicine. (2006). Crossing the quality chasm: The IOM Quality Health Care Initiative. Retrieved August 8, 2008, from http://www.iom.edu/CMS/8089.aspx

Irvine, D. (1998). Finding value in nursing care: A framework for quality improvement and clinical evaluation. *Nursing Economics,* 16(3), 110–118.

Jackson, S. E. (2006). The influence of managed care on U.S. baccalaureate nursing education programs. *Journal of Nursing Education,* 45(2), 67–74.

Jenkins, J., & Calzone, K. A. (2007). Establishing the essential nursing competencies for genetics and genomics. *Journal of Nursing Scholarship,* 39(1), 10–16.

Joint Commission. (2008). Sentinel event. Retrieved August 14, 2008, from http://www.jointcommission.org/SentinelEvents/

Joint Commission on Accreditation of Healthcare Organizations (JCAHO). (2005). Retrieved November 26, 2005, from http://jcpatientsafety.org

Kaiser Family Foundation. (2005). Trends and indicators in the changing health care marketplace. Retrieved June 14, 2008, from http://www.kff.org/insurance/7031/index.cfm

Kersbergen, A. L. (2000). Managed care shifts health care from an altruistic model to a business framework. *Nursing & Health Care Perspectives,* 21(2), 81–83.

Kirk, M. (2002). The impact of globalization and environmental change on health: Challenges for nurse education. *Nurse Education Today,* 22(1), 60–71.

Leapfrog Group. (2007). About us. Retrieved August 20, 2008, from http://www.leapfroggroup.org/about_us

Lichtig, L.K., Knauf, R.A., & Milholland, D.K. (1999). Some impacts of nursing on acute care hospital outcomes. *Journal of Nursing Administration,* 29(2), 25–33.

Lynam, L. (1994). Case management and critical pathways: Friend or foe. *Neonatal Network,* 13(8), 48–51.

McLaughlin, C., & Kaluzny, A. (2006). *Continuous Quality Improvement in Health Care: Theory, Implementations, and Applications,* 3rd ed. Mass.: Jones and Bartlett.

Menix, K. D. (2000). Educating to manage the accelerated change environment effectively: Part 1. *Journal for Nurses in Staff Development,* 16(6), 282–288.

National Center for Policy Analysis. (2008). Consumer-driven health care. Retrieved August 2, 2008, from http://cdhc.ncpa.org/

National Council of State Boards of Nursing. (2008). 2007 NCLEX fact sheet. Retrieved September 16, 2007, from https:// www.ncsbn.org/534.htm

National Patient Safety Foundation. (2003). About the foundation: Our definitions. Retrieved September 16, 2008, from http://www.npsf.org/au/

Nelson, M. (2002). Educating for professional nursing practice: Looking backward into the future. *Online Journal of Issues in Nursing,* May 31, 2002, nursingworld.org/ojin/topic18/ tpc18_3.htm. Retrieved May 27, 2002.

Nightingale, F., & Barnum, B.S. (1992). *Notes on Nursing: What It Is, and What It Is Not,* commemorative ed. Philadelphia: Lippincott-Raven.

O'Neill, E. H., & Pew Health Professions Commission. (1998). *Recreating Health Professional Practice for a New Century* San Francisco: Pew Health Professions Commission.

Physicians for a National Health Plan. (2008). Single-payer health insurance. Retrieved August 2, 2008, from http://www.pnhp.org/facts/single_payer_resources.php

Ritter-Teitel, J. (2002). The impact of restructuring on professional nursing practice. *Journal of Nursing Administration,* 32(1), 31–41.

Robert Wood Johnson Foundation. (2008). About us. Retrieved August 20, 2008, from http://www.rwjf.org/about/

Rogers, A.E., Hwang, W., Scott, L.D., Aiken, L.H., et al. (2004). The working hours of hospital staff nurses and patient safety:

Both errors and near errors are more likely to occur when hospital staff nurses work twelve or more hours at a stretch. *Health Affairs, 23*(4), 202–212.

Rosenthal, J. & Booth, M. (2005). Maximizing the use of state adverse event data to improve patient safety. Portland, Maine: National Academy for Stae Health Policy. Retreived August 14, 2008, from http://www.nashp.org/Files/Patient_Safety_GNL61_for_web.pdf

Schroeder, P., ed. *Monitoring and Evaluation in Nursing.* Gaithersburg, Md. Aspen.

Strickland, O. (1997). Challenges in measuring patient outcomes. *Nursing Clinics of North America, 32*, 495–512.

Swansburg, R., & Swansburg, R. (2002*). Introduction to Management and Leadership for Nurse Managers,* 3rd ed. Boston: Jones and Bartlett.

Trossman, S. (2006). Issues update. It's in the genes: The ANA and nurse leaders want RNs and students to practice with genetics and genomics in mind. *American Journal of Nursing,* 106(2), 74–75.

U.S. Department of Health and Human Services. (2001). Healthy People 2010: Access to quality care. Retrieved July 17, 2007, from http://www.healthypeople.gov/Document/HTML/Volume1/01Access.htm

U.S. Department of Health and Human Services. (2006). What is behind HRSA's projected supply, demand and shortage of registered nurses? Retrieved September 17, 2008, from ftp://ftp.hrsa.gov/bhpr/workforce/behindshortage.pdf

U.S. Department of Health and Human Services. (2008). About HHS. Retrieved August 20, 2008, from http://www.hhs.gov/

U.S. Department of Labor. (2008). Employment projections. Retrieved September 16, 2008, from http://www.bls.gov/emp/#outlook

Whitehead, D. K., Weiss, S. A., & Tappen, R.M. (2007). Essentials of nursing leadership and management, 4th ed. Philadelphia: F.A. Davis.

chapter **11**

Time Management

⊙ ○ ○ ○ ○ ○ ○ ○ ○ ○

OBJECTIVES

After reading this chapter, the student should be able to:

- Describe personal perceptions of time.
- Discuss the rationale for good time management skills.
- Set short- and long-term personal career goals.
- Analyze activities at work using a time log.
- Incorporate time management techniques into clinical practice.
- Organize work to make more effective use of available time.
- Set limits on the demands made on one's time.
- Create a personal calendar using a computerized calendar system.

Coming onto the unit, Celia, the evening charge nurse, already knew that a hectic day was in progress. Scattered throughout the unit were clues from the past 12 hours. Two patients on emergency department stretchers had been placed outside observation rooms already occupied by patients who were admitted the previous day in critical condition. Stationed in the middle of the hall was the code cart, with its drawers opened and electrocardiograph paper cascading down the sides. Approaching the nurses' station, Celia found Guillermo buried deep in paperwork. He glanced at her with a face that had exhaustion written all over it. His first words were, "Three of your RNs called in sick. I called staffing for additional help, but only one is available. Good luck!" Celia surveyed the unit, looked at the number of staff members available, and reviewed the patient acuity level of the unit. She decided not to let the situation upset her. She would take charge of her own time and reallocate the time of her staff. She began to reorganize her staff mentally according to their capabilities and alter the responsibilities of each member. Having taken steps to handle the problem, Celia felt ready to begin the shift.

Business executives, managers, students, and nurses know that time is a valuable resource. Time cannot be saved and used later, so it must be used now and wisely. As a new nurse, you may at times find yourself sinking in the "quicksand" of a time trap, knowing what needs to be done but just not having the necessary time to do it (Ferrett, 1996). In today's fast-paced health-care environment, time management skills are critical to a nurse's success. Learning to take charge of your time and to use it effectively and efficiently is the key to time management (Gonzalez, 1996). Many nurses believe they never have enough time to accomplish their tasks. Like the White Rabbit in *Alice in Wonderland*, they are constantly in a rush against time. Time management, simply, is organizing and monitoring time so that patient care tasks can be scheduled and implemented in a timely and organized fashion (Bos & Vaughn, 1998).

The Tyranny of Time

Newton stated that time was absolute and that it occurred whether the universe was there or not. Einstein theorized that time has no independent existence apart from the order of events by which

people measure it (Smith, 1994). It really does not matter which theory is correct because, for nurses, their professional and personal lives are guided by time.

How often do you look at your watch during the day? Do you divide your day into blocks of time? Do you steal a quick glance at the clock when you come home after putting in a full day's work? Do you mentally calculate the amount of time left to complete the day's tasks of grocery shopping, driving in a car pool, making dinner, and leaving again to take a class or attend a meeting? Calendars, clocks, watches, newspapers, television, and radio remind people of their position in time. Perception of time is important because it affects people's use of time and their response to time (Box 11-1).

Computers complete operations in a fraction of a second, and speeds can be measured to the nanosecond. Time clocks that record the minute employees enter and leave work are commonplace, and few excuses for being late are really considered acceptable. Timesheets and schedules are part of most health-caregivers' lives. Staff members are

---

box 11-1

Time Perception

Webber (1980) collected a number of interesting tests of people's perception of time. You may want to try several of these:

- Do you think of time more as a galloping horseman or a vast motionless ocean?
- Which of these words best describes time to you: sharp, active, empty, soothing, tense, cold, deep, clear, young, or sad?
- Is your watch fast or slow? (You can check it with the radio.)
- Ask a friend to help you with this test. Go into a quiet room without any work, reading material, radio, food, or other distractions. Have your friend call you after 10–20 minutes have elapsed. Try to guess how long you were in that room.

Webber test results interpreted. A person who has a circular concept of time would compare time with a vast ocean. A galloping horseman would be characteristic of a linear conception of time, emphasizing speed and forward motion. A person oriented to a fast tempo and achievement would describe time as clear, young, sharp, active, or tense rather than empty, soothing, sad, cold, or deep. These same fast-tempo people are likely to have fast watches and to overestimate the amount of time that they sat in a quiet room.

Adapted from Webber, R.A. (1980). Time Is Money! Tested Tactics That Conserve Time for Top Executives. *New York: Free Press.*

expected to follow precisely set schedules and meet deadlines for almost everything, from distributing medications to completing reports on time. Many agencies produce vast quantities of computer-generated data that can be analyzed to determine the amount of time spent on various activities.

Several fallacies exist regarding time management. One of the foremost is that time can be managed like other resources. Time is finite. There are only 24 hours in a day, so the amount of time available cannot be controlled, only how it is used (Brumm, 2004). Individual personality, culture, and environment interact to influence human perceptions of time (Matejka & Dunsing, 1988). Everybody has an internal tempo (Chappel, 1970). Some internal tempos are quicker than others. Environment also affects the way people respond to time. A fast-paced environment influences most people to work at a faster pace, despite their internal tempo. For individuals with a slower tempo, this pace can cause discomfort. If you are high-achievement–oriented, you are likely to have already set some career goals for yourself and to have a mental schedule of deadlines for reaching these goals ("go on to complete my bachelor of science in nursing in 4 years; a master of science in nursing in 6 years").

Many health-care professionals are linear, fast-tempo, achievement-oriented people. Simply working at a fast pace, however, is not necessarily equivalent to achieving a great deal. Much energy can be wasted in rushing around and stirring things up but actually accomplishing very little. This chapter looks at ways in which you can use your time and energy wisely to accomplish your goals.

How Do Nurses Spend Their Time?

Nurses are the largest group of health-care professionals. Because of the number of nurses needed and the shift variations, attention concerning the efficiency and effectiveness of their time management is needed. Efficient nurses deliver care in an organized manner that makes best use of time, resources, and effort. Effective care improves a situation.

Today's labor market for skilled health-care professionals remains tight. Institutions face new challenges, not of "trimming the fat, but compensate [sic] for loss of muscle" (Baldwin, 2002, p. 1). Current shortages of nurses, radiology technicians, pharmacists, and other health-care specialists show all the signs of a long-term problem. Health-care institutions need to change their thinking on how to manage work. Most are looking toward technology to help cope with staffing shortages (Baldwin, 2002). For example:

A new graduate worked in a medical intensive care unit from 7 a.m. to 3 p.m. and rotated every third week to 11 p.m. to 7 a.m., working 7 days straight before getting 2 days off. It was not difficult to remain awake during the entire shift the first night on duty, but each night thereafter staying awake became increasingly difficult. After taking and recording the 2 a.m. vital signs, the new graduate inevitably fell asleep at the nurses' station. He was so tired that he had to check and recheck patient medications and other procedures for fear of making a fatal error. He became so anxious over the possibility of injuring someone that sleep during the day became impossible. Because of his obsession with rechecking his work, he had difficulty completing tasks and was always behind at the end of the shift (of course, napping did not help his time management).

A number of studies have examined how nurses use their time, especially nurses in acute care. For example, a study by Arthur Andersen found that only 35% of nursing time is spent in direct patient care (including care planning, assessment teaching, and technical activities). Lundgren and Segesten (2001) found that this increases to 50% when an all-RN staff is involved in patient care delivery, as the nurses spent less time supervising non-nursing personnel.

Documentation accounts for another 20% of nursing time. The remainder of time is spent on transporting patients, processing transactions, performing administrative responsibilities, and undertaking hotel services (Brider, 1992). Categories may change from study to study, but the amount of time spent on direct patient care is usually less than half the workday. As hospitals continue to reevaluate the way they deliver health care, nurses are finding themselves more involved with tasks that are not directly patient-related, such as determining quality improvement, developing critical pathways, and so forth. These are added to their already existing patient care functions. The critical nursing shortage compounds this problem. The result is that, in some cases, nurses are able to meet only the highest-priority patient needs, particularly in certain clinical settings such as short-stay units or ambulatory care centers (Curry, 2002).

Any change in the distribution of time spent on various activities can have a considerable impact on patient care and on the organization's bottom line. Prescott (1991) offered the following example:

If more unit management responsibilities could be shifted from nurses to non-nursing personnel, about 48 minutes per nurse shift could be redirected to patient care. In a large hospital with 600 full-time nurses, the result would be an additional 307 hours of direct patient care per day. Calculating the results of this time-saving strategy in another way shows an even greater impact: the changes would contribute the equivalent of the work of 48 additional full-time nurses to direct patient care.

Many health-care institutions are considering integrating units with similar patient populations and having them managed by a non-nurse manager, someone with business and management expertise, not necessarily nursing skills. However, as a group, nurses respect managers who have nursing expertise and who are able to perform as nurses. They believe that a nurse-manager has a greater understanding of both patient and professional staff needs. To address these service concerns, many educational institutions have developed dual graduate degrees combining nursing and management.

Organizing Your Work

Setting Your Own Goals

It is difficult to decide how to spend your time because there are so many tasks that need time. A good first step is to take a look at the situation, and get an overview. Then ask yourself, "What are my goals?" Goals help clarify what you want and give you energy, direction, and focus. Once you know where you want to go, set priorities. This is not an easy task. Remember Alice's conversation with the Cheshire Cat in Lewis Carroll's *Alice in Wonderland:*

"Would you tell me please, which way I ought to go from here?" asked Alice.

"That depends a good deal on where you want to go to," said the Cat.

"I don't care where," said Alice.

"Then it doesn't matter which way you go," said the Cat (Carroll, 1907).

How can you get somewhere if you do not know where you want to go? It is important to explore your personal and career goals. This can help you make decisions about the future.

This concept can be applied to daily activities as well as help in career decisions. Ask yourself questions about what you want to accomplish over a particular period. Personal development skills include discipline, goal setting, time management and organizational skills, self monitoring, and a positive attitude toward the job (Bos & Vaughn, 1998). Many of the personal management and organizational skills related to the workplace focus on time management and scheduling. Most new nurses have the skills required to perform the job but lack the personal management skills necessary to get the job done, specifically when it comes to time management.

To help organize your time, set both short- and long-term goals. Short-term goals are those that you wish to accomplish within the near future. Setting up your day in an organized fashion is a short-term goal, as is scheduling a required medical errors or domestic violence course.

Long-term goals are those you wish to complete over a long time. Advanced education and career goals are examples. A good question to ask yourself is, "What do I see myself doing 5 years from now?" Every choice you make requires a different allocation of time (Moshovitz, 1993).

Alinore, a licensed practical nurse returning to school to obtain her associate's degree in nursing, faced a multitude of responsibilities. A wife, a mother of two toddlers, and a full-time staff member at a local hospital, Alinore suddenly found herself in a situation in which there just were not enough hours in a day. She became convinced that becoming a registered nurse was an unobtainable goal. When asked where she wanted to be in 5 years, she answered, "At this moment, I think, on an island in Tahiti!" Several instructors helped Alinore develop a time plan. First, she was asked to list what she did each day and how much time each task required. This list included basic child care, driving children to and from day care, shopping, cooking meals, cleaning, hours spent in the classroom, study hours, work hours, and time devoted to leisure. Once this was established, she was asked which tasks could be allocated to someone else (e.g., her husband), which tasks could be clustered (e.g., cooking for several days at a time), and which tasks could be shared. Alinore's husband was willing to assist with car pools, grocery shopping, and cleaning. Previously, Alinore never asked him for help. Cooking meals was clustered: Alinore made all the meals in 1 day and then froze and labeled them to be used later. This left time for other activities. Alinore graduated at the top of her class and subsequently completed her BSN. She became a clinical preceptor for other associate degree nursing students on a pediatric unit in a county hospital. She never did get to Tahiti, though.

Employers pay nurses for their time. Does that mean that nurses "sell" their time? If so, then nurses "own" their time. Looking at time from this perspective changes the point of view about time, as nurses then manage their own time to accomplish patient care tasks.

Time management means handling time with a measure of proficiency. Therefore, time management means meeting patient care needs skillfully during a nursing shift (Navuluri, 2001). Organizing work eliminates extra steps or serious delays in completing it. Organizing also reduces the amount of time spent in activities that are neither productive nor satisfying.

Working on the most difficult tasks when you have the most energy decreases frustration later in the day when you may be more tired and less efficient. To begin managing your time, develop a clear understanding of *how you use your time*. Creating a personal time inventory helps you estimate how much time you spend on typical activities. Keeping the inventory for a week gives a fairly accurate estimate of how you spend your time. The inventory also helps identify "time wasters" (Gahar, 2000).

MacKenzie (1990) identified 20 of the biggest time wasters. Some of these come directly from the work environment, whereas others are personal characteristics. To avoid time wasters, take control. It is important to prevent endless activities and other people controlling you (American Bar Association Career Resource Center, n.d.). Every day, set priorities to help you meet your goals. Ten frequent activities that infringe on time are in Box 11-2.

Lists

One of the most useful organizers is the "to do" list. You can make this list either at the end of every day or at the beginning of each day before you do anything else. Some people say they do it at the end of the day because something always interferes at the

---

box 11-2

Ten Frequent Activities That Infringe on Time

- Managing by crisis
- Telephone calls
- Poor planning
- Taking on too much
- Unexpected visitors
- Improper delegation
- Disorganization
- Inability to say no
- Procrastinating
- Meetings

Adapted from the ABA Career Resource Center, http://www.abanet.org/careercounsel/prelaw/5timeprelawtips.pdf

---

beginning of the next day. Do not include routine tasks because they will make the list too long and you will do them without the extra reminder.

If you are a team leader, place the unique tasks of the day on the list: team conference, telephone calls to families, discussion of a new project, or in-service demonstration of a new piece of equipment. You may also want to arrange these tasks in order of their priority, starting with those that must be done that day. Ask yourself the following questions regarding the tasks on the list (Moshovitz, 1993):

- What is the relative importance of each of these tasks?
- How much time will each task require?
- When must each task be completed?
- How much time and energy have to be devoted to these tasks?

If you find yourself postponing an item for several days, decide whether to give it top priority the next day or drop it from the list as an unnecessary task.

The list should be in a user-friendly form: on your electronic organizer, in your pocket, or on a clipboard. Checking the list several times a day quickly becomes a good habit. Computerized calendar-creator programs help in setting priorities and guiding daily activities. Many of these are found on the Internet or intranet of an institution. These programs can be set to appear on the desktop when you turn on your computer to give an overview of the day, week, or month. This calendar acts as an automated to-do list. Your daily list may become your most important time manager (Box 11-3).

Long-Term Planning Systems

At the beginning of the semester, students are told the examination dates and when papers will be due. Many students find it helpful to enter the dates on a semester-long calendar so they can be seen at a glance. Then the students can see when clusters of assignments are due at the same time. This allows for advance planning or perhaps requests to change dates or get extensions.

Personal digital assistants (PDAs), or hand-held organizers, have become quite popular. These devices allow both short-term and long-term scheduling. PDAs permit storing of personal notes and reminders, contact data, Internet access, and other program files. Hand-held devices permit synchronization with personal computers and Internet-based calendars.

Schedules and Blocks of Time

Without some type of schedule, you are more likely to drift through a day or bounce from one activity to another in a disorganized fashion. Assignment sheets, worksheets, flow sheets, and critical pathways are all designed to help you plan patient care and schedule your time effectively. The critical pathway is a guide to recommended treatments and optimal patient outcomes (see Chapter 10). *Assignment sheets* indicate the patients for whom each staff member is responsible. *Worksheets* are then created to organize the daily care that must be given to the assigned patients (see Chapter 9 for examples of worksheets). *Flow sheets* are lists of items that must be recorded for each patient.

Effective worksheets and flow sheets schedule and organize the day by providing reminders of various tasks and when they need to be done. The danger in using them, however, is that the more they divide the day into discrete segments, the more they fragment the work and discourage a holistic approach. If a worksheet becomes the focus of attention, the perspective of the whole and of the individuals who are your patients may be lost. Some activities must be done at a certain time. These activities structure the day or week to a great extent, and their timing may be out of your control. However, in every job there are tasks that can be done whenever you want to do them, as long as they are done.

In certain nursing jobs, reports and presentations are often required. For these activities, you may need to set aside blocks of time during which you can concentrate on the task. Trying to create and complete a report in 5- or 10-minute blocks of time is unrealistic. By the time you reorient yourself to the project, the time allotted is over, and nothing has been accomplished. Setting aside large blocks of time to do complex tasks is much more efficient.

Consider energy levels when beginning a big task. Start when levels are high and not at, say, 4:00 in the afternoon if that is when you find yourself winding down (Baldwin, 2002). For example, if you are a morning person, plan your demanding work in the morning. If you get energy spurts later in the morning or early afternoon, plan to work on larger or heavier tasks at that time. Nursing shifts may be designed in 8-, 10-, or 12-hour blocks. Many nurses working the night shifts (11 p.m. to 7 a.m. or 7 p.m. to 7 a.m.) find they have more energy a little later into their shift rather than at the beginning, whereas nurses working the day shifts (7 a.m. to 3 p.m. or 7 a.m. to 7 p.m.) find they have the most energy at the beginning of their shift. Also, learn to delegate tasks that do not require professional nursing skills.

Some people go to work early to have a block of uninterrupted time. Others take work home with them for the same reason. This extends the workday and cuts into leisure time. The higher your stress level, the less effective you will be on the job—do not bring your work home with you. You need some time off to recharge your batteries (Turkington, 1996).

Filing Systems

Filing systems are helpful for keeping track of important papers. All professionals need to maintain copies of licenses, certifications, continuing education credits, and current information about their specialty area. Keeping these organized in an easily retrievable system saves time and energy when you need to refer to them. Using color-coded folders is often helpful. Each color holds documents that are related to one another. For example, all continuing education credits might be placed in a blue folder, anything pertaining to licensure in a yellow folder, and so on.

Setting Limits

To set limits, it is necessary to identify your objectives and then arrange the actions needed to meet them in order of their priority (Haynes, 1991; Navuluri, 2001). The focus of time management exists on two levels: temporal and spatial. Nurses need to focus on patient care needs during the shift (temporal) or within the boundaries of the working environment (spatial).

Saying No

Saying no to low-priority demands on your time is an important but difficult part of setting limits. Assertiveness and determination are necessary for effective time management. Learn to say no tactfully at least once a day (Hammerschmidt & Meador, 1993). Patient care is a team effort. Effective time management requires you to look at other members of the team who may be able to take on the task.

The wisdom of time management is that you may have to let others help you while never giving up ownership of your time. In other words, although supervisors and managers tell you what to do, how you accomplish this remains up to you (Navuluri, 2001). Is it possible to say no to your supervisor or manager? It may not seem so at first, but many requests are negotiable. Requests sometimes are in conflict with career goals. Rather than sit on a committee in which you have no interest, respectfully decline, and volunteer for one that holds promise for you as well as meets the needs of your unit.

Can you refuse an assignment? Your manager may ask you to work overtime or to come in on your scheduled day off, but you can decline. You may not refuse to care for a group of patients or to take a report because you think the assignment is too difficult or unsafe. You may, however, discuss the situation with your supervisor and, together, work out alternatives. You can also confront the issue of understaffing by filing an unsafe staffing complaint. Failure to accept an assignment may result in accusations of abandonment.

Some people have difficulty saying no. Ambition keeps some people from declining any opportunity, no matter how overloaded they are. Many individuals are afraid of displeasing others and therefore feel obligated to take on continuously all types of additional assignments. Still others have such a great need to be needed that they continually give of themselves, not only to patients but also to their coworkers and supervisors. They fail to stop and replenish themselves, and then they become exhausted. Remember, no one can be all things to all people at all times without creating serious guilt, anger, bitterness, and disillusionment. "Anyone who says it's possible has never tried it" (Turkington, 1996, p. 9).

Eliminating Unnecessary Work

Some work has become so deeply embedded in one's routines that it appears essential, although it is really unnecessary. Some nursing routines fall into this category. Taking vital signs, giving baths, changing linens, changing dressings, performing irrigations, and doing similar basic tasks are more often done according to schedule rather than according to patient need, which may be much more or much less often than the routine specifies. Some of these tasks may appropriately be delegated to others:

- If patients are ambulatory, bed linens may not need to be changed daily. Incontinent and diaphoretic patients need to have fresh linens more frequently. Not all patients need a complete bed bath every day. Elderly patients have dry, fragile skin; giving them good mouth, facial, and perineal care may be all that is required on certain days. This should be included in the patient's care plan.
- Much paperwork is duplicative, and some is altogether unnecessary. For example, is it necessary to chart nursing interventions in two or three places on the patient record? Charting by exception, flow sheets, and computerized records are attempts to eliminate some of these problems.
- Socialization in the workplace is an important aspect in maintaining interpersonal relationships. When there is a social component to interactions in a group, the result is usually positive. However, too much socialization can reduce productivity. Use judgment in deciding when socializing is interfering with work.

You may create additional work for yourself without realizing it. How often do you walk back down the hall to obtain equipment when it all could have been gathered at one time? How many times do you walk to a patient's room instead of using the intercom, only to find that you need to go back to where you were to get what the patient needs? Is the staff providing personal care to patients who are well enough to meet some of these needs themselves?

Streamlining Your Work

Many tasks cannot be eliminated or delegated, but they can be done more efficiently. There are many sayings in time management that reflect the principle of streamlining work. "Work smarter, not harder" is a favorite one that should appeal to nurses facing increasing demands on time. "Never handle a piece of paper more than once" is a more specific one, reflecting the need to avoid procrastination in your work. "A stitch in time saves nine" reflects the extent to which preventive action saves time in the long run.

Avoiding Crisis Management

Crisis management occurs when people procrastinate or do not pay attention to their intuitions. The key to avoiding crises is to anticipate possible problems and intervene before they become overwhelming. As a new nurse, it may be difficult to anticipate everything; however, there are some things that you can do by organizing your day. Several methods of working smarter and not harder are:

- Gather materials, such as bed linen, for all of your patients at one time. As you go to each room, leave the linen so that it will be there when you need it.
- While giving a bed bath or providing other personal care, perform some of the aspects of the physical assessment, such as taking vital signs, skin assessment, and parts of the neurological and musculoskeletal assessment. Prevention is always a good idea.
- If a patient does not "look right," do not ignore your intuition. The patient is probably having a problem.
- If you are not sure about a treatment or medication, ask before you proceed. It is usually less time-consuming to prevent a problem than it is to resolve one.

- When you set aside time to do a specific task that has a high priority, stick to your schedule, and complete it.
- Do not allow interruptions while you are completing paperwork, such as transcribing orders.

What else can you do to streamline your work? A few general suggestions follow, but the first one, a time log, can assist you in developing others unique to your particular job. If you complete the log correctly, a few surprises about how you really spend your time are almost guaranteed.

Keeping a Time Log

Perception of time is elastic. People do not accurately estimate the time they spend on any particular task; people cannot rely on their memories for accurate information about how they spend their time. The time log is an objective source of information. Most people spend a much smaller amount of their time on productive activities than they estimate. Once you see how large amounts of your time are spent, you will be able to eliminate or reduce the time spent on nonproductive or minimally productive activities (Drucker, 1967; Robichaud, 1986).

For example, many nurses spend a great deal of time searching for or waiting for missing medications, equipment, or supplies. Before beginning patient care, assemble all the equipment and supplies you will need, and check the patient's medication drawer against the medication administration record so you can order anything that is missing before you begin.

Figure 11.1 is an example of a time log in which you enter your activities every half hour. This means that you will have to pay careful attention to what you are doing so that you can record it accurately. Do not postpone record-keeping; do it every 30 minutes. A 3-day sample may be enough for you to see a pattern emerging. It is suggested that you repeat the process again in 6 months, both because work situations change and to see if you have made any long-lasting changes in your use of time.

Reducing Interruptions

Everyone experiences interruptions. Some of these are welcome and necessary, but too many interfere with your work. A phone call from the laboratory with a critical value is a necessary interruption. Hobbs (1987) stated that necessary interruptions are not time wasters. Middle-level managers are interrupted every 8 minutes, and senior managers suffer

Activities	Comments
6:30	
7:00	
7:30	
8:00	
8:30	
9:00	
9:30	
10:00	
10:30	
11:00	
11:30	
12:00	
12:30	
1:00	
1:30	
2:00	
2:30	
3:00	
3:30	
4:00	
4:30	
5:00	
5:30	
6:00	
6:30	
7:00	

Figure 11.1 Time log. (Adapted from Robichaud, A.M. [1986]).

interruptions every 5 minutes. Patient-care managers—nurses—seem to be interrupted every minute. Interruptions need to be kept to a minimum or eliminated, if possible. Closing the door to a patient's room may reduce interruptions. You may have to ask visitors to wait a few minutes before you can answer their questions, although you must remain sensitive to their needs and return to them as soon as possible.

There is nothing wrong about asking a colleague who wants your assistance to wait a few minutes if you are engaged in another activity. Interruptions that occur when you are trying to pour medications or make calculations can cause errors. Physicians and other professionals often request nursing attention when nurses are involved with patient-care tasks. Find out if an unlicensed person may help. If not, ask the physician to wait, stating that you will be more than glad to help as soon as you complete what you are doing. Be courteous, but be firm; you are busy also.

Categorizing Activities

Clustering certain activities helps eliminate the feeling of bouncing from one unrelated task to another. It also makes your caregiving more holistic. You may, for example, find that documentation takes less time if you do it while you are still with the patient or immediately after seeing a patient. The information is still fresh in your mind, and you do not have to rely on notes or recall. Many health-care institutions have switched to computerized charting, with the computers placed at the bedside. This setup assists in documenting care and interventions while the nurse is still with the patient. Also, try to follow a task through to completion before beginning another.

Finding the Fastest Way

Many time-consuming tasks can be done more efficiently by automation. Narcotic delivery systems that deliver the correct dose and electronically record the dose, the name of the patient, and the name of the health-care personnel removing the medication are being used in many institutions. This system saves staff time in documentation and in performing a narcotic count at the end of each shift. Bar coding is another method used by health-care institutions. Bar coding allows for scanning certain types of patient data, decreasing the number of paper chart entries (Baldwin, 2002; Meyer, 1992).

Efficient systems do not have to be complex. Using a preprinted color-coded sticker system helps identify patients who must be without food or fluids (NPO) for tests or surgery, those who require 24-hour urine collections, or those who require special cultures. The information need not be written or entered repeatedly if stickers are used.

Everyone talks about the amount of time wasted by physicians, nurses, and other clinicians in looking for such things as patient charts, equipment, and even patients. Erica Drazen, vice president of First Consulting Group in Lexington, Massachusetts, suggested using more sophisticated wireless technology, similar to the car tracking systems used by law enforcement. Tiny transmitters can be activated from a central point to locate the items or individuals. Using electronic medical record systems decreases the amount of time spent looking for patient records. By using approved access codes, health-care personnel can obtain information from anywhere within the institution. This also minimizes time spent on paper charting.

Automating Repetitive Tasks

Developing techniques for repetitive tasks is similar to finding the fastest method, but it focuses on specific tasks that are repeated again and again, such as patient teaching.

Many patients come to the hospital or ambulatory center for surgery or invasive diagnostic tests for same-day treatment. This does not give nurses much teaching time. Using videotapes and pamphlets as teaching aids can reduce the time needed to share the information, allowing the nurse to be available to answer individual questions and create individual adaptations. Many facilities are using these techniques for cardiac rehabilitation, preoperative teaching, and infant care instruction. Computer-generated teaching and instruction guides permit patients to take the information home with them. This can decrease the number of phone calls requiring repetition of information.

The Rhythm Model for Time Management

Navuluri (2001) looked at time management in terms of a Rhythm Model—a PQRST pattern: Prioritize, Question, Recheck, Self-reliance, Treat. By prioritizing, you can accomplish the most important tasks first. Questioning permits you to look at events and tasks in terms of effectiveness, efficiency, and efficacy. Rechecking unfinished tasks quickly helps you to manage your time efficiently. Self-reliance allows you to know the difference between events that are within your control and those that are not, as well as realizing your limitations. No one knows better what you are capable of doing than you. Treats are part of life. It is okay to take a break or time out. It is important because doing so permits you to refresh. Table 11-1 summarizes the Rhythm Model for Time Management.

Conclusion

Time can be your best friend or worst enemy, depending on your perspective and how you manage it. It is important to identify how you feel about time and to assess your own time management skills. Nursing requires that numerous activities be performed within what often seems to be very brief periods. Remember that there are only so many hours in the day. Knowing this can create stress. No one works well "under pressure." Learn to delegate. Learn to say, "I would really like to help you; can it wait until I finish this?" Learn to say no. Most of all, learn how to make the most of your day by working effectively and efficiently. Finally, remember that 8 hours should be designated as sleep time and several more as personal or leisure ("time off") time.

table 11-1	
The Rhythm Model for Time Management	
PRIORITIZE	List tasks in order of importance.
	Remember that some tasks must occur at specific times, whereas others can occur at any time.
	Emergencies take precedence.
	Identify events controlled by you and events controlled by others.
	Use critical thinking skills to assign priorities.
QUESTION:	
EFFECTIVENESS	Did the task produce the desired outcome?
EFFICIENCY	How can I accomplish the plan with the least expenditure of time?
	Is there a way to break this down into simpler tasks?
EFFICACY	Do I have the skill and ability to obtain the desired effect?
RECHECK	Mentally and physically recheck an unfinished or delegated task.
SELF-RELIANCE	Identify those tasks that are within your control and those that are not.
	Use critical thinking skills and adaptability to revise priorities.
	"Go with the flow."
TREAT	Treat yourself to a break when you can.
	Treat yourself to time off.
	Treat yourself to an educational experience: Commit yourself to excellence.
	Treat others courteously and with respect.

Study Questions

1. Develop a personal time inventory. Identify your time wasters. How do you think you can eliminate these activities?

2. Create your own patient care worksheet. How does this worksheet help you organize your clinical day?

3. Keep a log of your clinical day. Which activities took the most time? Why? Which activities took the least time? What situations interfered with your work? What could you do to reduce the interference?

4. Identify a task that is done repeatedly in your clinical area. Think of a new, more efficient way to do that task. How could you implement this new routine? How could you evaluate its efficiency?

5. Consider how many interruptions you had during the day. How did you handle them? How did they interfere in your time management?

Case Study to Promote Critical Reasoning

Antonio was recently hired as a team leader for a busy cardiac step-down unit. Nursing responsibilities of the team leader, in addition to patient care, include meeting daily with team members, reviewing all admissions and discharges for acuity and length of stay, and documenting all patients who exceed length of stay and the reasons. At the end of each month, the team leaders are required to meet with unit managers to review the patient care load and team member performance. This is the last week of the month, and Antonio has a meeting with the unit manager at the end of the week. He is 2 weeks behind on staff evaluations and documentation of patients who exceeded length of stay. He is becoming very stressed over his team leader responsibilities.

1. Why do you think Antonio is feeling stressed?

2. Make a to-do list for Antonio.

3. Develop a time log for Antonio to use to analyze his activities.

4. How can Antonio organize and streamline his work?

References

American Bar Association Career Resource Center (n.d.). Identifying & conquering time wasters. Retrieved December 20, 2005, from abanet.org/careercounsel

Baldwin, F.D. (2002). Making do with less. *Healthcare Informatics,* pp. 1–7. Online, March 2002.

Bos, C.S., & Vaughn, S. (1998). *Strategies for Teaching Students With Learning and Behavioral Problems,* 4th ed. Boston: Allyn & Bacon.

Brider, P. (1992). The move to patient-focused care. *American Journal of Nursing,* 92(9), 27–33.

Brumm, J. (2004). Time can be on your side. *Nursing Spectrum.* http://nursingspectrum.com/StudentsCorner/StudentFeatures/TimeSide.htm.

Chappel, E.D. (1970). *Culture and Biological Man: Exploration in Behavioral Anthropology.* N.Y.: Holt, Rinehart, & Winston. (Reprinted as *The Biological Foundations of Individuality and Culture.* Huntingdon, N.Y.: Robert Krieger, 1979.)

Carroll, L. (1907). *Alice's Adventures in Wonderland.* Reprint 2002. N.Y.: North-South Books.

Curry, P. (March 25, 2002). Pressure cooker: Hospital's emphasis on productivity increases stress for nurses and patients. *Nurseweek News,* http://www.nurseweek. com

Drucker, P.E. (1967). *The Effective Executive.* N.Y.: Harper & Row.

Ferrett, S.K. (1996). *Connections: Study Skills for College and Career Success.* Chicago: Irwin Mirror Press.

Gahar, A. (2000). *Programming for College Students With Learning Disabilities.* (Grant No.: 84–078C) http://www.csbsju.edu

Gonzalez, S.I. (1996). Time management. *The Nursing Spectrum in Florida,* 6(17), 5.

Hammerschmidt, R., & Meador, C.K. (1993). *A Little Book of Nurses' Rules.* Philadelphia: Hanley & Belfus.

Haynes, M.E. (1991). *Practical Time Management.* Los Altos, Calif.: Crisp Publications.

Hobbs, S. (1987). Getting to grips with business plans, audit, and applications. *Nursing Standard.*

Lundgren, S., & Segesten, K. (2001). Nurses' use of time in a medical-surgical ward with all-RN staffing. *Journal of Nursing Management,* 9, 13–20.

MacKenzie, A. (1990). *The Time Trap.* N.Y.: American Management Association.

Matejka, J.K., & Dunsing, R.J. (1988). Time management: Changing some traditions. *Management World,* 17(2), 6–7.

Meyer, C. (1992). Equipment nurses like. *American Journal of Nursing,* 92(8), 32–38.

Moshovitz, R. (1993). *How to Organize Your Work and Your Life.* N.Y.: Doubleday.

Navuluri, R.B. (March 2001). Our time management in patient care. *Research for Nursing Practice,* 1–8.

Prescott, P.A. (1991). Changing how nurses spend their time. *Image,* 23(1), 23–28.

Robichaud, A.M. (1986). Time documentation of clinical nurse specialist activities. *Journal of Nursing Administration,* 16(1), 31–36.

Smith, H.W. (1994). *The Ten Natural Laws of Successful Time and Life Management: Proven Strategies for Increased Productivity and Inner Peace.* N.Y.: Warner Books.

Turkington, C.A. (1996). *Reflections for Working Women: Common Sense, Sage Advice, and Unconventional Wisdom.* N.Y.: McGraw-Hill.

Webber, R.A. (1980). *Time Is Money! Tested Tactics That Conserve Time for Top Executives.* N.Y.: Free Press.

3 unit

Professional Issues

chapter 12

Promoting a Healthy Workplace

○○○○○○○○○○○

OBJECTIVES

After reading this chapter, the student should be able to:

- Recognize the components of nurse job satisfaction.
- Describe quality indicators related to safety and quality.
- Recognize threats to safety in the workplace.
- Identify agencies responsible for overseeing workplace safety.
- Describe methods of dealing with violence in the workplace.
- Identify the role of the nurse in dealing with terrorism and other disasters.
- Recognize situations that may reflect sexual harassment.
- Make suggestions for improving the physical and social environment.
- Understand the American Nurses Association (ANA) Future Vision for Nursing.

Almost half our waking hours are spent in the workplace. For this reason alone, the quality of the workplace environment is a major concern. Yet, it is neglected to a surprising extent in many health-care organizations. It is neglected by administrators who would never allow peeling paint or poorly maintained equipment but who leave their staff, their most costly and valuable resource, unmaintained and unrefreshed. The "do more with less" thinking that has predominated many organizations places considerable pressure on staff and management alike (Chisholm, 1992). Improvement of the workplace environment is more difficult to accomplish under these circumstances, but it is more important than ever.

Much of the responsibility for enhancing the workplace rests with upper-level management, people who have the authority and resources to encourage organization-wide growth and change. Nurses, however, have begun to take more responsibility for identification of and problem solving for workplace issues. This chapter focuses on these issues, in addition to sexual harassment, impaired workers, enhancement of work-life quality, diversity, and disabled workers.

Workplace Safety

Safety is not a new concept in the workplace. The modern movement began during the Industrial Revolution. In 1913, the National Council for Industrial Safety (now the National Safety Council) was formed. The Occupational Safety and Health Act of 1970 created both the National Institute of Occupational Safety and Health (NIOSH) and the Occupational Safety and Health Administration (OSHA). The OSHA, part of the U.S. Department of Labor, is responsible for developing and enforcing workplace safety and health regulations. The NIOSH, part of the U.S. Department of Health and Human Services, provides research, information, education, and training in occupational safety and health. The National Safety Council (NSC) partners with the OSHA to provide training in a variety of safety initiatives. The NSC maintains that safety in the workplace is the responsibility of both the employer and the employee. The employer must ensure a safe, healthful work environment, and employees are accountable for knowing and following safety guidelines and standards (National Safety Council, 1992).

Threats to Safety

Working in a health-care facility is reported to be one of the most dangerous jobs in the United States. The Department of Labor reports that a health-care worker in a nursing facility is more likely to be injured on the job than a coal miner. Health and safety threats in the nursing workplace include infectious diseases, physical violence, ergonomic injuries related to the movement and repositioning of patients, exposure to hazardous chemicals and radiation, and sharps injuries (ANA, 2007).

Health care is the second-fastest-growing sector of the U.S. economy, employing more than 12 million workers. Women represent nearly 80% of the health-care workforce. Health-care workers face a wide range of hazards on the job, including needlestick injuries, back injuries, latex allergy, violence, and stress. Although it is possible to prevent or reduce health-care worker exposure to these hazards, health-care workers are experiencing increasing numbers of occupational injuries and illnesses; rates of occupational injury have risen over the past decade. By contrast, two of the most hazardous industries, agriculture and construction, are safer today than they were a decade ago. NIOSH-TIC-2 is a searchable bibliographical database of occupational safety and health publications, documents, grant reports, and journal articles supported in whole or in part by the NIOSH (cdc.gov/niosh/topics/healthcare/).

In spring 2001, a Florida nurse with 20 years' psychiatric nursing experience died of head and face trauma. Her assailant, a former wrestler, had been admitted involuntarily in the early morning to the private mental health–care facility. An investigation found that the facility did not have a policy on workplace violence and no method of summoning help in an emergency (Arbury, 2002).

Six hundred thousand to one million needlestick injuries occur annually to U.S. health-care workers. Percutaneous exposure is the principal route for human immunodeficiency virus (HIV) and hepatitis B and C virus transmission. Additionally, infections such as tuberculosis, syphilis, malaria, and herpes can be transmitted through needlesticks.

Threats to safety in the workplace vary from one setting to another and from one individual to another. A pregnant staff member may be more vulnerable to risks from radiation; staff members working in the emergency room of a large urban public hospital are at more risk for HIV and tuberculosis than the staff members working in the newborn nursery. All staff members have the right to be made aware of potential risks. No worker should feel intimidated or uncomfortable in the workplace.

Reducing Risk

OSHA

The Occupational Safety and Health Act of 1970 and the Mine Safety and Health Act of 1977 were the first federal guidelines and standards related to safe and healthful working conditions. Through these acts, the NIOSH and OSHA were formed. OSHA regulations apply to most U.S. employers that have one or more employees and that engage in businesses affecting commerce. Under OSHA regulations, the employer must comply with standards for providing a safe, healthful work environment. Employers are also required to keep records of all occupational (job-related) illnesses and accidents. Examples of occupational accidents and injuries include burns, chemical exposures, lacerations, hearing loss, respiratory exposure, musculoskeletal injuries, and exposure to infectious diseases.

OSHA regulations provide for workplace inspections that may be conducted with or without prior notification to the employer. However, catastrophic or fatal accidents and employee complaints may also trigger an OSHA inspection. OSHA encourages employers and employees to work together to identify and remove any workplace hazards before contacting the nearest OSHA area office. If the employee has not been able to resolve the safety or health issue, the employee may file a formal complaint, and an inspection will be ordered by the area OSHA director (U.S. Department of Labor, 1995). Any violations found are posted where all employees can view them. The employer has the right to contest the OSHA decision. The law also states that the employer cannot punish or discriminate against employees for exercising their rights related to job safety and health hazards or participating in OSHA inspections (U.S. Department of Labor, 1995).

OSHA inspections have focused especially on blood-borne pathogens, lifting and ergonomic (proper body alignment) guidelines, confined-space regulations, respiratory guidelines, and workplace violence. Since September 11, 2001, the OSHA has added protecting the worksite against terrorism (osha.gov). Table 12-1 lists the major categories of potential hazards found in hospitals as identified by the OSHA. The U.S. Department of Labor publishes fact sheets related to various OSHA guidelines and activities. They can be obtained from your employer, at the local public library, or via the Internet at osha.gov

table 12-1

Potential Hospital Hazards

Hazard	Definition	Examples
Biological	Infectious/biological agents such as bacteria, viruses, fungi, parasites	HIV, vancomycin-resistant enterococcus, methicillin-resistant *Staphylococcus aureus*, hepatitis B virus, tuberculosis
Chemical	Medications, solutions, and gases that are potentially toxic or irritating to the body system	Ethylene oxide, formaldehyde, glutaraldehyde, waste anesthetic gases, cytotoxic agents, pentamidine ribavirin
Psychological	Factors and situations encountered in or associated with the work environment that create or potentiate stress, emotional strain, and/or interpersonal problems	Stress, workplace violence, shiftwork, inadequate staffing, heavy workload, increased patient acuity
Physical	Agents that cause tissue trauma	Radiation, lasers, noise, electricity, extreme temperatures, workplace violence
Environmental, mechanical, biomedical	Factors in work environment that cause or lead to accidents, injuries, strain, or discomfort	Tripping hazards, unsafe or unguarded equipment, air quality, slippery floors, confined spaces, obstructed work areas or passageways, awkward postures, localized contact stresses, temperature extremes, repetitive motions, lifting and moving patients

Adapted from osha.gov/SLTC/healthcarefacilities/hazards

Centers for Disease Control and Prevention

The Centers for Disease Control and Prevention (CDC) is the lead federal agency for protecting the health and safety of citizens both at home and abroad. The CDC partners with other agencies throughout the nation to investigate health problems, conduct research, implement prevention strategies, and promote safe and healthy environments. The CDC publishes continuous updates of recommendations for prevention of HIV transmission in the workplace and universal precautions related to blood-borne pathogens; it also publishes the most recent information on other infectious diseases in the workplace, such as tuberculosis and hepatitis. Currently, the CDC is targeting public health emergency preparedness and response related to biological and chemical agents and threats (cdc.gov/). Information can be obtained by consulting the Mortality and Morbidity Weekly Report (MMWR) in the library, via the Internet (cdc.gov/health/diseases), or through the toll-free phone number (800-311-3435). Interested health-care workers can also be placed on the CDC's mailing list to receive any free publications.

NIOSH

The NIOSH is part of the CDC and is the federal agency responsible for conducting research and making recommendations for the prevention of work-related disease and injury. Occupational hazards for health-care workers continue to be enormous health and economic problems. According to statistics from the NIOSH, more than 6.1 million illnesses and injuries occur in the workplace yearly, with more than 2.9 million lost workdays attributed to occupational illnesses and injuries (cdc.gov/niosh/about).

Box 12-1 lists the most important federal laws enacted to protect individuals in the workplace.

ANA

When looking at agencies that are instrumental in dealing with workplace safety, the ANA must be included. The ANA is discussed more completely in Chapters 10 and 15. The ANA's history embodies advocacy for the nurse.

In 1999 the Commission on Workplace Advocacy was established as part of the ANA. The Commission consists of nine members, appointed

---

box 12-1

Federal Laws Enacted to Protect the Worker in the Workplace

- **Equal Pay Act of 1963:** Employers must provide equal pay for equal work, regardless of sex.
- **Title VII of Civil Rights Act of 1964:** Employees may not be discriminated against on the basis of race, color, religion, sex, or national origin.
- **Age Discrimination in Employment Act of 1967:** Private and public employers may not discriminate against persons 40 years of age or older except when a certain age group is a bona fide occupational qualification.
- **Pregnancy Discrimination Act of 1968:** Pregnant women cannot be discriminated against in employment benefits if they are able to perform job responsibilities.
- **Fair Credit Reporting Act of 1970:** Job applicants and employees have the right to know of the existence and content of any credit files maintained on them.
- **Vocational Rehabilitation Act of 1973:** An employer receiving financial assistance from the federal government may not discriminate against individuals with disabilities and must develop affirmative action plans to hire and promote individuals with disabilities.
- **Family Education Rights and Privacy Act—Buckley Amendment of 1974:** Educational institutions may not supply information about students without their consent.
- **Immigration Reform and Control Act of 1986:** Employers must screen employees for the right to work in the United States without discriminating on the basis of national origin.
- **Americans With Disabilities Act of 1990:** Persons with physical or mental disabilities or who are chronically ill cannot be discriminated against in the workplace. Employers must make "reasonable accommodations" to meet the needs of the disabled employee. These include such provisions as installing foot or hand controls; readjusting light switches, telephones, desks, tables, and computer equipment; providing access ramps and elevators; offering flexible work hours; and providing readers for blind employees.
- **Family Medical Leave Act of 1993:** Employers with 50 or more employees must provide up to 13 weeks of unpaid leave for family medical emergencies, childbirth, or adoption.
- **Needlestick Safety and Prevention Act of 2001:** This act directed the OSHA to revise the blood-borne pathogens standard to establish in greater detail requirements that employers identify and make use of effective and safer medical devices.

Adapted from Strader, M., & Decker, P. (1995). Role Transition to Patient Care Management. Norwalk, Conn.: Appleton and Lange; osha.gov/needlesticks/needlefact by the ANA Board of Directors, and represent constituent member associations. Additionally, state member associations often offer their own workplace advocacy information. Issues such as collective bargaining, workplace violence, mandatory overtime, staffing ratios, conflict management, delegation, ethical issues, compensation, needlestick safety, latex allergies, pollution prevention, and ergonomics are addressed.

The ANA Web site (www.nursingworld.org) keeps up-to-date information related to workplace advocacy and safety available to all nurses.

Joint Commission

The Joint Commission (JC) is an independent, nonprofit organization. Established more than 50 years ago, it is governed by a board that includes physicians, nurses, and consumers. The JC evaluates the quality and safety of care for more than 15,000 health-care organizations. To earn and maintain accreditation, organizations must have an extensive on-site review by a team of JC health-care professionals at least once every 3 years. Many of the national patient safety goals discussed in Chapter 10 were influenced by the safety of the health-care worker. For example, fatigue due to mandatory overtime has been identified as causing increased medication errors.

Institute of Medicine

The Institute of Medicine (IOM) is a private, nongovernmental organization that carries out studies at the request of many government agencies. The mission of the IOM is to improve the health of people everywhere; thus, the topics it studies are very broad (iom.edu). In 1996 the IOM began a quality initiative to assess the nation's health. Part of this initiative was the 2004 report: Keeping Patients Safe: Transforming the Work Environment of Nurses. The report identified concerns and issues related to organizational management, workforce deployment practices, work design, and organizational culture (Beyea, 2004). Each of these issues will be discussed in the section of this chapter on enhancing the quality of work life.

Programs

The primary objective of any workplace safety program is to protect staff members from harm and the organization from liability related to that harm.

The first step in development of a workplace safety program is to *recognize a potential hazard* and then take steps to control it. Based on OSHA regulations (U.S. Department of Labor, 1995), the employer must inform staff members of any potential health hazards and provide as much protection from these hazards as possible. In many cases, initial warnings come from the CDC, NIOSH, and other federal, state, and local agencies. For example, employers must provide tuberculosis testing and hepatitis B vaccine; protective equipment such as gloves, gowns, and masks; and immediate treatment after exposure for all staff members who may have contact with blood-borne pathogens. Employers are expected to remove hazards, educate employees, and establish institution-wide policies and procedures to protect their employees (Herring, 1994; Roche, 1993). Nurses who are not provided with latex gloves may refuse to participate in any activities involving blood or blood products. The employee cannot be subjected to discrimination in the workplace, and reasonable accommodations for safety against blood-borne pathogens must be provided. This may mean that the nurse with latex allergies is placed in an area where exposure to blood-borne pathogens is not an issue (Strader & Decker, 1995; U.S. Department of Labor, 1995). The OSHA also has information available on exposure to chemical or biological agents related to terrorism. Terrorism response exercises are conducted through OSHA to train health-care workers on responding to terrorism threats (http://www.osha.gov/). The second step in a workplace safety program is a *thorough assessment of the amount of risk entailed*. Staff members, for example, may become very fearful in situations that do not warrant such fear. For example:

Nancy Wu is the nurse manager on a busy geriatric unit. Most patients require total care: bathing, feeding, and positioning. She observed that several of the staff members working on the unit use poor body mechanics when lifting and moving the patients. In the last month, several of the staff members were referred to Employee Health for back pain. This week, she noticed that the patients seemed to remain in the same position for long periods and were rarely out of bed or in a chair for the entire day. When she confronted the staff, the response was the same from all of them: "I have to work for a living. I can't afford to risk a back injury for someone who may not live past the end of the week." Nancy was concerned about the care of the patients as well as the apparent lack of information her staff had about prevention of back injuries. She decided to seek assistance from the nurse practitioner in charge of Employee Health in order to develop a back injury prevention program.

Assessment of the workplace may require considerable data gathering to document the incidence of the problem and consultation with experts before a plan of action is drawn up. Health-care organizations often create formal committees, consisting of experts from within the institution and representatives from the affected departments, to assess these risks. It is important that staff members from various levels of the organization be allowed to offer input into an assessment of safety needs and risks.

The third step is to *create a plan* to provide optimal protection for staff members. It is not always a simple matter to protect staff members without interfering with the provision of patient care. For example, some devices that can be worn to prevent transmission of tuberculosis interfere with communication with the patient Some attempts have been made to limit visits or withdraw home health-care nurses from high-crime areas, but this leaves homebound patients without care (Nadwairski, 1992). A threat assessment team that evaluates problems and suggests appropriate actions may reduce the incidence and severity of problems due to violent behavior, but it may also increase employees' fear of violence if not handled well. Developing a safety plan includes the following:

- Seeking evidence-based practices and recommendations related to the problem
- Consulting federal, state, and local regulations
- Distinguishing real from imagined risks
- Seeking administrative support and enforcement for the plan
- Calculating costs of a program

The fourth and final stage in developing a workplace safety program is *implementing the program.* Educating the staff, providing the necessary safety supplies and equipment, and modifying the environment contribute to an effective program. Protecting patient and staff confidentiality and monitoring adherence to control and safety procedures should not be overlooked in the implementation stage (Jankowski, 1992).

An example of a safety program is the one for health-care workers exposed to HIV, instituted at the Department of Veterans Affairs Hospital, San Francisco (Armstrong, Gordon, & Santorella, 1995). An HIV exposure can be stressful for health-care workers and their loved ones. This employee assistance program includes up to 10 hour-long individual counseling sessions on the meaning and experience of this traumatic event. Additional counseling sessions for couples are also provided. Information about HIV and about dealing with acute stress reactions is provided. Counseling helps workers identify a plan to obtain assistance from their individual support systems, identify practice methods of dealing with blood-borne pathogens, and return to work. A systematic review related to needlestick injury provides evidence for the use of tissue adhesives.

In the past, the options for wound closure have been limited largely to sutures (needle and thread), staples, and adhesive tapes. Tissue adhesives (glues) offer the advantages that there are no sutures to remove later for the patient and no risk of needlestick injury to the health-care worker. The adhesive is applied over the surgical wound and holds the edges together until healing has occurred. Adhesives have been compared with alternative methods of surgical wound closure in eight randomized clinical trials involving 630 patients. There was no evidence of a difference in rates of wound dehiscence or infection after surgical incision closure with tissue adhesive, sutures, or adhesive tape. The recommendation from the evidence was that health-care providers may consider the use of tissue adhesives for the closure of incisions in the operating room, and a protocol was published in 2004 (Coulthard et al., 2004).

Violence

Violence in the workplace is a contemporary social issue. Newspapers and magazines have reported numerous violent incidents; one of six violent crimes occurs in the workplace, and homicide is the second leading cause of workplace death (Edwards, 1999). According to the Census of Fatal Occupational Injuries, there were 551 workplace homicides and 5703 workplace injuries in 2004. The rate of assaults on hospital workers is much higher than the rate of assaults for all private-sector industries. The Bureau of Labor Statistics measures the number of assaults resulting in injury per 10,000 full-time workers.

The overall private sector injury incidence rate is 2; the overall incidence rate for health service workers 9.3. Broken down further, the incidence rate for social service workers is 15, and the rate for nurses and personal care workers is 25 (bls.gov/news/release/cfoi.nr0).

The aggressor can be a disgruntled employee or employer, an unhappy significant other, or a person committing a random act of violence. Nurses have been identified as a group at risk for violence from patients, family members, and other staff members. Violence may also have negative organizational outcomes. Box 12-2 identifies some of the causes. Examples of violence include:

- **Threats.** Expressions of intent to cause harm, including verbal threats, threatening body language, and written threats
- **Physical assaults.** Slapping, beating, rape, homicide, and the use of weapons such as firearms, bombs, and knives
- **Muggings.** Assaults conducted by surprise with intent to rob (cdc.gov/niosh/pdfs/2002-101.pdf)

The circumstances surrounding health-care work contributes to workers' susceptibility to homicide and assault (Edwards, 1999; nursingworld.org/dlwa/osh/wp5; cdc.gov/niosh/pdfs/2002-101.pdf; www.osha.gov/)

- Prevalence of handguns and other weapons among patients, families, and friends
- Increased use of hospitals for criminal holds and violent individuals
- Increased number of acute and chronic mentally ill patients being released without follow-up care
- Health-care personnel having routine contact with the public in unrestricted areas
- Health-care personnel working alone or in small numbers
- Health-care personnel working late or until very early morning hours

box 12-2

Negative Organizational Outcomes Due to Workplace Violence

- Low worker morale
- Increased job stress
- Increased worker turnover
- Reduced trust of management
- Reduced trust of coworkers
- Hostile working environment

- Health-care personnel working in high-crime areas
- Health-care personnel working in buildings with poor security
- Health-care personnel treating weapon-carrying patients and families
- Health-care personnel working with inexperienced staff
- Health-care personnel working in units needing seclusion or restraint activities
- Health-care personnel transporting patients
- Patients waiting long times for service
- Overcrowded, uncomfortable waiting areas
- Health-care personnel lacking training and policies for managing crises

Nurses must know their workplace. For example (www/nursingworld.org/dlwa.osh/wp5?):

- How does violence from the surrounding community affect your workplace?
- Do services like trauma or acute psychiatric care increase the likelihood of violence?
- Does the facility's physical layout invite violence—for example, do doors open to the street? are waiting rooms cramped?
- How frequently do assaultive incidents, threats, and verbal abuse occur? where? who is involved? are incidents reported?
- Are current emergency response systems effective?
- Are post-assaultive treatment and support available to staff?
- Are staffing patterns sufficient? is the staff experienced?

Earlier in the chapter, the Florida nurse who was attacked and killed by a patient in April 2001 was mentioned. Although assaults that result in severe injury or death usually receive media coverage, most assaults on nurses by patients or coworkers are not reported by the nurse.

Ms. Jones works on the evening shift in the emergency department (ED) at a large urban hospital. The ED frequently receives patients who are victims of gunshot wounds, stabbings, and other gang-related incidents. Many of the patients entering the ED are high on alcohol or drugs. Ms. Jones has just interviewed a 21-year-old male patient who is awaiting treatment as a result of a fight after an evening of heavy drinking. Because his injuries have been determined not to be life-threatening, he had to wait to see a physician. "I'm tired of waiting. Let's get this show on the road," he screamed loudly as Ms. Jones walked by. "I'm sorry you have to wait, Mr. P., but the doctor is busy with another patient and will get to you as soon as possible." She handed him a cup of juice she had been bringing to another patient. He grabbed the cup, threw it in her face, and then grabbed her arm. Slamming her against the wall, he jumped off the stretcher and yelled obscenities at her. He continued to scream in her face until a security guard intervened.

Be aware of clues that may indicate a potential for violence (Box 12-3). These behaviors may occur in patients, family members, visitors, or even other staff members. Even patients with no history of violent behavior may react violently to medication or pain (Carroll & Sheverbush, 1996; Lanza & Carifio, 1991).

In the health-care industry, violence is underreported, and there are persistent misperceptions that assaults are part of the job and that the victim somehow caused the assault. Causes of underreporting may be a lack of institutional reporting policies and employee fear that the assault was a result of negligence or poor job performance (U.S. Department of Labor, 1995). Box 12-4 lists some of the faulty reasoning that leads to placing blame on the victim of the assault.

Actions to address violence in the workplace include (1) identifying the factors that contribute to violence and controlling as many as possible and (2) assessing staff attitudes and knowledge regarding violence in the workplace (Carroll & Sheverbush, 1996; Collins, 1994; Mahoney, 1991).

When you begin your new job, you may want to find out the policies and procedures related to

---

box 12-3

Behaviors Indicating a Potential for Violence

- History of violent behavior
- Delusional, paranoid, or suspicious speech
- Aggressive, threatening statements
- Rapid speech, angry tone of voice
- Pacing, tense posture, clenched fists, tightening jaw
- Alcohol or drug use
- Male gender, youth
- Policies that set unrealistic limits

Adapted from Kinkle, S. (1993). Violence in the ED: How to stop it before it starts. American Journal of Nursing, 93(7), 22–24; Carroll, C., & Sheverbush, J. (September 1996). Violence assessment in hospitals provides basis for action. American Nurse, 18.

---

box 12-4

When an Assault Occurs: Placing Blame on Victims

- **Victim gender:** Women receive more blame than men.
- **Subject gender:** Female victims receive more blame from women than men.
- **Severity:** The more severe the assault, the more often the victim is blamed.
- **Beliefs:** The world is a just place, and therefore the person deserves the misfortune.
- **Age of victim:** The older the victim, the more he or she is held to blame.

Adapted from Lanza, M.L., & Carifio, J. (1991). Blaming the victim: Complex (nonlinear) patterns of causal attribution by nurses in response to vignettes of a patient assaulting a nurse. Journal of Emergency Nursing, 17(5), 299–309.

---

violence in the workplace at your institution. Preventing an incident is better than having to intervene after violence has occurred. The following are suggestions to nurses about how to participate in workplace safety related to violence (nursingworld. org/osh/wp5/htm):

- *Participate in or initiate regular workplace assessments.* Identify unsafe areas and the factors within the organization that contribute to assaultive behavior, such as inadequate staffing, high-activity times of day, invasion of personal space, seclusion or restraint activities, and lack of experienced staff. Work with management to make and monitor changes.
- *Be alert for suspicious behavior* such as verbal expressions of anger and frustration, threatening body language, signs of drug or alcohol use, or presence of a weapon. Assess patients or suspicious workers, patients, and visitors for potential violence. Evaluate each situation for potential violence. Keep an open path for exiting.
- *Maintain behavior that helps to defuse anger.* Present a calm, caring attitude. Do not match threats, give orders, or present with behaviors that may be interpreted as aggressive. Acknowledge the person's feelings.
- *If you cannot defuse the situation,* then remove yourself from it quickly, call Security, and report the situation to management.
- *Know your patients.* Be aware of any history of violent behaviors, diagnoses of dementia, alcohol, or drug intoxication.

Box 12-5 lists some additional actions that can be taken to protect staff members and patients from violence in the workplace.

Steps Toward Increasing Protection From Workplace Violence

- Security personnel and escorts
- Panic buttons in medication rooms, stairwells, activity rooms, and nursing stations
- Bulletproof glass in reception, triage, and admitting areas
- Locked or key-coded access doors
- Closed-circuit television
- Metal detectors
- Use of beepers and/or cellular car phones
- Handheld alarms or noise devices
- Lighted parking lots
- Escort or buddy system
- Enforced wearing of photo identification badges

Adapted from Simonowitz, J. (1994). Violence in the workplace: You're entitled to protection. RN, 57(11), 61–63; nursingworld.org/dlwa/osh/wp6.

What if, in spite of all precautions, violence occurs? What should you do? You should:

- Report to your supervisor. Report threats as well as actual violence. Include a description of the situation; names of victims, witnesses, and perpetrators; and any other pertinent information.
- Call the police. Although the assault is in the workplace, nurses are entitled to the same rights as workers assaulted in another setting.
- Get medical attention. This includes medical care, counseling, and evaluation.
- Contact your collective bargaining unit or your state nurses association. Inform them if the problems persist.
- Be proactive. Get involved in policy making (nursingworld.org/ajn/2001/jul/issues).

Violence in the workplace can also be the result of horizontal violence or interactive workplace trauma. These terms denote a workplace that is infested with one or more "bullies." These bullies project domineering and aggressive behaviors toward others, usually when the other person is preoccupied or unaware. Individuals who desire to control others may use a variety of approaches, including verbal abuse, punishment, criticism, put-downs, and malicious gossip. Unfortunately, these individuals are often not identified during the employment interview. Bullies in the workplace may be coworkers, superiors, or subordinates. Regardless of their place on the organizational chart, bullies can cause a great deal of distress to others in the workplace. Barbara Broome (2008) states that bullies are like sharks. The shark tries to dominate the other fish and have

a superior presence. They attack aggressively, and when the victim bleeds, the victim becomes a fatality. Broome has suggestions for dealing with bullies in the workplace:

- Assume all identified "fish" are "sharks." Until you get to know people, do not make assumptions one way or the other.
- Do not "bleed." Crying or arguing only makes the bully more aggressive. Remove yourself from the presence of the shark.
- Admit it is difficult not to bleed, but know you can. Control your anger, and deal with facts only.
- Counter any aggression promptly. Recognize that aggression is often a prelude to an attack.
- Avoid ingratiating behaviors. You might believe that these will ward off the attack, but they will not, and you could still "lose your limb."
- Respond to all inappropriate behaviors appropriately. Bullies often believe that you will forget what they did in the last attack. Always respond appropriately.
- Make it known that the behavior is unacceptable and will not be tolerated. If the behavior continues, file a written complaint with Human Resources.

Sexual Harassment

A new supervisor on the unit needed to be hired. After months of interviewing, the candidate selected was a young male nurse whom the staff members jokingly described as "a blond Tom Cruise." The new supervisor was an instant hit with the predominantly female executives and staff members. However, he soon found himself on the receiving end of sexual jokes and innuendoes. He had been trying to prove himself a competent supervisor, with hopes of eventually moving up to a higher management position. He viewed the behavior of the female staff members and supervisors as undermining his credibility, in addition to being embarrassing and annoying. He attempted to have the unwelcome conduct stopped by discussing it with his boss, a female nurse manager. She told him jokingly that it was nothing more than "good-natured fun" and besides, "men can't be harassed by women" (Outwater, 1994).

In spite of the requirement for workplace education, sexual harassment remains one of the most persistent problems. The reasons are complex, but sex-role stereotypes and the unequal balance of power between men and women are major contributors. Unfortunately, underreporting of this problem is common, even though the emotional costs of anger, humiliation, and fear are high (nursingworld. org/dlwa/wpr/wp3/htm).

The laws that prohibit discrimination in the workplace are based on the Fifth and Fourteenth Amendments to the Constitution, mandating due process and equal protection under the law. The Equal Employment Opportunity Commission (EEOC) oversees the administration and enforcement of issues related to workplace equality. Although there may be exemptions from any law, it is important that nurses recognize that there is significant legislation that prohibits employers from making workplace decisions based on race, color, sex, age, disability, religion, or national origin. The employer may ask questions related to these issues but cannot make decisions about employment based on them. Behaviors that could be defined as sexual harassment are identified in Box 12-6. The EEOC issued a statement in 1980 that sexual harassment is a form of sex discrimination prohibited by Title VII of the Civil Rights Act of 1964. Two forms of sexual harassment are identified; both are based on the premise that the action is unwelcome sexual conduct:

1. **Quid pro quo.** Sexual favors are given in exchange for favorable job benefits or continuation of employment. The employee must demonstrate that he or she was required to endure unwelcome sexual advances to keep the job or job benefits and that rejection of these

behaviors would have resulted in deprivation of a job or benefits. Example: The administrator approaches a nurse for a date in exchange for a salary increase 3 months before the scheduled review.

2. **Hostile environment.** This is the most common sexual harassment claim and the most difficult to prove. The employee making the claim must prove that the harassment is based on gender and that it has affected conditions of employment or created an environment so offensive that the employee could not effectively discharge the responsibilities of the job (Outwater, 1994). In 1993, the Supreme Court ruled that a plaintiff is not required to prove any psychological injury to establish a harassment claim. If the environment could be shown to be hostile or abusive, then there was no further need to establish that it was also psychologically injurious. Although sexual harassment against women is more common, men can be victims as well.

Sexual harassment can cost an employer money, unfavorable publicity, expensive lawsuits, and large damage awards. Low morale caused by a hostile work environment can cause significant decreases in employee productivity, increased absenteeism, increases in sick leave and medical payments, and decreased job satisfaction.

In addition to Title VII, other legal protections include Title IX of the Education Amendments of 1972 and state fair employment statutes. Title IX of the Education Amendments of 1972 prohibits sex discrimination and sexual harassment in any educational program receiving financial assistance from the federal government. Students and employees are covered by this law. Most state fair employment statutes apply to public and private employers, employment agencies, and labor organizations. Often, state workers' compensation statutes provide remedies for employees who have been injured, either physically or psychologically, by sexual harassment in the workplace. Prohibition against sexual harassment in the workplace may also be included in collective bargaining agreements (nursingworld.org/ readroom/position/workplac/wkharass).

Addressing the issue of sexual harassment in the workplace is important. As an employee, be familiar with the policies and procedures related to reporting sexual harassment incidents. If you

---

box 12-6

Behaviors That Could Be Defined as Sexual Harassment

- Pressure to participate in sexual activities
- Asking about another person's sexual activities, fantasies, preferences
- Making sexual innuendoes, jokes, comments, or suggestive facial expressions
- Continuing to ask for a date after the other person has expressed disinterest
- Making sexual gestures with hands or body movements or showing sexual graffiti or visuals
- Making remarks about a person's gender or body

supervise other employees, regularly review your agency's policies and procedures. Seek appropriate guidance from your Human Resources personnel. If an employee approaches you with a complaint, then a confidential investigation of the charges should be initiated. Above all, do not dismiss any incidents or charges of sexual harassment involving yourself or others as "just having fun" or respond that "there is nothing anyone can do." Responses such as this can have serious consequences in the workplace (Outwater, 1994).

The ANA cites four tactics to fight sexual harassment (nursingworld.org/dlwa/wpr/wp3/htm):

1. **Confront.** Indicate immediately and clearly to the harasser that the attention is unwanted. If you are in a union facility, ask the nursing representative to accompany you.
2. **Report.** Report the incident immediately to your supervisor. If the harasser is your supervisor, report the incident to a higher authority. File a formal complaint, and follow the chain of command.
3. **Document.** Document the incident immediately while it is fresh in your mind—what happened, when and where it occurred, and how you responded. Name any witnesses. Keep thorough records, and keep them in a safe place away from work.
4. **Support.** Seek support from friends, relatives, and organizations such as your state nurses association. If you are a student, seek support from a trusted faculty member or advisor. Additionally, your employer has a responsibility to maintain a harassment-free workplace. You should expect your employer to demonstrate commitment to creating a harassment-free workplace, provide strong written policies prohibiting sexual harassment and describing how employees will be protected, and educate all employees verbally and in writing.

Latex Allergy

A nurse developed hives in 1987, nasal congestion in 1989, and asthma in 1992. She was diagnosed with latex allergy. Eventually she developed severe respiratory symptoms in the health-care environment even when she had no direct contact with latex. The nurse was forced to leave her occupation because of these health effects (Bauer et al., 1993).

A midwife initially suffered hives, nasal congestion, and conjunctivitis. Within a year, she developed asthma, and 2 years later she went into shock after a routine gynecological examination during which latex gloves were used. The midwife also suffered respiratory distress in latex-containing environments when she had no direct contact with latex products. She was unable to continue working (Bauer et al., 1993).

A physician with a history of seasonal allergies, runny nose, and eczema on his hands suffered severe runny nose, shortness of breath, and collapse minutes after putting on a pair of latex gloves. A cardiac arrest team successfully resuscitated him (Rosen et al., 1993).

Latex products are manufactured from the milky fluid of the rubber tree. Latex allergy was first identified in the late 1970s. It has become such a major health problem in the workplace that both the OSHA and the ANA have devoted Web sites to the problem. It is estimated that currently 8%–12% of health-care workers are sensitive to natural rubber latex products. Table 12-2 lists products commonly produced with latex.

Since the 1987 CDC recommendations for universal precautions, use of latex gloves has greatly increased exposure of health-care workers to natural rubber latex (NRL). The two major routes of exposure to NRL are skin and inhalation, particularly when glove powder acts as a carrier for NRL protein (OSHA latex alert: cdc.gov/niosh/latexalt). Reactions range from contact dermatitis, with scaling, drying, cracking, and blistering skin, to allergic contact dermatitis in the form of generalized hives. More serious reactions can progress to generalized urticaria, rhinitis, wheezing, swelling, shortness of breath, and anaphylaxis. According to the NIOSH, the most common reaction to latex products is irritant contact dermatitis, the development of dry, itchy, irritated areas on the skin, usually the hands. This reaction is caused by irritation from wearing gloves and by exposure to the powders added to them.

Allergic contact dermatitis (sometimes called *chemical sensitivity dermatitis*) results from the chemicals added to latex during harvesting, processing, or manufacturing. These chemicals can cause a skin rash similar to that of poison ivy. Neither irritant contact dermatitis nor chemical sensitivity dermatitis is a true allergy (cdc.gov/niosh/98-113).

table 12-2

Latex Equipment

Emergency Equipment	Personal Protective Equipment	Office Supplies	Hospital Supplies
Blood pressure cuffs	Gloves	Rubber bands	Anesthesia masks
Stethoscopes	Surgical masks	Erasers	Catheters
Disposable gloves	Goggles		Wound drains
Oral and nasal airways	Respirators		Injection ports
Endotracheal tubes	Rubber aprons		Rubber tops of multi-dose vials
Tourniquets			Dental dams
IV tubing			Hot water bottles
Syringes			Baby bottle nipples
Electrode pads			Pacifiers

Adapted from OSHA latex allergy: osha-slc.gov/SLTC/latexallergy/index; and OSHA latex alert: cdc.gov/niosh/latexalt?

Latex allergy should be suspected if an employee develops symptoms after latex exposures. A complete medical history can reveal latex sensitivity, and blood tests approved by the U.S. Food and Drug Administration are available to detect latex antibodies. Skin testing and glove-use tests are also available.

Compete latex avoidance is the most effective approach. Medications may reduce allergic symptoms, and special precautions are needed to prevent exposure during medical and dental care. Encourage employees with a latex allergy to wear a medical alert bracelet.

Decreasing the potential for development of latex allergy consists of reducing unnecessary exposure to NRL proteins for health-care workers. Many employees in a health-care setting, such as food handlers or gardeners, can use alternative gloves. If an employee must use NRL gloves, gloves with a lower protein content and those that are powder-free should be considered. Good housekeeping practices should be identified to remove latex-containing dust from the workplace. Employee education programs to ensure appropriate work practices and hand washing should be encouraged. Identification of employees with increased potential for latex allergies is not possible. However, clinical evidence indicates that certain workers may be at greater risk, including those with histories of allergies to pollens, grasses, and certain foods or plants (avocado, banana, kiwi, chestnut) and histories of multiple surgeries.

Decrease the potential for latex allergy problems (cdc.gov/niosh/98-113):

■ Evaluate any cases of hand dermatitis or other signs or symptoms of potential latex allergy.

■ Use latex-free procedure trays and crash carts.
■ Use nonlatex gloves for activities that do not involve contact with infectious materials.
■ Avoid using oil-based creams or lotions, which can cause glove deterioration.
■ Seek ongoing training and the latest information related to latex allergy.
■ Wash, rinse, and dry hands thoroughly after removing gloves or between glove changes.
■ Use powder-free gloves.

In spite of all precautions, what do you do if you develop a latex allergy? At this point, never wear latex gloves. Be aware of the following precautions (nursingworld.org/dlwa/osh/wp7):

■ Avoid all types of latex exposure.
■ Wear a medical alert bracelet.
■ Carry an Epi-kit with auto-injectible epinephrine.
■ Alert employers and colleagues to your latex sensitivity.
■ Carry nonlatex gloves.

OSHA "right to know" laws require employers to inform health-care workers of potentially dangerous substances in the workplace. For continuing information on latex allergies, see the NIOSH home page at cdc.gov/niosh

Patients as well as workers are at risk and should be screened for allergies. Patients with a history of hay fever, food allergies (especially to bananas, avocados, potatoes, tomatoes), asthma, or eczema can be at risk. Taking a thorough health history is vital. Treat any indication of potential latex sensitivity seriously (Society of Gastroenterology Nurses and Associates, 2001). As of 2006, most health-care personnel were well aware of issues related to latex allergies. In recent years, the number of new cases of latex allergy has decreased due to improved diagnostic methods, improved education, and more accurate labeling of medical devices. Although current research does not demonstrate whether the amount of allergen released during shipping and storage into medications from vials with rubber closures is sufficient to induce a systemic allergic reaction, nurses should take special precautions when patients are identified as high risk for latex allergies. The nursing staff should work closely with the pharmacy staff to follow universal one-stick-rule precautions, which assume that every pharmaceutical vial may contain a natural rubber latex closure, and the nurse should remain with any patient at the start of medication and keep frequent observations and vital signs for 2 hours (Hamilton et al., 2005).

Needlestick Injuries

In 1997 a 27-year-old nurse, Lisa Black, attended an in-service session on postexposure prophylaxis for needlesticks. A short time later, she was attempting to aspirate blood from a patient's intravenous line. The patient, in the advanced stages of acquired immunodeficiency syndrome, moved, and the needle went into Lisa's hand. Nine months later she tested positive for HIV and 3 months after that for hepatitis C. She continues to share her story with nurses everywhere in an effort to prevent this unfortunate accident from happening to one more nurse (Trossman, 1999a).

On April 18, 2001, the Needlestick Act, or revised Bloodborne Pathogens Standard, went into effect. The revised OSHA Bloodborne Pathogens Standard obligates employers to consider safer needle devices when they conduct their annual review of their exposure control plan. Frontline employees must be included in the annual review and updating of standards process. Stricter requirements are now in effect for annual review and updating to reflect changes in technology that eliminate or reduce exposure to bloodborne pathogens. JC surveyors are now asking if health-care organization leaders are familiar with the Needlestick Safety and Prevention Act and whether any action being taken to comply includes staff that use sharps and needles and are therefore at risk for injury. The law requires that these health-care workers and other staff be included in the review of safer devices as well as in making recommendations for replacement devices. (osha.gov/needlesticks/needlefaq;http://www.joint commission.org/SentinelEvents/SentinelEvent Alert/sea_22.htm)

Your Employer's Responsibility

According to the current OSHA requirements, your employer must provide you with the following (ANA, 1993; nursingworld.org/dlwa/osh/wp2):

- Free hepatitis B vaccine
- Protective equipment that fits you (gloves, gowns, goggles, masks)
- Immediate, confidential medical evaluation, treatment, and follow-up if you are exposed
- Implementation of universal precautions institution-wide
- Adequate sharps disposal
- Proper removal of hazards from the workplace
- Annual employee training

Many states have enacted their own laws related to blood-borne pathogen exposures. These laws may include some of the following requirements:

- Listing of safety devices as engineering controls
- Development of a list of available safety devices by the state for use by employers
- Development of a written exposure plan by employers and periodic review and updates
- Development of protocols for safety device identification and selection by employers and involvement by frontline workers in the process
- Development of a sharps injury log and reporting log information
- Development of methods to increase use of vaccines and personal protective equipment
- Waivers or exemptions from safety device use under certain circumstances (including patient and/or worker safety issues, use of alternative effective strategies, market unavailability, and so on)
- Placement of sharps containers in accessible positions
- Training for workers regarding safety device use (http://www.cdc.gov/niosh/topics/bbp/ ndl-law.htm)

Your Responsibility

What are your responsibilities related to this revised legislation? Each year your institution must review and update its blood-borne pathogen standards. You will need to take the time to learn new devices, and make certain that the current safety requirements are enforced with employees. Volunteer to participate in evaluation committees, or work on teams testing new devices. Follow these guidelines in your daily nursing practice (ANA, 1993; Brooke, 2001; nursingworld.org/dlwa/osh/wp2; Perry, 2001):

- Always use universal precautions.
- Use and dispose of sharps properly.
- Be immunized against hepatitis B.
- Immediately wash all exposed skin with soap and water.
- Flush affected eyes or mucous membranes with saline or water.
- Report all exposures according to your facility's protocol.
- If possible, know the HIV/hepatitis B virus status of your patient.
- Comply with postexposure follow-up.
- Support others who are exposed.
- Become active in the safety committee—be a change agent.
- Educate others.

Although health-care providers are aware of the need to use gloves as a protection against blood-borne pathogens, only one evidence-based summary has been reported regarding blood-borne pathogens and glove safety. The summary explored double gloving versus single gloving in reducing the number of infections. This includes postoperative wound infections or blood-borne infections in surgical patients and blood-borne infections in the surgical team and to determine if double gloving reduces the incidence of glove perforations compared with single gloving. A total of 18 randomized controlled trials met the inclusion criteria and were included in the review. There is clear evidence from this review that double gloving reduces the number of perforations to the innermost glove. There does not appear to be an increase in the number of perforations to the outermost glove when two pairs of gloves are worn. Korniewicz et al. (2004) participated in the first clinical trial to test the barrier integrity of nonlatex sterile surgical gloves after use in the operating room. During the 14-month study, more than 21,000 gloves were collected from more than 4000 surgical procedures. Based on results, Korniewicz et al. concluded that nonlatex or intact latex gloves provide adequate barrier protection but that nonlatex gloves may tear more frequently than latex during use.

Ergonomic Injuries

Occupational-related back injuries affect more than 75% of nurses over the lifetime of their career. Poor ergonomics is a safety factor for both nurses and patients, whose safe nursing care is already in jeopardy by the escalating nursing shortage (Durr, 2004).

Back Injuries

Back injuries are the most critical of ergonomic injuries. Annually, 12% of nurses leave the profession as a result of back injuries, and more than 52% complain of chronic back pain. Nursing aides, orderlies, and attendants ranked second and registered nurses sixth in a list of at-risk occupations for strains and sprains (DOL, 2002). The problem with lifting a patient is not just one of overcoming heavy weight. Size, shape, and deformities of the patient as well as balance and coordination, combativeness, uncooperativeness, and contractures must be considered. Any unpredictable movement or resistance from the patient can throw the nurse off balance quickly and result in a back injury. Environmental considerations such as space, equipment interference, and unadjustable beds, chairs, and commodes also contribute to back injury risk (Edlich, Woodard, & Haines, 2001).

This issue of back injuries and other ergonomic-related injuries has become so severe that in July 2001 the OSHA began to develop a comprehensive approach to ergonomics. Public forums, meetings with stakeholder groups and individuals, and written comments were analyzed. Out of this work, a four-pronged comprehensive approach to ergonomics was developed to include (osha.gov/ergonomics/ergofact02):

1. Task- or industry-specific written guidelines
2. Enforcement
3. Outreach/assistance
4. Research

The OSHA issued an ergonomics guideline for the nursing home industry on March 13, 2003. The back injury guide for health-care workers (dir.ca.gov/dosh/dosh_publications/backinj.pdf) and the OSHA guidelines for nursing homes (osha.gov/ergonomics/guidelines/nursinghome/index) are comprehensive resources. Although guidelines are less than legislated standards, the OSHA uses the General Duty Clause to cite employers for ergonomic hazards. Under this clause, employers must keep their workplaces free from recognized serious hazards, including ergonomic hazards. This requirement exists whether or not there are voluntary guidelines (osha.gov/ergonomics/FAQs-external).

The ANA, supported by the Johnson & Johnson Foundation, has begun a campaign entitled "Handle with Care." This initiative is aimed at preventing potentially career-ending back and other musculoskeletal injuries among nurses. Health-care facilities that have invested in these assistive patient handling programs report cost savings in thousands of dollars both for direct costs of back injuries and lost workdays (nursingworld.org/handlewithcare/factsheet). In addition, assistive patient handling equipment improves the quality care of patients. Dr. de Castro, senior staff specialist for occupational health and safety at the ANA, observes that such equipment:

- Improves the safety of the patient by decreasing the potential for manual patient-handling mishaps
- Increases patient comfort by taking away the human element of potentially awkward or forceful handlings
- Restores patient dignity, especially in situations when difficult handling situations impede on a person's privacy or self-esteem (de Castro, 2004)

The investment in a safe patient-handling program may seem daunting due to the cost of equipment such as mechanical lifts, transfer aids, and ergonomic beds and chairs. However, the cost savings in time, reduction of injuries, and lost workdays—as well as the improved quality of patient care—make this a sound return on investment.

Repetitive Stress Injuries

Repetitive stress injuries (RSIs) have been called the *workplace epidemic of the modern age.* RSIs usually affect people who spend long hours at computers, switchboards, and other worksites where repetitive motions are performed. The most common RSIs are carpal tunnel syndrome and mouse elbow. As technology expands in health-care facilities, the use of computers increases for all health-care personnel. Badly designed computer workstations present the highest risk of RSIs. Preventive measures (Krucoff, 2001) include the following:

- Keep the monitor screen straight ahead of you, about an arm's length away. Position the center of the screen where your gaze naturally falls.

- Align the keyboard so that your forearms, wrists, and hands are aligned parallel to the floor. Do not bend the hands back.
- Position the mouse directly next to you and on the same level as the keyboard.
- Keep thighs parallel to the floor as you sit on the chair. Feet should touch the floor, and the chair back should be ergonomically sound.
- Vary tasks. Avoid long sessions of sitting. Do not use excessive force when typing or clicking the mouse.
- Keep fingernails short, and use fingertips when typing.

Impaired Workers

Substance Abuse

Sue had been a nurse for 20 years. Current marital and family problems were affecting her at work. To ease the tension, she took a Xanax from a patient's medication drawer. This seemed to ease her tension. She continued to take medications, working her way up to narcotic analgesics.

Bill had begun weekend binge-drinking in college. Ten years later, he continues the habit several times during the month. He does not believe he is an alcoholic because he can "control" his drinking. After he begins showing up at work hung over and making medication errors, he is fired for the medication errors. At the exit interview, no mention is made of his drinking problem. The agency feared a lawsuit for defamation of character.

Mr. P., the unit manager, has noticed that Ms. J. has been late for work frequently. She arrives with a wrinkled uniform, dirty shoes, unkempt hair, and broken nails. Lately she has been overheard making terse remarks to patients such as, "Who do you think I am—your maid?," and spends longer and longer periods off the unit. The floor has a large number of surgical patients who receive intramuscular and oral medications for pain. Lately, Ms. J.'s patients continue to complain of pain even after medication administration has been charted. Ms. J. frequently forgets to waste her intramuscular narcotics in front of another nurse. Mr. P. is concerned that Ms. J. may be an impaired nurse.

As nursing education moved from the untrained nurse—embodied in the character of Sairey Gamp in the Dickens novel *Martin Chuzzlewit*—to the educated Florence Nightingale model, nurses were expected to be of good moral character. The problem of addiction among nurses was not discussed until the 1950s, with addicted nurses receiving little sympathy or treatment from their peers. Research on addicted medical professionals increased in the 1970s, followed by major help for nurses with addictive disease in 1980. At this time, the National Nurses' Society on Addictions (NNSA) task force and the ANA task force on addictions and psychological functions jointly passed a resolution calling for acknowledgment of the problem and guidelines for impaired nurse programs (Heise, 2003).

Alcohol and drug abuse continue to be major health problems in the United States. Health-care professionals are not immune to alcoholism or chemical dependency. In addition, various kinds of mental illnesses may also affect a nurse's ability to deliver safe, competent care. Impaired workers can adversely affect patient care, staff retention, morale, and management time as team members try to pick up the slack for the impaired worker (Damrosch & Scholler-Jaquish, 1993). The most common signs of impairment are (Blair, 2005; Damrosch & Scholler-Jaquish, 1993):

- Witnessed consumption of alcohol or other substances on the job
- Changes in dress, appearance, posture, gestures
- Slurred speech; abusive/incoherent language
- Reports of impairment or erratic behavior from patients and/or coworkers
- Witnessed unprofessional conduct
- Significant lack of attention to detail
- Witnessed theft of controlled substances
- When assigned patients routinely request pain medication within a short period of being medicated

Most employers and state boards of nursing have strict guidelines related to impaired nurses. Impaired-nurse programs, which are conducted by state boards of nursing, work with the employer to assist the impaired nurse to remain licensed while receiving help for the addiction problem. It is important that you become aware of workplace issues surrounding the impaired worker, signs and symptoms of impairment, and the policies and reporting procedures concerning an impaired worker. Compassion from coworkers and supervisors is of utmost importance in assisting the impaired worker to seek help (Damrosch & Scholler-Jaquish, 1993; Sloan & Vernarec, 2001).

The National Council of State Boards lists all state boards of nursing. Information on support programs for impaired nurses can be obtained from each state board (ncsbn.org/regulation/nursingpractice_npa_pennrn.asp).

Upholding the standards of the nursing profession is everyone's responsibility. Often coworkers, noticing a change in another's behavior, become protective and take on more work to ease the burden of their coworker. Although it is difficult to report a colleague, covering up or ignoring the problem can cause serious risks for the patient and the nurse. Many state boards make it mandatory for nurses to report suspected impaired coworkers; most states accept anonymous reports. In many states, state law requires hospitals and health-care providers to report impaired practitioners, but the law also grants immunity from civil liability if the report was made in good faith (Blair, 2005; Sloan & Vernarec, 2001).

Microbial Threats

Health-care workers are an at-risk group for several microbial threats. Severe acute respiratory syndromes (SARS) is a respiratory illness that has been reported in Asia, Europe, and North America. According to the World Health Organization, 8098 people worldwide became sick with SARS during the 2003 outbreak.

SARS begins with a high fever and mild respiratory symptoms. Other symptoms may include headache, an overall feeling of discomfort, and body aches. It is not uncommon for the person to have diarrhea and develop a dry cough. Most patients develop pneumonia. The virus that causes SARS is thought to be transmitted most readily by respiratory droplets. The virus can also spread when a person touches a surface or object contaminated with infectious droplets and then touches his or her mouth, nose, or eyes. In addition, it is possible that the SARS virus might spread more broadly through the air (airborne spread) or by other ways that are not known. The CDC provides current information on the handling of SARS in the workplace (cdc.gov).

Unlike the newer microbial threat SARS, tuberculosis (TB) was a leading cause of death among infectious diseases from the 19th into the mid-20th centuries. Although TB rates declined in the 1990s, they are currently on the rise as resources that were committed to fighting the disease were withdrawn. A more serious form of TB, mutidrug-resistant tuberculosis (MDR-TB) is on the rise. Nurses often come in contact with persons with active TB. At times, patients do not know they are infected until coming to the hospital with another complaint. As with SARS, the CDC provides current information and guidelines for dealing with TB in the workplace (cdc.gov/nchstp/tb/pubs/TB_HIVcoinfection/default).

Enhancing the Quality of Work Life

The continued nursing shortage enforces an awareness to "treat with kindness" the nurses who remain in the workforce.

Rotating Shifts

Safety in the workplace involves nurses working rotating shifts. Nurses who work permanently at night often readjust their sleep-wake cycle. However, even permanent night-workers may be subjected to continuous sleep deprivation. Nurses who randomly rotate shifts throw off their circadian rhythm. Fatigue, the primary complaint of these nurses, is the result of the body never getting the chance to adapt to changing sleep-wake cycles. The literature links some of the world's worst disasters, such as the Chernobyl nuclear reactor catastrophe and the Exxon Valdez oil spill, to rotating shift work and the changes in circadian rhythm. Other effects of shift work include a higher risk of miscarriage and premature labor, menstrual and digestive problems, and respiratory irritation. One of the most serious results of rotating night shifts is the increasing number of nurses affected by coronary heart disease (CHD). Studies indicate that nurses who rotate to nights for 6 years have a 70% greater risk of developing CHD than nurses who never rotated shifts due to the circadian effect of lowering of blood pressure and heart rate at night (Trossman, 1999b). Suggestions for nurses who rotate shifts:

- Try to schedule working the same shifts for an entire scheduling period instead of rotating different shifts in one schedule.
- Try to schedule to same days off within the schedule.
- If you become sleepy during the shift, take a walk or climb stairs.
- Limit caffeine intake, especially toward the end of the shift.
- If you work evenings or nights, do not eat a big meal at the end of the shift. This interferes with sleep.
- Try to sleep a continuous block of time instead of catching a few hours here and there.
- Make the room you are sleeping in as dark and noise-free as possible.
- Maintain good nutrition and an exercise program.
- Negotiate your schedule with your manager. If you and your colleagues feel strongly about eliminating rotating shifts, work together to make changes (Trossman, 1999b).

Mandatory Overtime

When nurses are forced routinely to work beyond their scheduled hours, they can suffer a range of emotional and physical effects. As patient acuity and workloads increase, nurses working overtime put both patients and nurses at greater risk. Mandatory overtime is seen by nurses as a control issue. Working overtime should be a choice, not a requirement. In some facilities, nurses are being threatened with dismissal or charge of patient abandonment if they refuse to participate in mandatory overtime (nursingworld.org/tan/98mayjun/ot).

The ANA presented the following message to the 107th Congress in 2001: "ANA opposes the use of mandatory overtime as a staffing tool. We urge you to support legislation that would ban the use of mandatory overtime through Medicare and Medicaid law. Nurses must be given the opportunity to refuse overtime if we believe that we are too fatigued to provide quality care" (nursingworld.org/gova/federal/legis/107/ovrtme). Dembe, Erickson, Delbros, and Banks (2005) analyzed the occurrence of occupational injury and illness between 1987 and 2000. After a review of 10,793 participants working at least 12 hours per day, working overtime was associated with a 23% increased work hazard and a 61% higher injury hazard rate compared with jobs without overtime. More recently, Rogers et al. (2004) found that nurses' error rates increase significantly during overtime, after 12 hours and over more than 60 hours per week. Currently, there are no regulations governing nurses' work hours. About half of staff nurses are scheduled routinely to work 12-hour shifts, and 85% of staff nurses routinely work longer than scheduled hours.

Staffing Ratios

Although some state nurses associations are calling for mandated staffing ratios, the issue is not clear-cut. What has become clear is that there is no "one size fits all" solution. In 2004 a review was conducted of peer-reviewed studies published between 1980 and 2003 of the effects of nurse staffing on patient, nurse employee, and hospital outcomes. The literature offered no support for specific nurse-patient ratios. However, findings from 12 key studies stood out, citing specific effects of nurse staffing on patient outcomes: incidences of failure to rescue, in-patient mortality, pnuemonia, urinary tract infections, and pressure ulcers. Effects of nurse staffing levels on nurse employee outcomes included needlestick injuries, nursing burnout, and nursing documentation, whereas hospital length of stay, financial outcomes, and direct nursing care were experienced by the hospital. Table 12-3 provides a matrix for staffing decision making.

Above all, the ANA recommends moving staffing away from an industrial model of measuring time and motion to a more professional model that examines factors needed to provide quality care. Changes in staffing levels should be based on analysis of nursing-sensitive indicators (nursingworld.org/readroom/stffprnc).

Using Unlicensed Assistive Personnel

Educational preparation and clinical experiences in practice for nurses differs for basic registered nurse (RN) education. The nursing shortage will continue to force health-care facilities to explore creative ways of providing safe and effective patient care. This will most likely include RNs working with not only licensed practical nurses (LPNs) but also with unlicensed assistive personnel (UAP). The legal regulation of nursing practice is defined by each state nursing practice act; however, the ANA believes that "curricula for all RN programs should include content on supervision, delegation, assignment, and legal aspects regarding nursing's utilization of assistive personnel" (nursingworld.org/readroom/position/uap/uaprned).

Hospital workforce issues will continue to be influenced by economic changes, managed care and insurance issues, media forces, and the nursing shortage. Linda Aiken has been researching relationships between positive patient, nurse, and agency outcomes and RN staffing, educational preparation, and organizational culture (Aiken, 2002, 2004). Nurses voice disillusionment with nursing practice and decreased loyalty to organizations. Nursing leaders in the 21st century must demonstrate a respect and value for their nursing staff, communicate effectively with all levels of the organization, maintain visibility, and establish participative decision making. As you move forward in your career, be part of the solution, not the problem (Ray, Turkel, & Marino, 2002).

Reporting Questionable Practices

Most employers have policies that encourage the reporting of behavior that may affect the workplace environment. Behaviors to report may include (ANA, 1994):

1. Endangering a patient's health or safety
2. Abusing authority
3. Violating laws, rules, regulations, or standards of professional ethics
4. Grossly wasting funds

The Code for Nurses (ANA, 2001) is very specific about nurses' responsibility to report questionable behavior that may affect the welfare of a patient:

When a nurse is aware of inappropriate or questionable practice in the provision of health care, concern should be expressed to the person carrying out the questionable practice and attention called to the possible detrimental effect on the patient's welfare. When factors in the health-care delivery system threaten the welfare of the patient, similar action should be directed to the responsible administrative person. If indicated, the practice should then be reported to the appropriate authority within the

table 12-3	
Matrix for Decision Making: Staffing	
Patients	Characteristics and number of patients requiring care
Intensity of Unit and Care	Intensity of individuals within and across the unit; variability of care; admissions, discharges, transfers, volume
Context	Architecture of unit; technology available
Expertise	Staff consistency, continuity, and cohesion; staff preparation and experience
Other	Quality improvement activities; nursing control of practice

Adapted from nursingworld.org/readroom/stffprnc

institution, agency, or larger system (ANA, 2001). The sources of various federal and state guidelines governing the workplace are listed in Box 12-7.

Protection by the agency should be afforded to both the accused and the person doing the reporting. *Whistleblower* is the term used for an employee who reports employer violations to an outside agency. Do not assume that doing the right thing will protect you. Speaking up could get you fired unless you are protected by a union contract or other formal employment agreement. In May 1994, the U.S. Supreme Court ruled that nurses who direct the work of other employees may be considered supervisors and therefore may not be covered by the protections guaranteed under the National Labor Relations Act. This ruling may cause nurses to have no protection from retaliation if they report illegal practices in the workplace (ANA, 1995b). The 1995 brochure from the ANA (1995a), *Protect Your Patients—Protect Your License,* states, "Be aware that reporting quality and safety issues may result in reprisals by an employer." Does this mean that you should never speak up? Case law, federal and state statutes, and the federal False Claims Act may afford a certain level of protection. Some states have whistleblower laws. They usually apply only to state employees or to certain types of workers. Although these laws may offer some protection, the most important point is to work through the employer's chain of command and internal procedures: (a) make sure that whistleblowing is addressed at your facility, either through a collective bargaining contract or workplace advocacy program; (b) contact your state nurses association to find out if your state offers whistleblower protection or has such legislation pending; (c) be

politically active by contacting your state legislators and urge them to support a pending bill or by educating your elected state officials on the need for such protection for all health-care workers; and (d) contact your U.S. congressional representatives and urge them to support the Patient Safety Act (nursingworld.org/tan/98janfeb/nlrbmass).

It is the responsibility of professional nurses to become acquainted with the state and federal regulations, standards of practice and professional performance, and agency protocols and practice guidelines governing their practice. Lack of knowledge will not protect you from ethical and legal obligations. Your state nurses association can help you seek information related to incompetent, unethical, or illegal practices. When you join your state association, you will gain access to an organization that has input into policies and procedures designed to protect the public.

Although the rights of disabled nurses are not usually considered "questionable practices," the ANA is concerned with those rights. The Americans With Disabilities Act, enacted in 1990, makes it unlawful to discriminate against a qualified individual with a disability. The employer is required to provide reasonable accommodations for the disabled person. A reasonable accommodation is a modification or adjustment to the job, work environment, work schedule, or work procedures that enable a qualified person with a disability to perform the job. Both you and your employer may see information from the Equal Employment Opportunity Commission (EEOC) for information (nursingworld.org/dlwa/wpr/wp6).

Terrorism and Other Disasters

Since the attacks on the World Trade Center and the Pentagon as well as the anthrax outbreaks and continued terrorist threats nationwide, concerns related to biological and chemical agents have surfaced. The CDC Web site (bt.cdc.gov/) supports ongoing information related to public health emergency preparedness and response. The ANA has published a position statement for employers on work release during a disaster. In addition, the ANA provides RNs with valuable information on how they can better care for their patients, protect themselves, and prepare their hospitals and communities to respond to acts of bioterrorism and natural disasters (nursingworld.org/news/disaster/). For example,

---

box 12-7

Laws Governing Health-Care Practices

- State nurse practice acts
- Federal and state health regulations
- State and federal pharmacy laws for controlled substances
- OSHA
- State medical records and communicable disease laws
- Environmental laws regulating hazardous waste and air and water quality
- CDC guidelines
- Federal and state antidiscrimination laws
- State clinical laboratory regulations
- JCAHO regulations

Adapted from American Nurses Association. (1994). Guidelines on Reporting Incompetent, Unethical, or Illegal Practices. *Washington, DC: ANA.*

many nurses worked with the ANA to provide support for the victims of Hurricane Katrina.

Your importance in emergency readiness and bioterrorism is important. Following are some suggestions for steps that can be implemented in the workplace (awhonn.org/HealthPolicyLegislative/BIOTERRORISMPREPAREDNESS/bioterrorismpreparedness):

- Know the evacuation procedures and routes in your facility.
- Develop your knowledge of the most likely and dangerous biochemical agents.
- Monitor for unusual disease patterns, and notify appropriate authorities as needed.
- Know the backup systems available for communication and staffing in the event of emergencies.
- Know the disaster policies and procedures in your facility as well as state and federal laws that pertain to licensed personnel.

Enhancing the Quality of Work Life

Both the social and physical aspects of a workplace can affect the way in which people work and how they feel about their jobs. The social aspects include working relationships, a climate that allows growth and creativity, and cultural diversity.

Social Environment

Working Relationships

Many aspects of the social environment received attention in earlier chapters. Team building, communicating effectively, and developing leadership skills are essential to the development of working relationships. The day-to-day interactions with one's peers and supervisors have a major impact on the quality of the workplace environment.

Support of One's Peers and Supervisors

Most employees feel keenly the difference between a supportive and a nonsupportive environment:

Ms. B. came to work already tired. Her baby was sick and had been awake most of the night. Her team expressed concern about the baby when she told them she had a difficult night. Each team member voluntarily took an extra patient so that Ms. B. could have a lighter assignment that day. When Ms. B. expressed her appreciation, her team leader said, "We know you would do the same for us." Ms. B. worked in a supportive environment.

Ms. G. came to work after a sleepless night. Her young son had been diagnosed with leukemia, and she was very worried about him. When she mentioned her concerns, her team leader interrupted her, saying, "Please leave your personal problems at home. We have a lot of work to do, and we expect you to do your share." Ms. G. worked in a nonsupportive environment.

Support from peers and supervisors involves professional concerns as well as personal ones. In a supportive environment, people are willing to make difficult decisions, take risks, and "go the extra mile" for team members and the organization. In contrast, in a nonsupportive environment, members are afraid to take risks, avoid making decisions, and usually limit their commitment.

Involvement in Decision Making

The importance of having a voice in the decisions made about one's work and patients cannot be overstated. Empowerment is a related phenomenon. It is a sense of having both the ability and the opportunity to act effectively (Kramer & Schmalenberg, 1993). Empowerment is the opposite of apathy and powerlessness. Many actions can be taken to empower nurses: remove barriers to their autonomy and to their participation in decision making, publicly express confidence in their capability and value, reward initiative and assertiveness, and provide role models who demonstrate confidence and competence. The following illustrates the difference between empowerment and powerlessness:

Soon after completing orientation, Nurse A heard a new nurse aide scolding a patient for soiling the bed. Nurse A did not know how incidents of potential verbal abuse were handled in this institution, so she reported it to the nurse manager. The nurse manager asked Nurse A several questions and thanked her for the information. The new aide was counseled immediately after their meeting. Nurse A noticed a positive change in the aide's manner with patients after this incident. Nurse A felt good about having contributed to a more effective patient care team. Nurse A felt empowered and will take action again when another occasion arises.

A colleague of Nurse B was an instructor at a community college. This colleague asked Nurse B if students would be welcome on her unit. "Of course," replied Nurse B. "I'll speak with my head nurse about it." When Nurse B did so, the response was that the unit was too busy to accommodate students. In addition, Nurse B received a verbal reprimand from the supervisor for overstepping her authority by discussing the placement of students. "All requests for student placement must be directed to the education department," she said. The supervisor directed Nurse B to write a letter of apology for having made an unauthorized commitment to the community college. Nurse B was afraid to make any decisions or public statements after this incident. Nurse B felt alienated and powerless.

Professional Growth and Innovation

The difference between a climate that encourages staff growth and creativity and one that does not can be quite subtle. In fact, many people are only partly aware, if at all, whether they work in an environment that fosters professional growth and learning. Yet the effect on the quality of the work done is pervasive, and it is an important factor in distinguishing the merely good health-care organization from the excellent health-care organization.

Much of the responsibility for staff development and promotion of innovation lies with upper-level management, people who can sponsor seminars, conduct organization-wide workshops, establish educational policies, promote career mobility, develop clinical ladders, initiate innovative projects, and reward suggestions.

Some of the ways in which first-line managers can develop and support a climate of professional growth are to encourage critical thinking, provide opportunities to take advantage of educational programs, encourage new ideas and projects, and reward professional growth.

Encourage Critical Thinking

If you ever find yourself or staff members saying, "Don't ask why. Just do it!" then you need to evaluate the type of climate in which you are functioning. An inquisitive frame of mind is relatively easy to suppress in a work environment. Patients and staff members quickly perceive a nurse's impatience or defensiveness when too many questions are raised. Their response will be to simply give up asking these questions.

On the other hand, if you support critical thinkers and act as a role model who adopts a questioning attitude, you can encourage others to do the same.

Seek Out Educational Opportunities

In most organizations, first-line managers do not have discretionary funds that can be allocated for educational purposes. However, they can usually support a staff member's request for educational leave or for financial support and often have a small budget that can be used for seminars or workshops.

Team leaders and nurse managers can make it either easier or more difficult for staff members to further their education. They can make things difficult for the staff member who is trying to balance work, home, and school responsibilities, or they can help lighten the load of the staff member who has to finish a paper or take an examination. Unsupportive supervisors have even attacked staff members who pursue further education, criticizing every minor error and blocking their advancement. Obviously, such behavior should be dealt with quickly by upper-level management because it is a serious inhibitor of staff development.

Encourage New Ideas

The increasingly rapid accumulation of knowledge in health care mandates continuous learning for safe practice. Intellectual curiosity is a hallmark of the professional.

Every move up the professional ladder should bring new challenges that enrich one's work (Roedel & Nystrom, 1987). As a professional, you can be a role model for an environment in which every staff member is both challenged and rewarded for meeting these challenges. Participating in brainstorming sessions, group conferences, and discussions encourages the generation of new ideas. Although new nurses may think they have nothing to offer, it is important for them to participate in activities that encourage them to look at fresh, new ideas.

Reward Professional Growth

A primary source of discontent in the workplace is lack of recognition. Positive feedback and recognition of contributions are important rewards. Everyone enjoys praise and recognition. A smile, a card or note, or a verbal "thank you" goes a long way with coworkers in recognizing a job well done. Staff recognition programs have also been identified as a means of increasing self-esteem, social gratification, morale, and job satisfaction (Hurst, Croker, & Bell, 1994).

Cultural Diversity

Ms. V. is beginning orientation as a new staff nurse. She has been told that part of her orientation will be a morning class on cultural diversity. She says to the Human Resources person in charge of orientation, "I don't think I need to attend that class. I treat all people as equal. Besides, anyone living in the United States has an obligation to learn the language and ways of those of us who were born here, not the other way around."

Mr. M. is a staff nurse on a medical–surgical unit. A young man with HIV infection has been admitted. He is scheduled for surgery in the morning and has requested that his significant other be present for the preoperative teaching. Mr. M. reluctantly agrees but mumbles under his breath to a coworker, "It wouldn't be so bad if they didn't throw their homosexuality around and act like an old married couple. Why can't he act like a man and get his own preop instructions?"

Diversity in health-care organizations includes ethnicity, race, culture, gender, lifestyle, primary language, age, physical capabilities, and career stages of employees. The composition of nurses in health care is changing to include more older workers, minorities, and men. Working with people who have different customs, traditions, communication styles, and beliefs can be exciting as well as challenging. An organization that fosters diversity encourages respect and understanding of human characteristics and acceptance of the similarities and differences that make us human.

Often, when stressful situations arise, gender, age, and culture can contribute to misunderstandings. Davidhizer, Dowd, and Giger (1999) identified six important factors in their model for understanding cultural diversity:

1. **Communication.** Communication and culture are closely bound. Culture is transmitted through communication, and culture influences how verbal and nonverbal communication is expressed. Vocabulary, voice qualities, intonation, rhythm, speed, silence, touch, body postures, eye movements, and pronunciation differ among cultural groups and vary among persons from similar cultures. Using respect as a central core to a relationship, everyone needs to assess personal beliefs and communication variables of others in the workplace.

2. **Space.** Personal space is the area that surrounds a person's body. The amount of personal space individuals prefer varies from person to person and from situation to situation. Cultural beliefs also influence a person's personal space comfort zone. In the workplace, an understanding of coworkers' comfort related to personal space is important. Often, this comfort is relayed in nonverbal rather than verbal communication.

3. **Social organization.** In most cultures, the family is the most important social organization. For some people, the importance of family supersedes that of other personal, work, or national causes; for example, caring for a sick child overrides the importance of being on time or even coming to work, regardless of staffing needs or policies. Because the health-care industry employs a large number of women, the value of the family becomes an important issue in the workplace.

4. **Time.** Time orientation is often related to culture, environment, and family experiences. Some cultures are more past-oriented and focus on maintaining traditions, with little interest in goals. People from cultures with more of a present and future orientation may be more likely to engage in activities, such as returning to school or receiving certifications that will enhance the future. Working with people who have different time orientations may cause difficulty in planning schedules and setting deadlines for the group.

5. **Environment control.** Environmental control consists of those activities that an individual plans for controlling nature. Environmental control is best understood through the psychological terms *internal* and *external locus of control*. Individuals with an external locus of control believe in fate or chance. People with an internal locus of control believe in developing plans and directing their environment. In the workplace, nurses are expected to operate from an internal locus of control. This approach may be different from what a person has grown up with or how a patient deals with illness.

6. **Biological variations.** More and more information is available to health-care workers about the variations among races in aspects such as body structure, skin color, genetic variations, susceptibility to disease, and psychological differences. The Joint Commission states that

cultural factors must be assessed in developing materials for patient education.

As you begin your career, be alert to the signs of cultural diversity or insensitivity where you work. Signs that increased sensitivity and responsiveness to the needs of a culturally diverse workforce are needed on your team or in your organization may include a greater proportion of minorities or women in lower-level jobs, lower career mobility and higher turnover rates in these groups, and acceptance or even approval of insensitivity and unfairness (Malone, 1993). Observe interaction patterns, such as where people sit in the cafeteria or how they cluster during coffee breaks. Are they mixing freely, or are there divisions by gender, race, language, or status in the organization (Moch & Diemert, 1987; Ward, 1992)? Other indications of an organization's diversity "fitness" include the following (Mitchell, 1995):

- The personnel mix reflects the current and potential population being served.
- Individual cultural preferences pertaining to issues of social distance, touching, voice volume and inflection, silence, and gestures are respected.
- There is awareness of special family and holiday celebrations important to people of different cultures.
- The organization communicates through action that people are individuals first and members of a particular culture second.

Effective management of cultural diversity requires considerable time and energy. Although organized cultural diversity programs are usually the responsibility of middle- and upper-level managers, you can play a part in raising awareness. You can be a culturally competent practitioner and a role model for others by becoming:

- Aware of and sensitive to your own culture-based preferences
- Willing to explore your own biases and values
- Knowledgeable about other cultures
- Respectful of and sensitive to diversity among individuals
- Skilled using and selecting culturally sensitive intervention strategies

Physical Environment

Attention to the physical environment of the workplace is not as well developed as to the social aspect, especially in nursing. The increasing focus on workplace ergonomics—such as modifications to various elements of the physical environment, including floors, chairs, desks, beds, and workstations, to decrease the incidence of back and upper extremity injuries—has already been discussed. The use of lighting, colors, and music to improve the workplace environment is increasing. Computer workstations designed to promote efficiency in the patient care unit are becoming commonplace. Relocation of supplies and substations closer to patient rooms to reduce the number of steps, improved visual and auditory scanning of patients from the nurses' station, better light and ventilation, a unified information system, and reduced need for patient transport are all possible with changes in the physical environment.

Health-care pollution is a more recently identified problem. Dioxin emissions, mercury, and battery waste are often not disposed properly in the hospital environment. Disinfectants, chemicals, waste anesthesia gases, and laser plumes that float in the air are other sources of pollution exposure for nurses. Nurses have a responsibility to be aware of these potential problems and identify areas in the hospital at risk. Rethinking product choices, such as avoiding the use of polyvinyl chloride or mercury products, providing convenient collection sites for battery and mercury waste, and making waste management education for employees mandatory are starts toward a more pollution-free environment (Slattery, 1998). The purchase of recycled paper and products, waste treatment choices that minimize toxic disinfectants, and waste disposal choices that reduce incineration to a maximum are needed. Nurses as professionals need to be aware of the consequences of the medical waste produced by the health sector, supporting continued education for both nurses and patients.

Conclusion

Workplace safety is an area of increasing concern. Staff members have a right to be informed of any potential risks in the workplace. Employers have a responsibility to provide adequate equipment and supplies to protect employees and to create programs and policies to inform employees about minimizing risks to the extent possible. Issues of workplace violence, sexual harassment, impaired workers, ergonomics and workplace injuries, and terrorism should be addressed to protect both employees and patients. The IOM and JCAHO patient safety initiatives will continue to affect the way nurses do business. Workplace issues related to nursing and positive patient outcomes will continue to be discussed.

A social environment that promotes professional growth and creativity and a physical environment that offers comfort and maximum work efficiency should be considered in improving the quality of work life. Cultural awareness, respect for the diversity of others, and increased contact between groups should be the goals of the workforce for the next century.

Many waking hours are spent in the workplace. It can offer a climate of companionship, professional growth, and excitement. Everyone is responsible for promoting a safe, healthy work environment for each other.

Study Questions

1. Why is it important for nurses to understand the major federal laws and agencies responsible to protect the individual in the workplace?

2. What actions can nurses take if they believe that OSHA guidelines are not being followed in the workplace?

3. What are nurses' responsibilities in dealing with the following workplace issues: transmission of blood-borne pathogens, violence, sexual harassment, and impaired coworkers?

4. What information do you need to obtain from your employer related to terrorism and other disasters?

5. What will you look for in the work environment that will support positive patient outcomes?

6. Discuss experiences you have had in your clinical rotations. Were the environments supportive or nonsupportive social environments? What recommendations would you make for improvement?

7. Review the ten areas of concern for *Nursing's Agenda for the Future*. Identify what contributions you will make now and in the future to support this agenda.

Case Study to Promote Critical Reasoning

You have been hired as a new RN on a busy pediatric unit in a large metropolitan hospital. The hospital provides services for a culturally diverse population, including African-American, Asian, and Hispanic people. Family members often attempt alternative healing practices specific to their culture and bring special foods from home to entice a sick child to eat. One of the more experienced nurses said to you, "We need to discourage these people from fooling with all this hocus pocus. We are trying to get their sick kid well in the time allowed under their managed care plans, and all this medicine-man stuff is only keeping the kid sick longer. Besides, all this stuff stinks up the rooms and brings in bugs." You have observed how important these healing rituals and foods are to the patients and families and believe that both the families and the children have benefited from this nontraditional approach to healing.

1. What are your feelings about nontraditional healing methods?

2. How should you respond to the experienced nurse?

3. How can you be a patient advocate without alienating your coworkers?

4. What could you do to assist your coworkers in becoming more culturally sensitive to their patients and families?

5. How can health-care facilities incorporate both Western and nontraditional medicine? Should they do this? Why or why not?

References

Aiken, L.H. (2004). Nurse Burnout and Patient Satisfaction, *Journal of the American Medical Association,* 42(2), 57–66.

Aiken, L.H., Clarke, S.P., Sloane, D.M., et al. (2002) Hospital nurse staffing and patient mortality, nurse burnout, and job dissatisfaction. *Journal of the American Medical Association,* 288(16), 1987–1991.

American Nurses Association. (2001). *Code for Nurses.* Washington, DC: ANA.

American Nurses Association. (1994). *Guidelines on Reporting Incompetent, Unethical, or Illegal Practices.* Washington, DC: ANA.

American Nurses Association. (1993). *HIV, Hepatitis-B, Hepatitis-C: Blood-Borne Diseases.* Washington, DC: ANA.

American Nurses Association. (1995a). *Protect Your Patients— Protect Your License.* Washington, DC: ANA.

American Nurses Association. (1995b). *The Supreme Court Has Issued the Ultimate Gag Order for Nurses.* Washington, DC: ANA.

American Nurses Association. (2007). *Occupational health.* Retrieved July 10, 2009, from http://www.nursingworld.org/MainMenuCategories/OccupationalandEnvironmental/occupationalhealth.aspx

Arbury, S. (2002). Healthcare workers at risk. *Job Safety and Health Care Quarterly,* 13(2), 30–31.

Armstrong, K., Gordon, R., & Santorella, G. (1995). Occupational exposure of healthcare workers to HIV. *Social Work in Health Care,* 21(3), 61–80.

Bauer, X., Ammon, J., Chen, Z., Beckman, W., et al. (1993). Health risk in hospitals through airborne allergens for patients pre-sensitized to latex. *Lancet,* 342, 1148–1149.

Beyea, S. (2004). A critical partnership-safety for nurses and patients. *AORN,* 79(6), 1299–1302.

Blair, D. (2005). Spot the signs of drug impairment. *Nursing Management,* 36(2), 20–21, 52.

Brooke, P. (2001). The legal realities of HIV exposure. *RN,* 64(12), 71–73.

Broome, B. (2008). Dealing with sharks and bullies in the workplace. *ABNF Journal,* winter 2008, 28–30.

Carroll, C., & Sheverbush, J. (September 1996). Violence assessment in hospitals provides basis for action. *American Nurse,* 18.

Centers for Disease Control and Prevention (CDC). (1992). Surveillance for occupationally acquired HIV infection— United States, 1981–1992. *MMWR,* 41(43), 823–825.

Chisholm, R.F. (1992). Quality of working life: A crucial management perspective for the year 2000. *Journal of Health and Human Resources Administration,* 15(1), 6–34.

Collins, J. (1994). Nurses' attitudes toward aggressive behavior following attendance at "The Prevention and Management of Aggressive Behavior Programme." *Journal of Advanced Nursing,* 20, 117–131.

Coulthard, P., Worthington, H., Esposito, M., van der Est, M., et al. (2004). Tissue adhesives for closures of surgical incisions. *Cochrane Database of Systemic Reviews,* Issue 2.

Damrosch, S., & Scholler-Jaquish, A. (1993). Nurses' experiences with impaired nurse coworkers. *Applied Nursing Research,* 6(4), 154–160.

Davidhizar, R., Dowd, S., Giger, J. (1999). Managing diversity in the healthcare workplace. *Health Care Supervisor,* 17(3), 51–62.

De Castro, A.B. (2004). Handle with care: The ANA campaign on work-related musculoskeletal injuries. Accessed April 13, 2008, from http://www.nursingworld.org/MainMenuCategories/ANAMarketplace/ANAPeriodicals/OJIN/TableofContents/Volume92004/Number3September30/HandleWithCare.aspx#USDL02

Dembe, A.E., Erickson, J.B., Delbros, R.G., & Banks, S.M. (2005). The impact of overtime and long work hours on occupational injuries and illness: New evidence from the U.S. *Occupational and Environmental Medicine,* 62(9), 588–597.

Durr, L. (2004). Commission on Workforce Issues: What nurses should expect in the workplace: The ANA Bill of Rights for Registered Nurses. *Virginia Nurses Today,* 12(2), 17.

Edlich, R., Woodard, C., & Haines, M. (2001). Disabling back injuries in nursing personnel. *Journal of Emergency Nursing,* 27(2), 150–155.

Edwards, R. (1999). Prevention of workplace violence. *Aspen's Advisor for Nurse Executives,* 14(8), 8–12.

Hamilton, R., Brown, R., Veltri, M., Feroli, R., et al. (2005). Administering pharaceuticals to latex allergy patients from vials containing natural rubber latex closures. *American Journal Health Systems Pharmacy,* 62, 1822–1827.

Heise, B. (2003). The historical context of addictions within the nursing profession. *Journal of Addictions Nursing,* 14, 117–124.

Herring, L.H. (1994). *Infection Control.* N.Y.: National League for Nursing.

Hurst, K.L., Croker, P.A., & Bell, S.K. (1994). How about a lollipop? A peer recognition program. *Nursing Management,* 25(9), 68–73.

Jankowski, C.B. (1992). Radiation protection for nurses: Regulations and guidelines. *Journal of Nursing Administration,* 22(22), 30–34.

Kinkle, S. (1993). Violence in the ED: How to stop it before it starts. *American Journal of Nursing,* 93(7), 22–24.

Korniewicz, M., Garzon, L., Seltzer, J., & Feinleib, M. (2004). Failure rates in nonlatex surgical gloves. *American Journal of Infection Control,* 32(5), 268–273.

Kramer, M., & Schmalenberg, C. (1993). Learning from success: Autonomy and empowerment. *Nursing Management,* 24(5), 58–64.

Krucoff, M. (2001). How to prevent repetitive stress injury in the workplace. *American Fitness,* 19(1), 31.

Lanza, M.L., & Carifio, J. (1991). Blaming the victim: Complex (nonlinear) patterns of causal attribution by nurses in response to vignettes of a patient assaulting a nurse. *Journal of Emergency Nursing,* 17(5), 299–309.

Mahoney, B. (1991). The extent, nature, and response to victimization of emergency nurses in Pennsylvania. *Journal of Emergency Nursing,* 17, 282–292.

Malone, B.L. (1993). Caring for culturally diverse racial groups: An administrative matter. *Nursing Administration Quarterly,* 17(2), 21–29.

Mitchell, A. (1995). Cultural diversity: The future, the market, and the rewards. *Caring,* 14(12), 44–48.

Moch, S.D., & Diemert, C.A. (1987). Health promotion within the nursing work environment. *Nursing Administration Quarterly,* 11(3), 9–12.

Nadwairski, J.A. (1992). Inner-city safety for home care providers. *Journal of Nursing Administration,* 22(9), 42–47.

National Safety Council. (1992). *Accident Prevention Manual for Business and Industry.* Chicago: National Safety Council.

Outwater, L.C. (1994). Sexual harassment issues. *Caring,* 13(5), 54–56, 58, 60.

Perry, J. (2001). Attention all nurses! New legislation puts safer sharps in your hands. *American Journal of Nursing,* 101(9), 24AA–24CC.

Ray, M., Turkel, M., & Marino, F. (2002). The transformative process for nursing in workforce redevelopment. *Nursing Administration Quarterly,* 26(2), 1–14.

Roche, E. (23 February 1993). Nurses' risks and their rights. *Vital Signs,* 3.

Roedel, R.S., & Nystrom, P.C. (1987). Clinical ladders and job enrichment. *Hospital Topics,* 65(2), 22–24.

Rogers, A.E., Hwang, W., Scott, L.D., Aiken, L.H., et al. (2004). The working hours of hospital staff nurses and patient safety: Both errors and near errors are more likely to occur when hospital staff nurses work twelve or more hours at a stretch. *Health Affairs* 23(4), 202–212.

Rosen, A., Isaacson, D., Brady, M., & Corey J.P. (1993). Hypersensitivity to latex in health care workers: Report of five cases. *Otolaryngology—Head and Neck Surgery,* 109, 731–734.

Simonowitz, J. (1994). Violence in the workplace: You're entitled to protection. *RN,* 57(11), 61–63.

Slattery, M. (September/October 1998). Caring for ourselves to care for our patients. *American Nurse,* 12–13.

Sloan, A., & Vernarec, E. (2001). Impaired nurses: Reclaiming careers. *Medical Economics,* 64(2), 58–64.

Society of Gastroenterology Nurses and Associates. (2001). Guidelines for preventing sensitivity and allergic reactions to natural rubber latex in the workplace. *Gastroenterology Nursing,* 24(2), 88–94.

Strader, M.K., & Decker, P.J. (1995). *Role Transition to Patient Care Management.* Norwalk, Conn.: Appleton & Lange.

Trossman, S. (May/June 1999a). When workplace threats become a reality. *American Nurse,* 1, 12.

Trossman, S. (September/October 1999b). Working 'round the clock. *American Nurse,* 1–2.

U.S. Department of Labor (OSHA). (1995). *Employee Workplace Rights and Responsibilities.* OSHA 95–35.

U.S. Department of Labor. Bureau of Labor Statistics. (2002). *Lost-work time injuries and illnesses: Characteristics and resulting time away from work, 2000.* April 10, 2002. Retrieved April 13, 2008, from ftp://ftp.bls.gov/pub/news.release/History/osh2.04102002.news.

Ward, L.B. (27 December 1992). In culturally diverse work place, language may alienate. *Miami Herald.*

chapter **13**
Work-Related Stress and Burnout

⊙ ○ ○ ○ ○ ○ ○ ○ ○ ○ ○

OBJECTIVES

After reading this chapter, the student should be able to:

- Identify signs and symptoms of stress, reality shock, and burnout.
- Describe the impact of stress, reality shock, and burnout on the individual and the health-care team.
- Evaluate his or her own and colleagues' stress levels.
- Develop strategies to manage personal and professional stresses.

Consider the Statistics

Fifty years ago, the term *personal anxiety* was never used to describe stress. In the decades since, stress has become the most common psychological complaint and a widespread health problem. In the last decade alone, approximately 28,000 studies have been published on the subject of stress and over 1000 studies on the subject of burnout (Pines, 2004, p. 66).

In the workplace, stress is usually defined from a "demand-perception-response" perspective—that stress is related to the perception of the demands being made on the individual as well as that individual's perception of the ability to meet those demands. When there is a mismatch between the two, the stress response is triggered. The stress threshold, or hardiness, depends on the individual's characteristics, experiences, coping mechanisms, and the circumstances of the event (McVicar, 2003).

The phrase "this is so stressful" is frequently used to describe negative work and personal situations. However, in reality, some stress responses are positive (eustress). The stress response is not a single event but a continuum, ranging from feeling of eustress to mild/moderate distress to severe distress. It is the severe and prolonged distress that causes people to "burn out" emotionally and experience serious physiological and psychological disturbances. Table 13-1 describes the continuum of the stress response.

Stress

Effects of Stress

Hans Selye first explored the concept of stress in the 1930s. Selye (1956) defined *stress* as the non-specific response of the body to any demands made on it. His description of the general adaptation syndrome (GAS) has had an enormous influence on our present-day notions about stress and its effect on people. The GAS consists of three stages:

1. **Alarm.** The body awakens to the stressor, and there is a slight change below the normal level of resistance.
2. **Resistance.** The body adjusts to the stressor and tries to restore balance.
3. **Exhaustion.** As the stressor continues, the body energy falls below the normal level of resistance, and illness may occur.

Most people think of stress as work pressure, rush-hour traffic, or sick children. These are triggers to the stress response, the actual body reaction to the daily factors mentioned. As identified by Selye, *stress* is the fight-or-flight response in the body, caused by adrenaline and other stress hormones, causing physiological changes such as increased heart rate and blood pressure, faster breathing, dilated pupils, increased blood sugar, and dry mouth.

Currently, stress is assessed on four levels: environmental, social, physiological, and psychological. *Environmental stressors* include weather, pollens, noise, traffic, and pollution. *Social stressors* include deadlines, finances, work responsibilities and interactions, and multiple demands on time and attention. *Physiological stressors* include illness, aging, injuries, lack of exercise, poor nutrition, and inadequate sleep. *Psychological stressors* are thoughts: how the brain interprets changes in the environment and the body and determines when the body turns on the fight-or-flight response (Davis, Eshelman, & McCay, 2000).

Epidemiological research has shown that long-term stress contributes to cardiovascular disease, hypertension, ulcers, substance abuse, immune system disorders, emotional disturbances, and job-related injuries (Crawford, 1993; Lusk, 1993).

Responses to Stress

"Whether the stress you experience is the result of major life changes or the cumulative effect of minor everyday hassles, it is how you respond to these experiences that determines the impact stress will have on your life" (Davis, Eshelman, & McCay, 2000).

Some people manage potentially stressful events more effectively than others (Crawford, 1993; Teague, 1992). Perceptions of events and the subsequent stress responses vary considerably from one person to another. A patient crisis that one nurse considers stressful, for example, may not seem stressful to a coworker. The following is an example:

A new graduate was employed on a busy telemetry floor. Often, when patients were admitted, they were in acute distress, with shortness of breath, diaphoresis, and chest pain. Family members were distraught and anxious. Each time the new graduate had to admit a patient, she experienced a "sick-to-the-stomach" feeling, tightness in the chest and throat, and difficulty concentrating.

table 13-1

Stress Continuum

	Eustress	Distress	Severe Distress
Psychological	Fear/excitement	Feelings of uneasiness, apprehension, sadness, depression, pessimism, listlessness	Burnout
		Lack of self-esteem	Emotional exhaustion/depersonalization and disengagement
		Increased level of arousal/mental acuity	Isolation
		Negative attitude	
		Increased use of alcohol/smoking/drugs	
		Decreased interest in sexual activity	
		Procrastination/unable to complete tasks	
Physiological	Autonomic nervous system response: increased blood pressure/heart rate; increased metabolic rate; release of cortisol; quicker reaction times	Prolonged elevated blood pressure/pulse	Clinical hypertension
		Indigestion	Coronary artery disease
		Bowel disturbances	Gastric disorders
		Weight gain or loss	Menstrual problems
		Reduced immunity	
		Fatigue/low energy	
		Poor sleep habits	
		Headache	
		Trembling hands, fingers, body	
		Dry mouth and throat	
Individual response	**Adaptive**	Varies among individuals but usually ***maladaptive***	Varies among individuals but usually ***severely maladaptive,*** possible life-threatening
	Increased alertness	Absenteeism	
	Focus totally on the situation	Apathy	
	Able to respond to changes quickly	Cynicism	
	Callousness	Defensiveness	
	Energized for fight or flight preparation		

Adapted from Martin, K. (May 1993). To cope with stress. *Nursing 93, 39–41, with permission;* Goliszek, A. (1992). Sixty-Six Second Stress Management: The Quickest Way to Relax and Ease Anxiety. *Far Hills, N.J.: New Horizon; and McVicar, A. (2003). Workplace stress in nursing: A literature review. Journal of Advanced Nursing, 44(6), 633–642.*

She was afraid that she would miss something important and that the patient would die during the admission. The more experienced nurses seemed to handle each admission with ease, even when the patient's physical condition was severely compromised.

Selye also differentiated between "good" stress and "bad" stress. In 1974, Selye stated: "Stress is the spice of life. Since stress is associated with all types of activity, we could not avoid most of it only by never doing anything" (Lenson, 2001, p. 5). Good stress can push people to perform better and accomplish more. What makes an event

"good stress" or "bad stress"? Lenson identified seven factors:

1. People can exert a high level of control over the outcomes of good stresses. With bad stresses, there is little or no control.
2. Positive feelings are experienced in processing good stress. With bad stress, negative or ambivalent feelings occur.
3. Good stress helps achieve positive goals. No desirable outcomes occur with bad stress.
4. There is a feeling of eagerness when anticipating the work that needs to be done to process the good stressors.

5. Bad stress leaves feelings of exhaustion and avoidance.

6. Good stress helps growth; bad stress is limiting. Good stress improves interpersonal relationships; bad stress makes these relationships worse.

7. Processing all stress requires human action.

The Real World

Today's health-care system has adopted the corporate mindset. Both the new graduate and the seasoned professional continue to experience redesigning, changing staffing models, complex documentation requirements, continued nursing shortages, and the expectation that work does not end when the employee goes home (Trossman, 1999). Most agencies expect new graduates to come to the work setting able to organize their work, set priorities, and provide leadership to ancillary personnel. New graduates often say, "I had no idea that nursing would be this demanding." Even though nursing programs of study are designed to help students prepare for the demands of the work setting, new nurses still need to continue to learn on the job. In fact, experienced nurses say that what they learned in school is only the beginning; school provided them with the fundamental knowledge and skills needed to continue to grow and develop as they practice nursing in various capacities and work settings. Graduation signals not the end of learning but the beginning of a journey toward becoming an expert nurse (Benner, 1984).

Right now you are probably thinking, "Nothing can be more stressful than going to school. I can't wait to go to work and not have to study for tests, go to the clinical agency for my assignment, do patient care plans," and so forth. In most associate degree programs, students are assigned to care for one to three patients a day, working up to six or seven patients under a preceptor's supervision by the end of their program. Compare this with your "next clinical rotation," your first real job as a nurse. You may work 7–10 days in a row on 8- to 12-hour shifts, caring for 10 or more patients. You may also have to supervise several technicians or licensed practical nurses. These drastic changes from school to employment cause many to experience *reality shock* (Kraeger & Walker, 1993; Kramer, 1981).

Initial Concerns

The first few weeks on a new job are the "honeymoon" phase. The new employee is excited and enthusiastic about the new position. Coworkers usually go out of their way to make the new person feel welcome and overlook any problems that arise. But honeymoons do not last forever. The new graduate is soon expected to behave like everyone else and discovers that expectations for a professional employed in an organization are quite different from expectations for a student in school. Those behaviors that brought rewards in school are not necessarily valued by the organization. In fact, some of them are criticized. The new graduate who is not prepared for this change feels confused, shocked, angry, and disillusioned. The tension of the situation can become almost unbearable if it is not resolved. Table 13-2 provides a list of ongoing and newer workplace stresses

Graduate nurses in the first 3 months of employment identified concerns related to skills, personal and professional roles, patient care management, the

table 13-2

Stress in the Workplace

Ongoing Sources	Newer Sources
Conflict with physicians	Terrorism
Work overload/ work devalued	Changes in technology
Role conflict	Downsizing
Ineffective, hostile, incompetent supervisors and/or peers	Constant changes in nursing care delivery
	Work/home conflicts
Lack of personal job fit; inadequate preparation, recognition, or clear job description	Elder and child care issues
	Workplace violence
Poor work control, fear and uncertainty related to career progress	Lawsuits related to job stress
Age, gender, racial, religious discrimination	Demands of accreditation/ compliance issues
Dealing with death and dying patients/ families	Pressure for immediate results
Salary	Colleagues' inexperience

Adapted from DeFrank, R., & Ivancevich, J. (1998). Stress on the job: An executive update. Academy of Management Executives, 12(3), 55; *McVicar, A. (2003). Workplace stress in nursing: A literature review.* Journal of Advanced Nursing, 44(6), 633–642; *and Hall, D. (2004). Work-related stress of registered nurses in a hospital setting.* Journal for Nurses in Staff Development, 20(1), 6–14.

shocks of bad experiences, the affirmations of good experiences, constructive evaluation, knowledge of the unit routine, and priorities of school versus work (Godinez, Schweiger, Gruver, & Ryan, 1999; Heslop, 2001).

Well-supervised orientation programs are very helpful for newly licensed nurses. In this era of the nursing shortage, the orientation program may be cut short and the new nurse required to function on his or her own very quickly. One way to minimize initial work stress is to ask questions about the orientation program: How long will it be? Whom will I be working with? When will I be on my own? What happens if at the end of the orientation I still need more assistance?

Differences in Expectations

The enthusiasm and eagerness of the first new job quickly disappear as reality sets in. Regardless of the career one chooses, there is no perfect job. The problem begins when reality and expectations collide. After 2 or 3 months, the new nurse begins to experience a formal separation from being a student and embraces the professional reality of the nursing role. To cope with reality, several facts of work life need to be recognized (Goliszek, 1992, pp. 36, 46):

1. Expectations are usually distortions of reality. Unless you accept this and react positively, you will go through life experiencing disappointment. *As a student, you had only two or three patients to care for, and you are very surprised to hear on your first full day of orientation that you have five patients. Although you did hear the nurses talking about their caseload while you were a student, you expected to continue to have two or three patients for at least the next 4 months.*

2. To some extent, you need to fit yourself into your work, not fit the work to suit your needs or demands. Having a positive attitude helps to maintain flexibility and a sense of humor. *Your first position is at a physician's office. The physician is ready to retire, and his patient load is dwindling. You wanted to apply for a position in acute care, but you have a very active social life and did not want to work weekends. The current position is not very challenging, and you are concerned that you might be unemployed soon. You are starting to miss the acute care environment. Go back to your SWOT analysis. Evaluate your*

current strengths, weaknesses, opportunities, and threats. Where do you see yourself in 1 year? 5 years? How will you fit yourself into your work to meet your goals?

3. The way you perceive events on the job will influence how you feel about your work. Your attitude will affect whether work is a pleasant or unpleasant experience. Health care is not easy. *Sick people can be cranky and demanding. Health-care agencies continue to want to do more with less. How you perceive your contribution to the healthcare system will definitely influence your reality.*

4. Feelings of helplessness and powerlessness at work cause frustration and unrelieved job stress. If you go to work every day feeling that you do not make a difference, it is time to reevaluate your position and your goals.

What are these differences in expectations? Kramer (1981), who studied reality shock for many years, found a number of them, which are listed in Table 13-3.

Ideally, health care should be comprehensive. It should meet not only all of a patient's needs but also be delivered in a way that considers the patient as a whole person, a member of a particular family that has certain unique characteristics and needs, and a member of a particular community. Most health-care professionals, however, are not employed to provide comprehensive, holistic care. Instead, they are asked to give medications, provide counseling, make home visits, or prepare someone for surgery, but rarely to do all these things. These tasks are divided among different people, each a specialist, for the sake of efficiency rather than continuity or effectiveness.

table 13-3

Professional Ideals and Work Realities

Professional Ideals	Work Realities
Comprehensive, holistic care	Mechanistic, fragmented care
Emphasis on quality of care	Emphasis on efficiency
Explicit expectations	Implicit (unstated) expectations
Balanced, frequent feedback	Intermittent, often negative feedback
Assignments that "make sense"	

Adapted from Kramer, M. (January 27–28, 1981). Coping with reality shock. Workshop presented at Jackson Memorial Hospital, Miami, Fla.

When efficiency is the goal, the speed and amount of work done are rewarded rather than the quality of the work. This creates a conflict for the new graduate, who while in school was allowed to take as much time as needed to provide good care.

Expectations are also communicated in different ways. In school, an effort is made to provide explicit directions so that students know what they are expected to accomplish. In many work settings, however, instructions on the job are brief, and many expectations are left unspoken. New graduates who are not aware of these expectations may find that they have unknowingly left tasks undone or are considered inept by coworkers. The following is an example:

Brenda, a new graduate, was assigned to give medications to all her team's patients. Because this was a fairly light assignment, she spent some time looking up the medications and explaining their actions to the patients receiving them. Brenda also straightened up the medicine room and filled out the order forms, which she thought would please the task-oriented team leader. At the end of the day, Brenda reported these activities with some satisfaction to the team leader. She expected the team leader to be pleased with the way she used the time. Instead, the team leader looked annoyed and told her that whoever passes out medications always does the blood pressures as well and that the other nurse on the team, who had a heavier assignment, had to do them. Also, because supplies were always ordered on Fridays for the weekend, it would have to be done again tomorrow, so Brenda had in fact wasted her time.

Additional Pressures on the New Graduate

The first job a person takes after finishing school is often considered a proving ground where newly gained knowledge and skills are tested. Many people set up mental tests for themselves that they feel must be passed before they can be confident of their ability to function. Passing these self-tests also confirms achievement of identity as a practitioner rather than a student.

At the same time, new graduates are undergoing testing by their coworkers, who are also interested in finding out whether the new graduate can handle the job. The new graduate is entering a new group, and the group will decide whether to accept this new member. The group is usually reasonable, but sometimes new graduates are given tasks they are not ready to handle. If this happens, Kramer

(1981) recommended that new graduates refuse to take the test rather than fail it. Another opportunity for proving themselves will soon come along.

Additional problems, such as dealing with resistant staff members, cultural differences, and age differences, may also occur. Above all, the experience of loss is frequently described by new graduates. Losses are described as the following (Boychuk, 2001):

- The ideal world of caring and curing they had come to know through their education
- Their innocence
- The familiarity of academia
- The protection of clinical supervision by nursing instructors
- Externally set boundaries of care and safety
- A sense of collegiality and trusted relationships with peers
- Grounded feedback

Resolving the Problem

Before considering ways to resolve these problems, some less successful ways of coping with these problems are listed.

- **Abandon professional goals.** When faced with reality shock, some new graduates abandon their professional goals and adopt the organization's operative goals as their own. This eliminates their conflict but leaves them less effective caregivers. It also puts the needs of the organization before their needs or the needs of the patient and reinforces operative goals that might better be challenged and changed.
- **Give up professional ideals.** Others give up their professional ideals but do not adopt the organization's goals or any others to replace them. This has a deadening effect; they become automatons, believing in nothing related to their work except doing what is necessary to earn a day's pay.
- **Leave the profession.** Those who do not give up their professional ideals try to find an organization that will support them. Unfortunately, a significant proportion of those who do not want to give up their professional ideals escape these conflicts by leaving their jobs and abandoning their profession. Kramer and Schmalenberg (1993) stated that there would be fewer shortages of nurses if more health-care organizations met these ideals.

Instead of focusing on the bad stress, new nurses can meet the transition to professional nursing by adapting to good stress:

- **Develop a professional identity.** Opportunities to challenge one's competence and develop an identity as a professional can begin in school. Success in meeting these challenges can immunize the new graduate against the loss of confidence that accompanies reality shock.
- **Learn about the organization.** The new graduate who understands how organizations operate will not be as shocked as the naïve individual. When you begin a new job, it is important to learn as much as you can about the organization and how it really operates. This not only saves you some surprises but also gives you some ideas about how to work within the system and how to make the system work for you.
- **Use your energy wisely.** Keep in mind that much energy goes into learning a new job. You may see many things that you think need to be changed, but you need to recognize that to implement change requires your time and energy. It is a good idea to make a list of these things so that you do not forget them later when you have become socialized into the system and have some time and energy to invest in change.
- **Communicate effectively.** Deal with the problems that can arise with coworkers. The same interpersonal skills you use in communicating with patients can be effective in dealing with your coworkers.
- **Seek feedback often and persistently.** Seeking feedback not only provides you with needed information but also pushes the people you work with to be more specific about their expectations of you.
- **Develop a support network.** Identify colleagues who have held onto their professional ideals with whom you can share your problems and the work of improving the organization. Their recognition of your work can keep you going when rewards from the organization are meager. A support network is a source of strength when resisting pressure to give up professional ideals and a source of power when attempting to bring about change. Developing your skills can help to prevent the problems of reality shock.
- **Find a mentor.** A mentor is someone more experienced within or outside the organization who provides career development support, such as coaching, sponsoring advancement, providing challenging assignments, protecting protégés from adversity, and promoting positive visibility. Mentors provide guidance to new graduates as they change from student to professional nurse. Mentors can also assume psychosocial functions, such as personal support, friendship, acceptance, role modeling, and counseling. Many organizations have preceptors for the new employee. In many instances, the preceptor will become your mentor. However, the mentor role is much more encompassing than the preceptor role. The mentor relationship is a voluntary one and is built on mutual respect and development of the mentee. Table 13-4 identifies responsibilities of the mentor and mentee in this relationship (Scheetz, 2000; Simonetti & Ariss, 1999).

You have made it through the first 6 months of employment, and you are finally starting to feel like a "real" nurse. You are beginning to realize that a stress-free work environment is probably impossible to achieve. Shift work, overtime, distraught families, staff shortages, and pressure to do more with less continue to contribute to the stresses placed on nurses. An inability to deal with this continued stress will eventually lead to burnout.

table 13-4	
Mentor and Mentee Responsibilities	
Mentor Responsibilities	**Mentee Responsibilities**
Has excellent communication and listening skills	Demonstrates eagerness to learn
Shows sensitivity to needs of nurses, patients, and workplace	Participates actively in the relationship by keeping all appointments and commitments
Able to encourage excellence in others	Seeks feedback and uses it to modify behaviors
Able to share and provide counsel	Demonstrates flexibility and an ability to change
Exhibits good decision-making skills	Is open in the relationship with mentor
Shows an understanding of power and politics	Demonstrates an ability to move toward independence
Demonstrates trustworthiness	Able to evaluate choices and outcomes

Burnout

Definition

The ultimate result of unmediated job stress is burnout. The term *burnout* became a favorite buzz-word of the 1980s and continues to be part of today's vocabulary. Herbert Freudenberger formally identified it as a leadership concern in 1974. The literature on job stress and burnout continues to grow as new books, articles, workshops, and videos appear regularly. A useful definition of burnout is the "progressive deterioration in work and other performance resulting from increasing difficulties in coping with high and continuing levels of job-related stress and professional frustration" (Paine, 1984, p. 1).

More than 20 years of research on nursing work environments point to personal, job, and organizational factors that contribute to dissatisfaction and ultimately burnout (McLennan, 2005). Ultimately, nurse burnout affects patients' satisfaction with their nursing care. A survey of 820 nurses and 621 patients in 20 hospitals across the United States (Vahey et al., 2004) showed that units characterized by nurses as having adequate staff, good administrative support for nursing care, and good relations between physicians and nurses were twice as likely as other units to report high satisfaction with nursing care. The level of nurse burnout on these units also affected patient satisfaction.

Much of the burnout experienced by nurses has been attributed to the frustration that arises because care cannot be delivered in the ideal manner nurses learned in school. For those whose greatest satisfaction comes from caring for patients, anything that interferes with providing the highest quality care causes work stress and feelings of failure.

People who expect to derive a sense of significance from their work enter their professions with high hopes and motivation and relate to their work as a calling. When they feel that they have failed, that their work is meaningless, that they make no difference in the world, they start feeling helpless and hopeless and eventually burn out (Pines, 2004, p. 67).

The often unrealistic and sometimes sexist image of nurses in the media adds to this frustration. Neither the school ideal nor the media image is realistic, but either may make nurses feel dissatisfied with themselves and their jobs, keeping stress levels high (Corley et al., 1994; Fielding & Weaver,

1994; Grant, 1993; Hendrickson, Knickman, & Finkler, 1994; Kovner-Malkin, 1993; Nakata & Saylor, 1994; Pines, 2004; Skubak, Earls, & Botos, 1994).

Sharon had wanted to be a nurse for as long as she could remember. She married early, had three children, and put her dreams of being a nurse on hold. Now her children are grown, and she finally realized her dream by graduating last year from the local community college with a nursing degree. However, she has been overwhelmed at work, critical of coworkers and patients, and argumentative with supervisors. She is having difficulty adapting to the restructuring changes at her hospital and goes home angry and frustrated every day. She cannot stop working for financial reasons but is seriously thinking of quitting nursing and taking some computer classes. "I'm tired of dealing with people. Maybe machines will be more friendly and predictable." Sharon is experiencing burnout.

Aspects

Goliszek (1992) identified four stages of the burnout syndrome:

1. **High expectations and idealism.** At the first stage, the individual is enthusiastic, dedicated, and committed to the job and exhibits a high energy level and a positive attitude.
2. **Pessimism and early job dissatisfaction.** In the second stage, frustration, disillusionment, or boredom with the job develops, and the individual begins to exhibit the physical and psychological symptoms of stress.
3. **Withdrawal and isolation.** As the individual moves into the third stage, anger, hostility, and negativism are exhibited. The physical and psychological stress symptoms worsen. Through stage three, simple changes in job goals, attitudes, and behaviors may reverse the burnout process.
4. **Irreversible detachment and loss of interest.** As the physical and emotional stress symptoms become severe, the individual exhibits low self-esteem, chronic absenteeism, cynicism, and total negativism. Once the individual has moved into this stage and remains there for any length of time, burnout is inevitable.

Regardless of the cause, experiencing burnout leaves an individual emotionally and physically exhausted.

Stressors Leading to Burnout

Personal Factors

Some of the personal factors influencing job stress and burnout are age, gender, number of children, education, experience, and favored coping style. For example, the fact that many nurses are single parents raising families alone adds to the demands of already difficult days at work. Married nurses may have the additional stress of dual-career homes, causing even more stress in coordinating work and vacation schedules as well as day-care problems. Baby boomers are finding they need to care for elderly parents along with their children (DeFrank & Ivancevich, 1998). Competitive, impatient, and hostile personality traits have also been associated with emotional exhaustion and subsequent burnout (Borman, 1993). Most experienced nurses state that they separate their home from work when dealing with work-related stressors and that they try but usually fail to leave their work-related stressors in the workplace (Hall, 2004).

Job-Related Conditions

Job-related stress is broadly defined by the National Institute for Occupational Safety and Health as the "harmful physical and emotional responses that occur when the requirements of the job do not match the capabilities, resources, or needs of the worker" (http://www.cdc.gov/niosh/homepage.html). Since the prior edition of this text, the threat of terrorism has been added to the list of job-related conditions that contribute to job-related stress. Box 13-1 lists some of these conditions, which were discussed in Chapter 12.

Human Service Occupations

People who work in human service organizations consistently report lower levels of job satisfaction than do people working in other types of organizations. Much of the stress experienced by nurses is related to the nature of their work: continued intensive, intimate contact with people who often have serious and sometimes fatal physical, mental, emotional, and/or social problems. Efforts to save patients or help them achieve a peaceful ending to their lives are not always successful. Despite nurses' best efforts, many patients get worse, not better. Some return to their destructive behaviors; others do not recover and die. The continued loss of patients alone can lead to burnout. Even exposure

box 13-1

Five Sources of Job Stress That Can Lead to Burnout

1. **Intrinsic factors.** Characteristics of the job itself, such as the multiple aspects of complex patient care that many nurses provide; lack of autonomy
2. **Organizational variables.** Characteristics of the organization, such as limited financial resources, staffing, workload, models of care delivery
3. **Reward system.** The way in which employees are rewarded or punished, particularly if these are obviously unfair
4. **Human resources system.** In particular, the number and availability of opportunities for staff development, salary and benefits, organizational policies
5. **Leadership.** The way in which managers relate to their staff, particularly if they are unrealistic, uncaring, or unfair; communication patterns with supervisors and coworkers

Adapted from Carr, K., & Kazanowski, M. (1994). Factors affecting job satisfaction of nurses who work in long-term care. Journal of Advanced Nursing, 19, 878–883; Crawford, S. (1993). Job stress and occupational health nursing. American Association of Occupational Health Nurses Journal, 41, 522–529; Duquette, A., Sandhu, B., & Beaudet, L. (1994). Factors related to nursing burnout: A review of empirical knowledge. Issues in Mental Health Nursing, 15, 337–358; and Best, M., & Thurston, N. (2004). Measuring nurse job satisfaction, Journal of Nursing Administration, 34(6), 283–290.

to medicinal and antiseptic substances, unpleasant sights, and high noise levels can cause stress for some people. Health-care providers experiencing burnout may become cynical and even hostile toward their coworkers and colleagues (Carr & Kazanowski, 1994; Dionne-Proulx & Pepin, 1993; Goodell & Van Ess Coeling, 1994; Stechmiller & Yarandi, 1993; Tumulty, Jernigan, & Kohut, 1994).

In some instances, human service professionals also experience lower pay, longer hours, and more extensive regulation than do professionals in other fields. Inadequate advancement opportunities for women and minorities in lower-status, lower-paid positions are apparent in many health-care areas.

Conflicting Demands

Meeting work-related responsibilities and maintaining a family and personal life can increase stress when there is insufficient time or energy for all of these. As mentioned in the section on personal factors, both the single and the married parent are at risk because of the conflicting demands of their personal and work lives. The perception of balance in one's life is a personal one.

There appear to be some differences in the way that men and women find a comfortable balance.

Men often define themselves in terms of their separateness and their career progress; women are more likely to define themselves through attachment and connections with other people. Women who try to focus on occupational achievement and pursue personal attachments at the same time are likely to experience conflict in both their work and personal lives. In addition, society evaluates the behaviors of working adult men and women differently. "When a man disrupts work for his family, he is considered a good family man, while a woman disrupting work for family risks having her professional commitment questioned" (Borman, 1993, p. 1).

Closely tied to conflicting demands is the decision to come to work when ill. Nurses who come to work when ill describe tension associated with making this decision: tension between the nurse and the supervisor, tension between the nurse and the team members, and tension within the nurse due to responsibilities to self and others. As you move forward in your career, be proactive in working with team members and your supervisors in helping yourself and others find balance in the workplace (Crout, Change, & Cioffi, 2005).

Technology

Decisions related to changes in technology are often made without input from employees. These same employees are then required to adapt and cope with the changes. How many of the following changes have you had to adapt to: e-mail, voice mail, fax machines, computerized charting, desktop computers, cellular phones? Often, employees feel that their role has become secondary to technology (DeFrank & Ivancevich, 1998).

Lack of Balance in Life

When personal interests and satisfactions are limited to work, a person is more susceptible to burnout; trouble at work becomes trouble with that individual's whole life. A job can become the center of someone's world, and that world can become very small. Two ways out of this are to set limits on the commitment to work and to expand the number of satisfying activities and relationships outside of work.

Many people in the helping professions have difficulty setting limits on their commitment. This is fine if they enjoy working extra hours and taking calls at night and on weekends, but if it exhausts them, then they need to stop doing it or risk serious burnout. For example, when you are asked to work another double shift or the third weekend in a row, you can say no. At the same time as you are setting limits at work, you can expand your outside activities so that you live in a large world in which a blow to one part can be cushioned by support from other parts. If you are the team leader or nurse manager, you also need to recognize and accept staff members' need to do this as well. Ask yourself the following questions:

- Do I exercise at least three times weekly?
- Do I have several close friends I see regularly?
- Do I have a plan for my life and career that I have told someone about?
- Do I have strong spiritual values that I carry out in practice regularly?
- Do I have some strong personal interests that I regularly enjoy?

Studies have shown that the two best indicators of customer satisfaction are related to employee satisfaction and employee work-life balance. Well-rounded employees have a different perspective on life and are perceived by employers as more trustworthy and more grounded in reality. You do not have to give up your personal life to excel in your professional life (Farren, 1999).

Consequences

Certain combinations of personal and organizational factors can increase the likelihood of burnout. Finding the right fit between your preferences and the characteristics of the organization for which you work can be keys to preventing burnout. Health care demands adaptable, innovative, competent employees who care about their patients, desire to continue learning, and try to remain productive despite constant challenges. Unfortunately, these are the same individuals who are prone to burnout if preventive action is not taken (Lickman, Simms, & Greene, 1993; McGee-Cooper, 1993).

Burnout has financial, physical, emotional, and social implications for the professional, the patients, and the organization. Burnout can happen to anyone, not just to people with a history of emotional problems. In fact, it is not considered an emotional disturbance in the sense that depression is; instead, it is considered a reaction to sustained organizational stressors (Duquette, Sandhu, & Beaudet, 1994).

The shortage of professional nurses is predicted to continue for at least another 10 years. Two of the main causes of the shortage are individuals not entering the profession and nurses leaving. As discussed, one reason for leaving is burnout. A recent study of 106 nurses demonstrated that the three dimensions of burnout (emotional exhaustion, depersonalization, and personal accomplishment) were correlated with work excitement. Work excitement is defined as "personal enthusiasm and commitment for work evidenced by creativity, receptivity to learning, and ability to see opportunity in everyday situations (Sadovich, 2005, p. 91). Work excitement factors include: work arrangements, variable work experiences, the work environment, and growth and development opportunities. As you pursue your nursing career, consider looking for positions that support a favorable work environment.

A Buffer Against Burnout

The idea that personal hardiness provides a buffer against burnout has been explored in recent years. Hardiness includes the following:

- A sense of personal control rather than powerlessness
- Commitment to work and life's activities rather than alienation
- Seeing life's demands and changes as challenges rather than as threats

The hardiness that comes from having this perspective leads to the use of adaptive coping responses, such as optimism, effective use of support systems, and healthy lifestyle habits (Duquette, Sandhu, & Beaudet, 1994; Nowak & Pentkowski, 1994). In addition, letting go of guilt, fear of change, and the self-blaming, "wallowing-in-the-problem" syndrome will help you buffer yourself against burnout (Lenson, 2001).

Ask yourself, "What can I possibly do as a new graduate? I don't even have a job yet, let alone understand the politics of health-care organizations." It is never too early to understand yourself—what triggers stressful situations for you, how you respond to stress, and how you manage it.

Stress Management

Although you cannot always control the demands placed on you, you can learn to manage your reactions to them and to make healthy lifestyle choices that better prepare you to meet those demands.

ABCs of Stress Management

Frances Johnston (1994) suggested using the ABCs of stress management (awareness, belief, and commitment) in order to have as constructive a response to stress as possible (Box 13-2).

Awareness

How do you know that you are under stress and may be beginning to burn out? The key is being honest with yourself. Asking yourself the questions in Box 13-3 and answering them honestly is one way to assess your personal risk. To analyze your responses to stress further, you may also want to answer the questions in Box 13-4. The answers to these questions require some thought. You do not have to share your answers with others unless you want to, but you do need to be completely honest with yourself when you answer them or the exercise will not be worth the time spent on it. Try to determine the sources of your stress (Goliszek, 1992):

- Is it the *time of day* you do the activity?
- Is it the *reason* you do the activity?
- Is it the *way* you do the activity?
- Is it the *amount of time* you need to do the activity?

Another suggestion is to keep a stress diary. People often have "flash points" that send stress levels skyrocketing. Keeping a stress diary often helps in identifying these triggers. Identify the date, time, situation, scale (on a scale from 1 to 10), symptoms, reaction, and efficiency (on a scale from 1 to 10, how well did you cope with this stressor?). What was your reaction? Did you solve the problem, quietly seethe, or become reactionary? After 2 weeks, analyze the diary, and reflect on where and when your highest stress levels occured. Keep your stress diary for as long as you think necessary in order to identify personal stress triggers and patterns of behavior (Bruce, 2007).

---

box 13-2

ABCs of Stress Management

Become **Aware** of your own responses to stress and the consequences of too much stress.

Believe that you can change your perspective and your behavior.

Commit yourself to take action to prevent conflicts that cause stress, to learn techniques that help you cope in situations over which you have no control, and to understand that you can choose how to react in stressful situations.

Assessing Your Risk for Burnout

Do you feel more fatigued than energetic?

Do you work harder but accomplish less?

Do you feel cynical or disenchanted most of the time?

Do you often feel sad or cry for no apparent reason?

Do you feel hostile, negative, or angry at work?

Are you short-tempered? Do you withdraw from friends or coworkers?

Do you forget appointments or deadlines? Do you frequently misplace personal items?

Are you becoming insensitive, irritable, and short-tempered?

Do you experience physical symptoms such as headaches or stomachaches?

Do you feel like avoiding people?

Do you laugh less? Feel joy less often?

Are you interested in sex?

Do you crave junk food more often?

Do you skip meals?

Have your sleep patterns changed?

Do you take more medication than usual? Do you use alcohol or other substances to alter your mood?

Do you feel guilty when your work is not perfect?

Are you questioning whether the job is right for you?

Do you feel as though no one cares what kind of work you do?

Do you constantly push yourself to do better, yet feel frustrated that there is no time to do what you want to do?

Do you feel as if you are on a treadmill all day?

Do you use holidays, weekends, or vacation time to catch up?

Do you feel as if you are "burning the candle at both ends"?

Adapted from Golin, M., Buchlin, M., & Diamond, D. (1991). Secrets of Executive Success. Emmaus, Pa.: Rodale Press; and Goliszek, A. (1992). Sixty-Six Second Stress Management: The Quickest Way to Relax and Ease Anxiety. Far Hills, N.J.: New Horizon.

Questions for Self-Assessment

What does the term *health* mean to me?

What prevents me from living this definition of health?

Is health important to me?

Where do I find support?

Which coping methods work best for me?

What tasks cause me to feel pressured?

Can I reorganize, reduce, or eliminate these tasks?

Can I delegate or rearrange any of my family responsibilities?

Can I say no to less important demands?

What are my hopes for the future in terms of (1) career (2) finances (3) spiritual life and physical needs (4) family relationships (5) social relationships?

What do I think others expect of me?

How do I feel about these expectations?

What is really important to me?

Can I prioritize in order to have balance in my life?

Commitment

As you move forward to *C,* you will need to make a commitment to continuing to work on stress recognition and reduction. Once you have recognized the warning signs of stress and impending burnout and have gained some insight into your personal needs and reactions to stress, it is time to find the stress management techniques that are right for you.

The stress management techniques in the next section are divided into physical and mental health management for ease in reading and remembering them. However, bear in mind that this is really an artificial division and that mind and body interact continuously. Stress affects both mind and body, and you need to care for both if you are going to be successful in managing stress and preventing burnout.

Physical Health Management

Nurses spend much of their time teaching their patients the basics of keeping themselves healthy. However, many fail to apply these principles in their own lives. Some of the most important aspects of health promotion and stress reduction are reviewed in this section: deep breathing, good posture, rest, relaxation, proper nutrition, and exercise (Davidhizar, 1994; Posen, 2000; Wolinski, 1993).

Deep Breathing

Most of the time, people use only 45% of their lung capacity when they breathe. Remember all the times you instructed your patients to "take a few

Belief

Now that you have done the *A* part of stress management, you are ready to move on to *B,* which is belief in yourself. Your relationship with your inner self may be the most important relationship of all. Building your self-image and self-esteem will enable you to block out negativism (Davidhizar, 1994). You must also believe that your destiny is not inevitable but that change is possible. Be honest with yourself. Truly value your life. Ask yourself, "If I could live 1 more month, what would I do?"—and start doing it (Johnston, 1994).

deep breaths"? Practice taking a few slow, deep, "belly" breaths. When faced with a stressful situation, people often hold their breath for a few seconds. This reduces the amount of oxygen delivered to the brain and causes them to feel more anxious. Anxiety can lead to faulty reasoning and a feeling of losing control. Often you can calm yourself by taking a few deep breaths. Try it right now. Don't you feel better already?

Good Posture

A common response to pressure is to slump down into your chair, tensing your upper torso and abdominal muscles. Again, this restricts blood flow and the amount of oxygen reaching your brain. Instead of slumping, imagine a hook on top of your head pulling up your spine; relax your abdomen, and look up. Now, shrug your shoulders a few times to loosen the muscles, and picture a sunny day at the beach or a walk in the woods. Do you feel more relaxed?

Rest

Sleep needs vary with the individual. Find out how much sleep you need, and work on arranging your activities so that you get enough sleep. Fatigue in the human body is no different than fatigue in anything else. Starting out small, a fatigue fracture may remain unnoticed until a catastrophic failure occurs. Several studies indicate the consequences of fatigue:

- Subjects who had gone 17–19 hours without sleep ranked on testing as equal or worse than someone with a blood alcohol level of 0.05%.
- 24% of 2259 adults surveyed cited fatigue as the primary reason for a recent visit to a physician.
- 16%–60% of all traffic accidents are related to fatigue.

Fatigue is a multidimensional symptom. Origins of fatigue may be biological, psychological, and/or behavioral in nature. What can you do to ward off workplace fatigue?

1. Spot the pattern. Be aware of a weakened state or decrease in strength, an interruption in the ability to perform activities of daily living, or an overabundance in conditions or behaviors that contribute to fatigue such as physical or mental stress, sleep loss, or drug use.
2. Identify precursors. Are you pushing yourself continuously beyond the healthy limits of your physical and/or mental capabilities? You are bound to encounter fatigue.
3. Recognize the signs. Emotional outbursts, clumsiness, loss of sensory motor control, weariness, and exhaustion may indicate fatigue.
4. Discern the results. Physical and mental disorders, physical injuries, collapse, and even death may be the catastrophic consequences of fatigue. Be aware of the symptoms of fatigue in yourself and others. Plan how to care for yourself. Be supportive of your coworkers to safeguard against fatigue in others (Smith, 2004).

Relaxation and Time Out

Many people have found that relaxation with guided imagery or other forms of meditation decreases the physiological and psychological impact of chronic stress. Guided imagery has been used in competitions for many years, in golf, ice skating, baseball, and other sports. Research studies have shown that creation of a mental image of the desired results enhances one's ability to reach the goal. Positive behavior or goal attainment is enhanced even more if you imagine the details of the process of achieving your desired outcome (Vines, 1994). Box 13-5 lists useful relaxation techniques.

Imagine taking the National Council License Examination. You sit down at the computer, take a few deep breaths, and begin. Visualize yourself reading the questions, smiling as you identify the correct answer, and hitting the Enter key after recording your answer. You complete the examination, feeling confident that you were successful. A week later, you go to your mailbox and find a letter waiting for you: "Congratulations, you have passed the test and are now a licensed registered nurse." You imagine telling your family and friends. What an exciting moment!

box 13-5
Useful Relaxation Techniques
Guided imagery
Yoga
Transcendental meditation
Relaxation tapes or music
Favorite sports or hobbies
Quiet corners or favorite places

Taking breaks and time out during the day for a short walk or a refreshment (not caffeine) break or just to daydream can help de-stress you. Just as people have circadian rhythms during the night, circadian rhythms function during the day. These cycles are peaks of energy, with troughs of low energy. Watching for these low-energy cycles and taking breaks at that time will help keep stress from building up.

Proper Nutrition

New research results endorsing the benefits of healthful eating habits seem to appear almost daily. Although the various authorities may prescribe somewhat different regimens, ultimately it appears that too little or too much of any nutrient can be harmful. Many people do not realize that simply decreasing or discontinuing caffeine can help decrease a stress reaction in the body. Some general guidelines for good nutrition are in Box 13-6.

Exercise

Regular aerobic exercise for 20 minutes three times a week is recommended for most people. The exercise may be walking, swimming, jogging, bicycling, stair-stepping, or low-impact aerobics. Whichever you choose, work at a pace that is comfortable for you and increase it gradually as you become conditioned. Do not overdo it. The experience should leave you feeling invigorated, not exhausted.

The physiological benefits of exercise are well known. Exercise may not eliminate the stressors in

life, but it is an important element in a healthy lifestyle. Exercise has been shown to improve people's mood and to induce a state of relaxation through the reduction of physiological tension. Regular exercise decreases the energy from the fight-or-flight response discussed at the beginning of this chapter.

Exercise can also be a useful distraction, allowing time to regroup before entering a stressful situation again (Long & Flood, 1993). It is important to choose an exercise that you enjoy doing and that fits into your lifestyle. Perhaps you could walk to work every day or pedal an exercise bicycle during your favorite television program. It is not necessary to join an expensive club or to buy elaborate equipment or clothing to begin an exercise program. It is necessary to get up and get moving, however.

Some people recommend an organized exercise program to obtain the most benefit. For some, however, the cost or time required may actually contribute to their stress. For others, the organized program is an excellent motivator. Find out what works for you.

Keep your exercise plan reasonable. Plan for the long term, not just until you get past your next performance evaluation or lose that extra five pounds.

Mental Health Management

Mental health management begins with *taking responsibility for your own thoughts and attitudes.* Do not allow self-defeating thoughts to dominate your thinking. You may have to remind yourself to stop thinking that you have to be perfect all the time. You may also have to adjust your expectations and become more realistic. Do you always have to be in control? Does everything have to be perfect? Do you have a difficult time delegating? Are you constantly frustrated because of the way you perceive situations? If you answer yes to many of these questions, you may be setting yourself up for failure, resentment, low self-esteem, and burnout. Give yourself positive strokes, even if no one else does (Davidhizar, 1994; Posen, 2000; Wolinski, 1993).

Realistic Expectations

One of the most common stressors in life is having unrealistic expectations. Expecting family members, coworkers, and your employer to be perfect and meet your every demand on your time schedule is setting yourself up for undue stress.

---

box 13-6

Guidelines for Good Nutrition

Eat smaller, more frequent, meals for energy. Six small meals are more beneficial than three large ones.

Eat foods that are high in complex carbohydrates, contain adequate protein, and are low in fat content. Beware of fad diets!

Eat at least five servings of fruits and vegetables daily.

Avoid highly processed foods.

Avoid caffeine.

Use salt and sugar sparingly.

Drink plenty of water.

Make sure you take enough vitamins, including C, B, E, beta carotene, and calcium; and minerals, including copper, manganese, zinc, magnesium, and potassium.

Adapted from Bowers, R. (1993). Stress and your health. National Women's Health Report, 15(3), 6.

Reframing

Reframing is looking at a situation in many different ways. When you can reframe stressful situations, they often become less stressful or at least more understandable. If you have an extremely heavy workday and believe it is due to the fact that your nurse manager created it for personal reasons, the day becomes much more stressful than if you realize that, unfortunately, all institutions are short-staffed.

Humor

Laughter relieves tension. Humor is a good way to reduce stress both for yourself and your patients. Remember, however, that humor is very individual, and what may be funny to you may be hurtful to your patient or coworker.

Social Support

Much research has been done to show that the presence of social support and the quality of relationships can significantly influence how quickly people become ill and how quickly they recover. A sense of belonging and community, an environment where people believe they can share their feelings without fear of condemnation or ridicule, helps to maintain a sense of well-being. Having friends with whom to share hopes, dreams, fears, and concerns and with whom to laugh and cry is paramount to mental health and stress management. In the work environment, coworkers who are trusted and respected become part of social support systems (Wolinski, 1993). Box 13-7 lists some additional tips for coping with work stress.

Nurses are professional caregivers. Many years ago, Carl Rogers (1977) said that you cannot care for others until you have taken care of yourself. The word *selfish* may bring to mind someone who is greedy, self-centered, and egotistical; however, to take care of yourself you have to become *creatively selfish*. Learn to nurture yourself so that you will be better able to nurture others.

Stress reduction, relaxation techniques, exercise, and good nutrition are all helpful in keeping energy levels high. Although they can prepare people to cope with the stresses of a job, they are not solutions to the conflicts that lead to reality shock and burnout. It is more effective to resolve the problem than to treat the symptoms (Lee & Ashforth, 1993). Box 13-8 lists the keys already discussed to physical and mental health management.

---

box 13-7

Coping With Daily Work Stress

Spend time on outside interests, and take time for yourself.

Increase professional knowledge.

Identify problem-solving resources.

Identify realistic expectations for your position. Make sure you understand what is expected of you; ask questions if anything is unclear.

Assess the rewards your work can realistically deliver.

Develop good communication skills, and treat coworkers with respect.

Join rap sessions with coworkers. Be part of the solution, not part of the problem.

Do not exceed your limits—you do not always have to say yes.

Deal with other people's anger by asking yourself, "Whose problem is this?"

Recognize that you can teach other people how to treat you.

---

box 13-8

Keys to Physical and Mental Health Management

Deep breathing

Posture

Rest

Relaxation

Nutrition

Exercise

Realistic expectations

Reframing

Humor

Social support

Organizational Approaches to Job Stress

The nursing shortage phenomenon has cause many organizations to address issues of stress on the job as a method of recruitment and retention. Organizational change and stress management are useful approaches for preventing stress at work. The National Institute for Occupational Safety and Health has identified factors that lead to a healthy, low-stress workplace (Judkins, Reid, & Furlow, 2006; Sauter et al., 1999):

- Employee recognition for performance
- Opportunities for career development
- An organizational culture that values the individual
- Management decisions that are aligned with organizational values

■ Collaborative practice and shared governance models

In 2002, Dr. Linda Aiken and her colleagues identified a relationship between staffing, mortality, nurse burnout, and job dissatisfaction (Aiken et al., 2002). With each additional patient assigned to a nurse, the following occurred:

■ A 30-day mortality increase of 7%
■ Failure-to-rescue rate increase of 7%
■ Nursing job dissatisfaction increase of 15%
■ Burnout rate increase of 23%
■ 43% of nurses surveyed were suffering from burnout

Conclusion

You already know that the work of nursing is not easy and may sometimes be very stressful. Yet nursing is also a profession filled with a great deal of personal and professional satisfaction. Periodically ask yourself the questions designed to help you assess your stress level and risk for burnout, and review the stress management techniques described in this chapter.

There is no one right way to manage stress and avoid burnout. Rather, by managing small segments of each day, you will learn to identify and manage your stress. This chapter contains many reminders to help you de-stress during the day (Box 13-9). You can also help your colleagues do the same. If you find yourself in danger of job burnout during your career, you will have learned how to bring yourself back to a healthy, balanced position.

Ultimately, you are in control. Every day you are faced with choices. By gaining power over your choices and the stress they cause, you empower yourself. Instead of being preoccupied with the past or the future, acknowledge the present moment, and say to yourself (Davidson, 1999):

■ I choose to relish my days.
■ I choose to enjoy this moment.
■ I choose to be fully present to others.
■ I choose to fully engage in the activity at hand.
■ I choose to proceed at a measured, effective pace.
■ I choose to acknowledge all I have achieved so far.

---

box 13-9

Ten Daily De-Stress Reminders

Express yourself! Communicate your feelings and emotions to friends and colleagues to avoid isolation and share perspectives. Sometimes, another opinion helps you see the situation in a different light.

Take time off. Taking breaks, or doing something unrelated to work, will help you feel refreshed as you begin work again.

Understand your individual energy patterns. Are you a morning or an afternoon person? Schedule stressful duties during times when you are most energetic.

Do one stressful activity at a time. Although this may take advanced planning, avoiding more than one stressful situation at a time will make you feel more in control and satisfied with your accomplishments.

Exercise! Physical exercise builds physical and emotional resilience. Do not put physical activities "on the back burner" as you become busy.

Tackle big projects one piece at a time. Having control of one part of a project at a time will help you to avoid feeling overwhelmed and out of control.

Delegate if possible. If you can delegate and share in problem solving, do so. Not only will your load be lighter, but others will be able to participate in decision making.

It's okay to say no. Do not take on every extra assignment or special project.

Be work-smart. Improve your work skills with new technologies and ideas. Take advantage of additional job training.

Relax. Find time each day to consciously relax and reflect on the positive energies you need to cope with stressful situations more readily.

Adapted from Bowers, R. (1993). Stress and your health. National Women's Health Report, 15(3), 6.

■ I choose to focus on where I am and what I am doing.
■ I choose to acknowledge that this is the only moment in which I can take action.

People cannot live in a problem-free world, but they can learn how to handle stress. Using the suggestions in this chapter, you will be able to adopt a healthier personal and professional lifestyle. The self-assessment worksheet on DavisPlus, entitled "Coping with Stress," can help you manage stress and help you understand your responses better. The worksheet on DavisPlus, entitled "Values Clarification," will help you identify how to begin to change taking into account what is most important to you.

Evidence-Based Practice

Faragher, E., Cass, M., & Cooper, C. (2003). The relationship between job satisfaction and health: A meta-analysis. *Journal of Occupational and Environmental Medicine*, 62, 105–112.

This systematic review and meta-analysis, completed in 2003, consisted of 500 studies of job satisfaction with 267,995 employees in a large variety of organizations, It demonstrated a strong correlation between job satisfaction and mental and physical health. Aspects of mental health, i.e., burnout, lowered self-esteem, anxiety, and depression, were identified. Cardiovascular disease was the main physical illness showing a correlation between job satisfaction and physical health. These relationships demonstrated that job satisfaction level is an important factor influencing health of workers.

Additional studies can be found in:

Ekstedt, M. (2005). Lived experiences of the time preceding burnout. *Journal of Advanced Nursing*, 49(1), 59–67.

Ruggeriero, J. (2005). Health, work variables, and job satisfaction among nurses. *Journal of Nursing Administration*, 35(5), 254–263.

Study Questions

1. Discuss the characteristics of health-care organizations that may lead to burnout among nurses. Which of these have you observed in your clinical rotations? How could they be changed or eliminated?

2. How can a new graduate adequately prepare for reality shock? Based on your responses to the questions in Boxes 13-3 and 13-4, what plans will you make to prepare yourself for your new role?

3. What qualities would you look for in a mentor? What qualities would you demonstrate as a mentee? Can you identify someone you know who might become a mentor to you?

4. How are the signs of stress, reality shock, and burnout related?

5. How can you help colleagues deal with their stress? What if a colleague does not recognize that he/she is under stress? What might you do to guide your colleague?

6. Identify the physical and psychological signs and symptoms you exhibit during stress. What sources of stress are most likely to affect you? How do you deal with these signs and symptoms?

7. Develop a plan to manage stress on a long-term basis.

Case Study to Promote Critical Reasoning

Shawna, a new staff member, has been working from 7 a.m. to 3 p.m. on an infectious disease floor since obtaining her RN license 4 months ago. Most of the staff members with whom she works with have been there since the unit opened 5 years ago. On a typical day, the staffing consists of a nurse manager, two RNs, an LPN, and one technician for approximately 40 patients. Most patients are HIV-positive with multisystem failure. Many are severely debilitated and need help with their activities of daily living. Although the staff members encourage family members and loved ones to help, most of them are unavailable because they work during the day. Several days a week, the nursing students from Shawna's community college program are assigned to the floor.

Tina, the nurse manager, does not participate in any direct patient care, saying that she is "too busy at the desk." Laverne, the other RN, says the unit depresses her and that she has requested a transfer to pediatrics. Lynn, the LPN, wants to "give meds" because she is "sick of the patients' constant whining," and Sheila, the technician, is "just plain exhausted." Lately, Shawna has noticed that the other staff members seem to avoid the nursing students and reply to their questions with annoyed, short answers. Shawna is feeling alone and overwhelmed and goes home at night worrying about the patients, who need more care and attention. She is afraid to ask Tina for more help because she does not want to be considered incompetent or a complainer. When she confided in Lynn about her concerns, Lynn replied, "Get real—no one here cares about the patients or us. All they care about is the bottom line! Why did a smart girl like you choose nursing in the first place?"

1. What is happening on this unit in leadership terms?

2. Identify the major problems and the factors that contributed to these problems.

3. What factors might have contributed to the behaviors exhibited by Tina, Lynn, and Sheila?

4. How would you feel if you were Shawna?

5. Is there anything Shawna can do for herself, for the patients, and for the staff members?

6. What do you think Tina, the nurse manager, should do?

7. How is the nurse manager reacting to the changes in her staff members?

8. What is the responsibility of administration?

9. How are the patients affected by the behaviors exhibited by all staff members?

References

Aiken, L.H., Clarke, S.P., Slane, D.M., Sochalski, J., et al. (2002). Hospital nurse staffing and patient mortality, nurse burnout, and job dissatisfaction. *Journal of the American Medical Association*, 288(16), 1989-1993.

Benner, P. (1984). *From Novice to Expert.* Menlo Park, Calif.: Addison-Wesley.

Best, M., & Thurston, N. (2004). Measuring nurse job satisfaction, *Journal of Nursing Administration*, 34(6), 283–290.

Borman, J. (1993). Chief nurse executives balance their work and personal lives. *Nursing Administration Quarterly*, 18(1), 30–39.

Bowers, R. (1993). Stress and your health. *National Women's Health Report*, 15(3), 6.

Boychuk, J. (2001). Out in the real world: Newly graduated nurses in acute-care speak out. *Journal of Nursing Administration*, 31, 426–439.

Bruce, M. (2007). Keep a stress diary. *Nursing Standard*, 22(5), 64.

Carr, K., & Kazanowski, M. (1994). Factors affecting job satisfaction of nurses who work in long-term care. *Journal of Advanced Nursing*, 19, 878–883.

Corley, M., Farley, B., Geddes, N., Goodloe, L., et al. (1994). The clinical ladder: Impact on nurse satisfaction and turnover. *Journal of Nursing Administration*, 24(2), 42–48.

Crawford, S. (1993). Job stress and occupational health nursing. *American Association of Occupational Health Nurses Journal*, 41, 522–529.

Crout, L., Change, E., & Cioffi, J. (2005). Why do registered nurses work when ill? *Journal of Nursing Administration*, 35(1), 23–28.

Davidhizar, R. (1994). Stress can make you or break you. *Advance Practice Nurse*, 10(1), 17.

Davidson, J. (1999). *Managing Stress*, 2nd ed. N.Y.: Pearson Education Macmillan Company.

Davis, M., Eshelman, E., & McCay, M. (2000). *The Relaxation and Stress Reduction Workbook*, 5th ed. Calif.: New Harbinger Publications.

DeFrank, R., & Ivancevich, J. (1998). Stress on the job: An executive update. *Academy of Management Executives*, 12(3), 55.

Dionne-Proulx, J., & Pepin, R. (1993). Stress management in the nursing profession. *Journal of Nursing Management*, 1, 75–81.

Duquette, A., Sandhu, B., & Beaudet, L. (1994). Factors related to nursing burnout: A review of empirical knowledge. *Issues in Mental Health Nursing*, 15, 337–358.

Faragher, E., Cass, M., & Cooper, C. (2003). The relationship between job satisfaction and health: A meta-analysis. *Journal of Occupational and Environmental Medicine*, 62, 105–112.

Farren, C. (1999). Stress and productivity: What tips the scale? *Strategy and Leadership*, 27(1), 36.

Fielding, J., & Weaver, S. (1994). A comparison of hospital and community-based mental health nurses: Perceptions of their work environment and psychological health. *Journal of Advanced Nursing*, 19, 1196–1204.

Freudenberger, H.J. (1974). Staff burn-out. *Journal of Social Issues*, 30(1), 159.

Godinez, G., Schweiger, J., Gruver, J., & Ryan, P. (1999). Role transition from graduate to staff nurse: A qualitative analysis. *Journal for Nurses in Staff Development*, 15(3), 97–110.

Golin, M., Buchlin, M., & Diamond, D. (1991). *Secrets of Executive Success.* Emmaus, Pa.: Rodale Press.

Goliszek, A. (1992). *Sixty-Six Second Stress Management: The Quickest Way to Relax and Ease Anxiety.* Far Hills, N.J.: New Horizon.

Goodell, T., & Van Ess Coeling, H. (1994). Outcomes of nurses' job satisfaction. *Journal of Nursing Administration*, 24(11), 36–41.

Grant, P. (1993). Manage nurse stress and increase potential at the bedside. *Nursing Administration Quarterly*, 18(1), 16–22.

Hall, D. (2004). Work-related stress of registered nurses in a hospital setting. *Journal for Nurses in Staff Development*, 20(1), 6–14.

Heslop, L. (2001). Undergraduate student nurses: Expectations and their self-reported preparedness for the graduate year role. *Journal of Advanced Nursing*, 36, 626–634.

Johnston, F. (May-June 1994). Stress can kill. *Today's OR Nurse,* 5–6.

Judkins, S., Reid, B., & Furlow, L. (2006). Hardiness training among nurse managers: Building a healthy workplace. *Journal of Continuing Education in Nursing,* 37(5), 202–207.

Kovner, C., Hendrickson, G., Knickman, J., & Finkler, S. (1994). Nurse care delivery models and nurse satisfaction. *Nursing Administration Quarterly,* 19(1), 74–85.

Kraeger, M., & Walker, K. (1993). Attrition, burnout, job dissatisfaction and occupational therapy manager. *Occupational Therapy in Health Care,* 8(4), 47–61.

Kramer, M. (January 27–28, 1981). Coping with reality shock. Workshop presented at Jackson Memorial Hospital, Miami, FL.

Kramer, M., & Schmalenberg, C. (1993). Learning from success: Autonomy and empowerment. *Nursing Management,* 24(5), 58–64.

Lee, R.T., & Ashforth, B.E. (1993). A further examination of managerial burnout: Toward an integrated model. *Journal of Organizational Behavior,* 14(1), 3–20.

Lenson, B. (2001). *Good Stress—Bad Stress.* N.Y.: Marlowe and Company.

Lickman, P., Simms, L., & Greene, C. (1993). Learning environment: The catalyst for work excitement. *Journal of Continuing Education in Nursing,* 24, 211–216.

Long, B., & Flood, K. (1993). Coping with work stress: Psychological benefits of exercise. *Work and Stress,* 7(2), 109–119.

Lusk, S. (1993). Job stress. *American Association of Occupational Health Nurses Journal,* 41, 601–606.

Malkin, K.F. (1993). Primary nursing: Job satisfaction and staff retention. *Journal of Nursing Management,* 1, 119–124.

Martin, K. (May 1993). To cope with stress. *Nursing* 93, 39–41.

McGee-Cooper, A. (September-October 1993). Shifting from high stress to high energy. *Imprint,* 93(5), 61–69.

McLennan, M. (2005). Nurses' views on work enabling factors. *Journal of Nursing Administration,* 35(6), 311–318.

McVicar, A. (2003). Workplace stress in nursing. A literature review. *Journal of Advanced Nursing,* 44(6), 633–642.

Nakata, J., & Saylor, C. (1994). Management style and staff nurse satisfaction in a changing environment. *Nursing Administration Quarterly,* 18(3), 51–57

National Institute for Occupational Safety and Health (NIOSH) Accessed July 27, 2002, at http://www.cdc.gov/niosh/homepage.html

Nowak, K., & Pentkowski, A. (1994). Lifestyle habits, substance use, and predictors of job burnout in professional women. *Work and Stress,* 8(1), 19–35.

Paine, W.S. (1984). Professional burnout: Some major costs. *Family and Community Health,* 6(4), 1–11.

Pines, A. (2004). Adult attachment styles and their relationship to burnout: A preliminary, cross-cultural investigation. *Work & Stress,* 18(1), 66–80.

Posen, D. (2000). Stress management for patient and physician. http://www.mentalhealth.com/mag1/p51-str.html

Rogers, C. (1977). *Carl Rogers on Personal Power.* N.Y.: Dell.

Sadovich, J. (2005). Work excitement in nursing: An examination between work excitement and burnout. *Nursing Economics,* 23(2), 91–96.

Sauter, S., Murphy, L, Colligan, M., Swanson, N., et al. (1999). *Stress at Work* (NIOSH Pub. No. 99-101). Accessed September 24, 2007, at http://www.cdc.gov/niosh/stresswk.html

Scheetz, L.J. (2000). *Nursing Faculty Secrets.* Philadelphia: Hanley & Belfus.

Selye, H. (1956). *The Stress of Life.* N.Y.: McGraw-Hill.

Simonetti, J., & Ariss, S. (1999). The role of a mentor. *Business Horizons,* 42(6), 56–73.

Skubak, K., Earls, N., & Botos, M. (1994). Shared governance: Getting it started. *Nursing Management,* 25(5), 80I-J, 80N, 80P.

Smith, B. (October 2004). Test your stamina for workplace fatigue. *Nursing Management,* 38–40.

Stechmiller, J., & Yarandi, H. (1993). Predictors of burnout in critical care nurses. *Heart Lung,* 22, 534–540.

Teague, J.B. (1992). The relationship between various coping styles and burnout among nurses. *Dissertation Abstracts International,* 1994.

Trossman, S. (July/August 1999). Stress! It's everywhere! And it can be managed! *American Nurse,* 1.

Tumulty, G., Jernigan, E., & Kohut, G. (1994). The impact of perceived work environment on job satisfaction of hospital staff nurses. *Applied Nursing Research,* 7(2), 84–90.

Vahey, D., Aiken, L., Sloane, D., Clarke, S. et al. (2004). Nurse burnout and patient satisfaction. *Medical Care,* 42(2), II-57-II-66.

Vines, S. (1994). Relaxation with guided imagery, *American Association of Occupational Health Nurses Journal,* 42, 206–213.

Wolinski, K. (1993). Self-awareness, self-renewal, self management. *AORN Journal,* 58, 721–730.

○●○○○○○○○○○

OBJECTIVES

After reading this chapter, the student should be able to:

- Evaluate personal strengths, weaknesses, opportunities, and threats using a SWOT analysis.
- Develop a résumé including objectives, qualifications, skills experience, work history, education, and training.
- Compose job search letters including cover letter, thank-you letter, and acceptance and rejection letters.
- Discuss components of the interview process.
- Discuss the factors involved in selecting the right position.
- Explain why the first year is critical to planning a career.

The National Center for Health Workforce Analysis at Health Resources and Services Administration has projected a growing shortage of registered nurses (RNs) over the next 15 years, with a 12% shortage by 2010 and a 20% shortage by 2015 (http://bhpr.hrsa.gov/healthworkforce/nursingshortage/tech_report/default.htm). This continued shortage of RNs will allow you to have many choices and opportunities as a professional nurse. By now you have invested considerable time, expense, and emotion into preparing for your new career. Your educational preparation, technical and clinical expertise, interpersonal and management skills, personal interests and needs, and commitment to the nursing profession will contribute to meeting your career goals. Successful nurses view nursing as a lifetime pursuit, not as an occupational stepping stone.

This chapter deals with the most important endeavor: finding and keeping your first nursing position. The chapter begins with planning your initial search; developing a strengths, weaknesses, opportunities, and threats (SWOT) analysis; searching for available positions; and researching organizations. Also included is a section on writing a résumé and employment-related information about the interview process and selecting the first position.

Getting Started

By now at least one person has said to you, "Nurses will never be out of a job." This statement is only one of several career myths. These myths include the following:

1. "Good workers do not get fired." They may not get fired, but many good workers have lost their positions during restructuring and downsizing.
2. "Well-paying jobs are available without a college degree." Even if entrance into a career path does not require a college education, the potential for career advancement is minimal without that degree. In many health-care agencies, a baccalaureate degree in nursing is required for an initial management position.
3. "Go to work for a good company, and move up the career ladder." This statement assumes that people move up the career ladder due to longevity in the organization. In reality, the responsibility for career advancement rests on the employee, not the employer.

4. "Find the 'hot' industry, and you will always be in demand." Nursing is projected to continue to be one of the "hottest industries" well into the next decade. A nurse who performs poorly will never be successful, no matter what the demand.

Many students attending college today are adults with family, work, and personal responsibilities. On graduating with an associate degree in nursing, you may still have student loans and continued responsibilities for supporting a family. If this is so, you may be so focused on job security and a steady source of income that the idea of career planning has not even entered your mind. You might even assume that your goal is just to "get the first job." The correct goal is to find a job that fits *you*, one that is a good first step on the path to a lifelong career in nursing. It is also not too early to begin formal planning of your career. You will most likely work well in excess of 70,000 hours in a lifetime outside the home. Do you want to spend all this time devoted to a career that is not fulfilling?

SWOT Analysis

Many students assume their first position will be as a staff nurse on a medical-surgical floor. They see themselves as "putting in their year" and then moving on to what they really want to do. However, as the health-care system continues to evolve and reallocate resources, this may no longer be the automatic first step for new graduates. Instead, new graduates should focus on long-term career goals and the different avenues by which they can be reached.

Many times, your past experiences will be an asset in presenting your abilities for a particular position. A SWOT analysis plan, borrowed from the corporate world, can guide you through your own internal strengths and weaknesses as well as external opportunities and threats that may help or hinder your job search and career planning. The SWOT analysis is an in-depth look at what will make you happy in your work. Although you have already made the decision to pursue nursing, knowing your strengths and weaknesses can help you select the work setting that will be satisfying personally (Ellis, 1999). Your SWOT analysis may include the following factors (Pratt, 1994):

Strengths
■ Relevant work experience
■ Advanced education

- Product knowledge
- Good communication and people skills
- Computer skills
- Self-managed learning skills
- Flexibility

Weaknesses

- Poor communication and people skills
- Inflexibility
- Lack of interest in further training
- Difficulty adapting to change
- Inability to see health care as a business

Opportunities

- Expanding markets in health care
- New applications of technology
- New products and diversification
- Increasing at-risk populations
- Nursing shortage

Threats

- Increased competition among health-care facilities
- Changes in government regulation

Take some time to personalize the preceding SWOT analysis. What are *your* strengths? What are the things *you* are not so good at? What weaknesses do *you* need to minimize, or what strengths do *you* need to develop as you begin your job search? What opportunities and threats exist in the health-care community *you* are considering? Doing a SWOT analysis will help you make an initial assessment of the job market. It can be used again after you narrow your search for that first nursing position.

In addition to completing a SWOT analysis, there are several other tools that can help you learn more about yourself. Two of the most common are the Strong Interest Inventory (SII) and the Myers-Briggs Type Indicator (MBTI). The SII compares the individual's interests with the interests of those who are successful in a large number of occupational fields in the areas of (1) work styles, (2) learning environment, (3) leadership style, and (4) risk-taking/adventure. Completing this inventory can help you discover what work environment might be best suited to your interests.

The MBTI is a widely used indicator of personality patterns. This self-report inventory provides information about individual psychological-type preferences on four dimensions:

1. Extroversion (E) or Introversion (I)
2. Sensing (S) or Intuition (N)
3. Thinking (T) or Feeling (F)
4. Judging (J) or Perceiving (P)

Although there are many factors that influence behaviors and attitudes, the MBTI summarizes underlying patterns and behaviors common to most people. Both tools should be administered and interpreted by a qualified practitioner. Most university and career counseling centers are able to administer them. If you are unsure of just where you fit in the workplace, you might explore these tests with your college or university or take it online at http://www.myersbriggs.org/

Beginning the Search

Even with a nationwide nursing shortage, hospital mergers, emphasis on increased staff productivity, budget crises, staffing shifts, and changes in job market availability affect the numbers and types of nurses employed in various facilities and agencies. Instead of focusing on long-term job security, the career-secure employee focuses on becoming a career survivalist. A career survivalist focuses on the person, not the position. Consider the following career survivalist strategies (Waymon & Baber, 1999):

- **Be self-employed psychologically.** Your career belongs to you, not to the person who signs your paycheck. Security and advancement on the job are up to you. Security may be elusive, but opportunities for nurses are growing every day.
- **Learn for employability.** Take personal responsibility for your career success. Learn not only for your current position but also for your next position. Employability in health care today means learning technology tools, job-specific technical skills, and people skills such as the ability to negotiate, coach, work in teams, and make presentations.
- **Plan for your financial future.** Ask yourself, "How can I spend less, earn more, and manage better?" Often, people make job decisions based on financial decisions, which makes them feel trapped instead of secure.
- **Develop multiple options.** The career survivalist looks at multiple options constantly. Moving up is only one option. Being aware of emerging

trends in nursing, adjacent fields, lateral moves, and special projects presents other options.

■ **Build a safety net.** Networking is extremely important to the career survivalist. Joining professional organizations, taking time to build long-term nursing relationships, and getting to know other career survivalists will make your career path more enjoyable and successful.

What do employers think you need to be ready to work for them? In addition to passing the National Council Licensure Examination (NCLEX), employers cite the following skills as desirable in job candidates (Shingleton, 1994):

Oral and Written Communication Skills

■ Ability to assume responsibility
■ Interpersonal skills
■ Proficiency in field of study/technical competence
■ Teamwork ability
■ Willingness to work hard
■ Leadership abilities
■ Motivation, initiative, and flexibility
■ Critical thinking and analytical skills
■ Computer knowledge
■ Problem-solving and decision-making abilities
■ Self-discipline
■ Organizational skills

Active job searches may include looking in a variety of places (Beatty, 1991; Hunsaker, 2001):

■ Public employment agencies
■ Private employment agencies
■ Human resource departments
■ Information from friends or relatives
■ Newspapers; professional journals
■ College and university career centers
■ Career and job fairs
■ Internet Web sites
■ Other professionals (networking)

In recent years, three trends have emerged related to recruiting. First, employers are using more creativity by using alternative sources to increase diversity of employees. They commonly have advertisements in minority newspapers and magazines and recruit nurses at minority organizations. Second, employers are using more temporary help as a way to evaluate potential employees. Nursing staffing agencies are common in most areas of the county. Third, the Internet is being used more frequently for advertising and recruitment (Hunsaker, 2001).

Regardless of where you begin your search, explore the market vigorously and thoroughly. Looking only in the classified ads on Sunday morning is a limited search. Instead, speak to everyone you know about your job search. Encourage classmates and colleagues to share contacts with you, and do the same for them. Also, when possible, try to speak directly with the person who is looking for a nurse when you hear of a possible opening. The people in Human Resources (Personnel) offices may reject a candidate on a technicality that a nurse manager would realize does not affect that person's ability to handle the job if he or she is otherwise a good match for the position. For example, experience in day surgery prepares a person to work in other surgery-related settings, but a human resources interviewer may not know this.

Try to obtain as much information as you can about the available position. Is there a match between your skills and interests and the position? Ask yourself whether you are applying for this position because you really want it or just to gain interview experience. Be careful about going through the interview process and receiving job offers only to turn them down. Employers may share information with one another, and you could end up being denied the position you really want. Regardless of where you explore potential opportunities, use these "pearls of wisdom" from career nurses:

■ Know yourself.
■ Seek out mentors and wise people.
■ Be a risk taker.
■ Never, ever stop learning.
■ Understand the business of health care.
■ Involve yourself in community and professional organizations.
■ Network.
■ Understand diversity.
■ Be an effective communicator.
■ Set short- and long-term goals, and strive continually to achieve them.

Researching Your Potential Employer

You have spent time taking a look at yourself and the climate of the health-care job market. You have narrowed your choices to the organizations that really interest you. Now is the time to find out as much as possible about these organizations.

Ownership of the company may be public or private, foreign or American. The company may be local or regional, a small corporation or a division of a much larger corporation. Depending on the size and ownership of the company, information may be obtained from the public library, chamber of commerce, government offices, or company Web site. A telephone call or letter to the corporate office or local human resources department may also generate valuable information on organizations of interest (Crowther, 1994). Has the organization recently gone through a merger, a reorganization, or downsizing? Information from current and past employees is valuable and may provide you with more details about whether the organization might be suitable for you. Be wary of gossip and half-truths that may emerge, however, because they may discourage you from applying to an excellent health-care facility. In other words, if you hear something negative about an organization, investigate it for yourself. Often, individuals jump at work opportunities before doing a complete assessment of the culture and politics of the institution.

The first step in assessing the culture is to review a copy of the company's mission statement. The mission statement reflects what the institution considers important to its public image. What are the core values of the institution?

The department of nursing's philosophy and objectives indicate how the department defines nursing; they identify what the department's important goals are for nursing. The nursing philosophy and goals should reflect the mission of the organization. Where is nursing administration on the organizational chart of the institution? To whom does the chief nursing administrator report? Although much of this information may not be obtained until an interview, a preview of how the institution views itself and the value it places on nursing will help you to decide if your philosophy of health care and nursing is compatible with that of a particular organization. To find out more about a specific health-care facility, you can (Zedlitz, 2003):

- Talk to nurses currently employed at the facility.
- Access the Internet Web site for information on the mission, philosophy, and services.
- Check the library for newspaper and magazine articles related to the facility.

Writing a Résumé

Your résumé is your personal data sheet and self-advertisement. It is the first impression the recruiter or your potential employer will have of you. With the résumé you are selling yourself: your skills, talents, and abilities. You may decide to prepare your own résumé or have it prepared by a professional service. Regardless of who prepares it, the purpose of a résumé is to get a job interview. Many people dislike the idea of writing a résumé. After all, how can you sum up your entire career in a single page? You want to scream at the printed page, "Hey, I'm bigger than that! Look at all I have to offer!" However, this one-page summary has to work well enough to get you the position you want. Chestnut (1999) summarized résumé writing by stating, "Lighten up. Although a very important piece to the puzzle in your job search, a résumé is not the only ammunition. What's between your ears is what will ultimately lead you to your next career" (p. 28). Box 14-1 summarizes reasons for preparing a well-considered, up-to-date résumé.

Although you labor intensively over preparing your résumé, most job applications live or die within 10–30 seconds as the receptionist or applications examiner decides whether your résumé should be forwarded to the next step or rejected. The initial screening is usually done by

---

box 14-1

Reasons for Preparing a Résumé

Assists in completing an employment application quickly and accurately

Demonstrates your potential

Focuses on your strongest points

Gives you credit for all your achievements

Identifies you as organized, prepared, and serious about the job search

Serves as a reminder and adds to your self-confidence during the interview

Provides initial introduction to potential employers in seeking the interview

Serves as a guide for the interviewer

Functions as a tool to distribute to others who are willing to assist you in a job search

Adapted from Marino, K. (2000). Resumes for the Health Care Professional. N.Y.: John Wiley & Sons; and Zedlitz, R. (2003). How to Get a Job in Health Care. N.Y.: Delmar Learning.

non-nursing personnel. Some beginning helpful tips include: (Marino, 2000):

- Keep the résumé to one or two pages. Do not use smaller fonts to cram more information on the page. Proofread, proofread, proofread. Typing errors, misspelled words, and poor grammar can damage your chances of obtaining an interview. Do not substitute quantity of words for quality.
- Your educational background goes at the end of the résumé, unless you are a recent graduate and your degree is stronger than your experience or you are applying for a job at an educational institution.
- State your objective. Although you know very well what position you are seeking, the receptionist doing the initial screening does not want to take the time to determine this. Tailor your resume to the insitution and position to which you are applying.
- Employers care about what you can do for them and your potential future success with their company. Your résumé must answer that question.

Essentials of a Résumé

Résumés most frequently follow one of four formats: standard, chronological, functional, or a combination. Regardless of the type of résumé, basic elements of personal information, education, work experience, qualifications for the position, and references should be included (Marino, 2000; Zedlitz, 2003):

- **Standard.** The standard résumé is organized by categories. By clearly stating your personal information, job objective, work experience, education and work skills, memberships, honors, and special skills, the employer can easily have a "snapshot" of the person requesting entrance into the workforce. This is a useful résumé for first-time employees or recent graduates.
- **Chronological.** The chronological résumé lists work experiences in order of time, with the most recent experience listed first. This style is useful in showing stable employment without gaps or many job changes. The objective and qualifications are listed at the top.
- **Functional**. The functional résumé also lists work experience but in order of importance to your job objective. List the most important work-related experience first. This is a useful format when you have gaps in employment or

lack direct experience related to your objective. Figure 14.1 shows a functional résumé that could be used for seeking initial employment as an RN.
- **Combination**. The combination résumé is a popular format, listing work experience directly related to the position but in a chronological order.

Most professional recruiters and placement services agree on the following tips in preparing a résumé (Anderson, 1992; Rodriguez & Robertson, 1992):

- *Make sure your résumé is readable.* Is the type large enough for easy reading? Are paragraphs indented or bullets used to set off information, or does the entire page look like a gray blur? Using bold headings and appropriate spacing can offer relief from lines of gray type, but be careful not to get so carried away with graphics that your résumé becomes a new art form. The latest trends with résumé writing are using fonts such as Ariel or Century New Gothic over the standard Times New Roman (James, 2003). The paper should be an appropriate color such as cream, white, or off-white. Use easily readable fonts and a laser printer. If a good computer and printer are not available, most printing services prepare résumés at a reasonable cost.
- *Make sure the important facts are easy to spot.* Education, current employment, responsibilities, and facts to support the experience you have gained from previous positions are important. Put the strongest statements at the beginning. Avoid excessive use of the word "I." If you are a new nursing graduate and have little or no job experience, list your educational background first. Remember that positions you held before you entered nursing can frequently support experience that will be relevant in your nursing career. Be sure you let your prospective employer know how you can be contacted.
- *Do a spelling and grammar check.* Use simple terms, action verbs, and descriptive words. Check your finished résumé for spelling, style, and grammar errors. If you are not sure how something sounds, get another opinion.
- *Follow the don'ts.* Do not include pictures, fancy binders, salary information, or hobbies (unless they have contributed to your work experience). Do not include personal information such as weight, marital status, and number of children.

Delores Wheatley
5734 Foster Road
Middleton, Indiana 46204
(907) 123-4567

Objective: Position as staff registered nurse on medical-surgical unit

HIGHLIGHTS OF QUALIFICATIONS
High School Diploma, 2004
Coral Ridge High School
Dolphin Beach, Florida

Associate of Science Degree in Nursing, 2009
Howard Community College (HCC)
Middleton, Indiana
Currently enrolled in the following courses at HCC:
30-hour IV certification course
8-hour phlebotomy course
16-hour 12-lead EKG course

EXPERIENCE
Volunteer, Association for the Blind, 2001-2004
Nursing Assistant, Howard Community Hospital, 2004-2007
  (summer employment)
Special Olympics Committee, 2007-2008

QUALIFICATIONS
Experience with blind and disabled children
Pediatric inpatient experience
Ability to work as part of an interdisciplinary team
Experience with families in crisis

Figure 14.1 Sample functional résumé.

Do not repeat information just to make the résumé longer. A good résumé is concise and focuses on your strengths and accomplishments.

No matter which format you use, it is essential to include the following (Parker, 1989):

- A clearly stated job objective.
- Highlighted qualifications.
- Directly relevant skills experience.
- Chronological work history.
- Relevant education and training.

How to Begin

Start by writing down every applicable point you can think of in the preceding five categories. Work history is usually the easiest place to begin. Arrange your work history in reverse chronological order, listing your current job first. Account for all your employable years. Short lapses in employment are acceptable, but give a brief explanation for longer periods (e.g., "maternity leave"). Include employer, dates worked (years only, e.g., 2001–2002), city, and state for each employer you list. Briefly describe the duties and responsibilities of each position. Emphasize your accomplishments, any special techniques you learned, or changes you implemented. Use action verbs, such as those listed in Table 14-1, to describe your accomplishments. Also cite any special awards or committee chairs. If a previous position was not in the health field, try to relate your duties and accomplishments to the position you are seeking.

Education

Next, focus on your education. Include the name and location of every educational institution you attended; the dates you attended; and the degree, diploma, or certification attained. Start with your most recent degree. It is not necessary to include your license number because you will give a copy of the license when you begin employment. If you are still waiting to take the NCLEX, you need to indicate when you are scheduled for the examination. If you are seeking additional training, such as for intravenous certification, include only what is relevant to your job objective.

Your Objective

It is now time to write your job objective. Write a clear, brief job objective. To accomplish this, ask yourself: what do I want to do? for or with whom? when? at what level of responsibility? For example (Parker, 1989):

- **What:** RN
- **For whom:** Pediatric patients
- **Where:** Large metropolitan hospital
- **At what level:** Staff

A new graduate's objective might read: "Position as staff nurse on a pediatric unit" or "Graduate nurse position on a pediatric unit." Do not include phrases such as "advancing to neonatal intensive care unit." Employers are trying to fill current openings and do not want be considered a stepping stone in your career.

Skills and Experience

Relevant skills and experience are included in your résumé not to describe your past but to present a "word picture of you in your proposed new job, created out of the best of your past experience" (Parker, 1989, p. 13; Impollonia, 2004). Begin by jotting down the major skills required for the position you are seeking. Include five or six major skills such as:

- Administration/management
- Teamwork/problem solving
- Patient relations
- Specialty proficiency
- Technical skills

Other

Academic honors, publications, research, and membership in professional organizations may be included. Were you active in your school's student nurses association? A church or community organization? Were you on the dean's list? What if you were "just a housewife" for many years? First, do an attitude adjustment: you were not "just a housewife" but a family manager. Explore your role in work-related terms such as *community volunteer, personal relations, fund raising, counseling,* or *teaching.* A

---

table 14-1

Action Verbs

Management Skills	Communication Skills	Accomplishments	Helping Skills
Attained	Collaborated	Achieved	Assessed
Developed	Convinced	Adapted	Assisted
Improved	Developed	Coordinated	Clarified
Increased	Enlisted	Developed	Demonstrated
Organized	Formulated	Expanded	Diagnosed
Planned	Negotiated	Facilitated	Expedited
Recommended	Promoted	Implemented	Facilitated
Strengthened	Reconciled	Improved	Motivated
Supervised	Recruited	Instructed	Represented
		Reduced (losses)	
		Resolved (problems)	
		Restored	

Adapted from Parker, Y. (1989). The Damn Good Résumé Guide. Berkeley, Calif.: Ten Speed Press.

college career office, women's center, or professional résumé service can offer you assistance with analyzing the skills and talents you shared with your family and community. A student who lacks work experience has options as well. Examples of non-work experiences that show marketable skills include (Eubanks, 1991; Parker, 1989):

- Working on the school paper or yearbook
- Serving in the student government
- Leadership positions in clubs, bands, church activities
- Community volunteer
- Coaching sports or tutoring children in academic areas

After you have jotted down everything relevant about yourself, develop the highlights of your qualifications. This area could also be called the summary of qualifications or just summary. These are immodest one-liners designed to let your prospective employer know that you are qualified and talented and the best choice for the position. A typical group of highlights might include (Parker, 1989):

- Relevant experience
- Formal training and credentials, if relevant
- Significant accomplishments, very briefly stated
- One or two outstanding skills or abilities
- A reference to your values, commitment, or philosophy, if appropriate

A new graduate's highlights could read:

- 5 years of experience as a licensed practical nurse in a large nursing home
- Excellent patient/family relationship skills
- Experience with chronic psychiatric patients
- Strong teamwork and communication skills
- Special certification in rehabilitation and reambulation strategies

Tailor the résumé to the job you are seeking. Include only relevant information, such as internships, summer jobs, inter-semester experiences, and volunteer work. Even if your previous experience is not directly related to nursing, your previous work experience can show transferable skills, motivation, and your potential to be a great employee.

Regardless of how wonderful you sound on paper, if the résumé itself is not high quality, it may end up in a trash can. As well, let your prospective employer know whether you have an answering machine or fax for leaving messages.

Job Search Letters

The most common job search letters are the cover letter, thank-you letter, and acceptance letter. Job search letters should be linked to you SWOT analysis. Regardless of their specific purpose, letters should follow basic writing principles (Banis, 1994):

- State the purpose of your letter.
- State the most important items first, and support them with facts.
- Keep the letter organized.
- Group similar items together in a paragraph, and then organize the paragraphs to flow logically.

Business letters are formal, but they can also be personal and warm but professional.

- Avoid sending an identical form letter to everyone. Instead, personalize each letter to fit each individual situation.
- As you write the letter, keep it work-centered and employment-centered, not self-centered.
- Be direct and brief. Keep your letter to one page.
- Use the active voice and action verbs and have a positive, optimistic tone.
- If possible, address your letters to a specific individual, using the correct title and business address. Letters addressed to "To Whom It May Concern" do not indicate much research or interest in your prospective employer.
- A timely (rapid) response demonstrates your knowledge of how to do business.
- Be honest. Use specific examples and evidence from your experience to support your claims.

Cover Letter

You have spent time carefully preparing the résumé that best sells you to your prospective employer. The cover letter will be your introduction. If it is true that first impressions are lasting ones, the cover letter will have a significant impact on your prospective employer. The purposes of the cover letter include (Beatty, 1989):

- Acting as a transmittal letter for your résumé
- Presenting you and your credentials to the prospective employer
- Generating interest in interviewing you

Regardless of whether your cover letter will be read first by human resources personnel or by the individual nurse manager, the effectiveness of your cover letter cannot be overemphasized. A poor cover letter can eliminate you from the selection process before you even have an opportunity to compete. A sloppy, unorganized cover letter and résumé may suggest you are sloppy and unorganized at work. A lengthy, wordy cover letter may suggest a verbose, unfocused individual (Beatty, 1991). The cover letter should include the following (Anderson, 1992):

- **State your purpose in applying and your interest in a specific position.** Also identify how you learned about the position.
- **Emphasize your strongest qualifications that match the requirements for the position.** Provide evidence of experience and accomplishments that relate to the available position, and refer to your enclosed résumé.
- **Sell yourself.** Convince this employer that you have the qualifications and motivation to perform in this position.
- **Express appreciation to the reader for consideration.**

If possible, address your cover letter to a specific person. If you do not have a name, call the health-care facility, and obtain the name of the human resources supervisor. If you do not have a name, create a greeting by adding the word "manager" so that your greeting reads: Dear Human Resources Manager or Dear Personnel Manager (Zedlitz, 2003, p. 19). Figure 14.2 is an example of a cover letter.

Thank-You Letter

Thank-you letters are important but seldom used tools in a job search. You should send a thank-you letter to everyone who has helped in any way in your job search. As stated earlier, promptness is important. Thank-you letters should be sent out within 24 hours to anyone who has interviewed you. The letter (Banis, 1994, p. 4) should be used to:

- Express appreciation
- Reemphasize your qualifications and the match between your qualifications and the available position
- Restate your interest in the position
- Provide any supplemental information not previously stated

Figure 14.3 is a sample thank-you letter.

Acceptance Letter

Write an acceptance letter to accept an offered position; confirm the terms of employment, such as salary and starting date; and reiterate the employer's decision to hire you. The acceptance letter often follows a telephone conversation in which the terms of employment are discussed. Figure 14.4 is a sample acceptance letter.

Rejection Letter

Although not as common as the first three job search letters, you should send a rejection letter if you are declining an employment offer. When rejecting an employment offer, indicate that you have given the offer careful consideration but have decided that the position does not fit your career objectives and interests at this time. As with your other letters, thank the employer for his or her consideration and offer. Figure 14.5 is a sample rejection letter.

Using the Internet

It is not uncommon to search the Internet for positions. Numerous sites either post positions or assist potential employees in matching their skills with available employment. More and more corporations are using the Internet to reach wider audiences. If you use the Internet in your search, it is always wise to follow up with a hard copy of your résumé if an address is listed. Mention in your cover letter that you sent your résumé via the Internet and the date you did so. If you are using an Internet-based service, follow up with an e-mail to ensure that your résumé was received. Table 14-2 summarized the major "do's and don'ts" when using the Internet to job search.

The Interview Process

Initial Interview

Your first interview may be with the nurse manager, someone in the human resources office, or an interviewer at a job fair or even over the telephone. Regardless of with whom or where you interview, preparation is the key to success.

You began the first step in the preparation process with your SWOT analysis. If you did not obtain any of the following information regarding your prospective employer at that time, it is imperative that you do it now (Impollonia, 2004):

- Key people in the organization
- Number of patients and employees
- Types of services provided
- Reputation in the community

5734 Foster Road
Middleton, Indiana 46204

April 15, 2009

Ms. Martha Berrero
Human Resources Manager
All Care Nursing Center
4431 Lakeside Drive
Middleton, Indiana 46204

Dear Ms. Berrero:

I am applying for the registered nurse position that was advertised in the *Fort Lauderdale News* on April 14. The position seems to fit very well with my education, experience, and career interests.

Your position requires interest and experience in caring for the elderly and in IV certification. In addition to my clinical experience in the nursing program at Howard Community College (HCC), I worked as a certified nursing assistant at Howard Community Hospital 25 hours/week during the 2 years I was enrolled in the HCC nursing program. My responsibilities included assisting the elderly clients with activities of daily living, including special range-of-motion and reambulation exercises. The experience of serving as a team member under the supervision of the registered nurse and physical therapist has been invaluable. I am currently enrolled in several continuing education courses at HCC. My enclosed résumé provides more details about my qualifications and education.

My background and career goals seem to match your job requirements. I am confident that I can perform the duties of a registered nurse at All Care Nursing Center. I am genuinely interested in pursuing a nursing career in care of the aging. Your agency has an excellent reputation in the community, and your parent company is likewise highly respected.

I am requesting a personal interview to discuss the possibilities of employment. I will call you during the week of April 21 to request an appointment. Should you need to reach me, please call 907-123-4567 or e-mail me at dwheatley@bellspot.com. My telephone has an answering machine. I will return your call or e-mail promptly.

Thank you for your consideration. I look forward to talking with you.

Sincerely yours,

Delores Wheatley

Delores Wheatley

Figure 14.2 Sample cover letter.

- Recent mergers and acquisitions
- The prospective employer's Web site for current news releases

You also need to review your qualifications for the position. What does your interviewer want to know about you? Consider the following:

- Why should I hire you?
- What kind of employee will you be?
- Will you get things done?
- How much will you cost the company?

- How long will you stay?
- What have you not told us about your weaknesses?

Answering Questions

The interviewer may ask background questions, professional questions, and personal questions. If you are especially nervous about interviewing, role-play your interview with a friend or family member acting as the interviewer. Have this person help you evaluate not just what you say but how you say it.

5734 Foster Road
Middleton, Indiana 46204

April 27, 2009

Ms. Martha Berrero
Human Resources Manager
All Care Nursing Center
4431 Lakeside Drive
Middleton, Indiana 46204

Dear Ms. Berrero:

Thank you very much for interviewing me yesterday for the registered nurse position at All Care Nursing Center. I enjoyed meeting you and learning more about the role of the registered nurse in long-term care with Jefferson Corporation.

My enthusiasm for the position and my interest in working with the elderly have increased as a result of the interview. I believe that my education and experience in long-term care fit with the job requirements. I know that currently I can make a contribution to the care of the residents and over time I hope to qualify as a nursing team leader.

I wish to reiterate my strong interest in working with you and your staff. I know that All Care Nursing Center can provide the kind of opportunities I am seeking. Please call me at 907-123-4567 if I can provide you with any additional information.

Again, thank you for the interview and for considering me for the registered nurse position.

Sincerely yours,

Delores Wheatley

Delores Wheatley

Figure 14.3 Sample thank-you letter.

Voice inflection, eye contact, and friendliness are demonstrations of your enthusiasm for the position (Costlow, 1999).

Whatever the questions, know your key points, and be able to explain in the interview why the company will be glad it hired you, say, 4 years from now. Never criticize your current employer before you leave. Personal and professional integrity will follow you from position to position. Many companies count on personal references when hiring, including those of faculty and administrators from your nursing program. When leaving positions you held during school or on graduating from your program, it is wise not to take parting shots at someone. Doing a professional program evaluation is fine, but "taking cheap shots" at faculty or other employees is unacceptable (Costlow, 1999).

Background Questions

Background questions usually relate to information on your résumé. If you have no nursing experience, relate your prior school and work experience and other accomplishments in relevant ways to the position you are seeking without going through your entire autobiography with the interviewer. You may be asked to expand on the information in your

5734 Foster Road
Middleton, Indiana 46204

May 2, 2009

Ms. Martha Berrero
Human Resources Manager
All Care Nursing Center
4431 Lakeside Drive
Middleton, Indiana 46204

Dear Ms. Berrero:

I am writing to confirm my acceptance of your employment offer of May 1. I am delighted to be joining All Care Nursing Center. I feel confident that I can make a significant contribution to your team, and I appreciate the opportunity you have offered me.

As we discussed, I will report to the Personnel Office at 8 a.m. on May 15 for new employee orientation. I will have the medical examination, employee, and insurance forms completed when I arrive. I understand that the starting salary will be $33.10/hour with full benefits beginning May 15. Overtime salary in excess of 40 hours/week will be paid if you request overtime hours.

I appreciate your confidence in me and look forward to joining your team.

Sincerely yours,

Delores Wheatley

Delores Wheatley

Figure 14.4 Sample acceptance letter.

résumé about your formal nursing education. Here is your opportunity to relate specific courses or clinical experiences you enjoyed, academic honors you received, and extracurricular activities or research projects you pursued. The background questions are an invitation for employers to get to know you. Be careful not to appear inconsistent with this information and what you say later.

Professional Questions

Many recruiters are looking for specifics, especially those related to skills and knowledge needed in the position available. They may start with questions related to your education, career goals, strengths, weaknesses, nursing philosophy, style, and abilities. Interviewers often open their questioning with words such as "review," "tell me," "explain," and "describe," followed by such phrases as "How did you do it?" or "Why did you do it that way?" (Mascolini & Supnick, 1993). How successful will you be with these types of questions?

When answering "how would you describe" questions, it is especially important that you remain specific. Cite your own experiences, and relate these behaviors to a demonstrated skill or strength.

5734 Foster Road
Middleton, Indiana 46204

May 2, 2009

Ms. Martha Berrero
Human Resources Manager
All Care Nursing Center
4431 Lakeside Drive
Middleton, Indiana 46204

Dear Ms. Berrero:

Thank you for offering me the position of staff nurse with All Care Nursing Center. I appreciate your taking the time to give me such extensive information about the position.

There are many aspects of the position that appeal to me. Jefferson Corporation is an excellent provider of health care services throughout this area and nationwide. However, after giving it much thought, I have decided to accept another position and must therefore decline your offer.

Again, thank you for your consideration and the courtesy extended to me. I enjoyed meeting you and your staff.

Sincerely yours,

Delores Wheatley

Delores Wheatley

Figure 14.5 Sample rejection letter.

Examples of questions in this area include the following (Bischof, 1993):

- **What is your philosophy of nursing?** This question is asked frequently. Your response should relate to the position you are seeking.
- **What is your greatest weakness? Your greatest strength?** Do not be afraid to present a weakness, but present it to your best advantage, making it sound like a desirable characteristic. Even better, discuss a weakness that is already apparent such as lack of nursing experience, stating that you recognize your lack of nursing experience but that your own work or management experience has taught you skills that will assist you in this position. These skills might include organization, time management, team spirit, and communication. If you are asked for both strengths and weaknesses, start with your weakness, and end on a positive note with your strengths. Do not be too modest, but do not exaggerate. Relate your strengths to the prospective position. Skills such as interpersonal relationships, organization, and leadership are usually broad enough to fit most positions.

table 14-2

Do's and Don'ts of Internet Job Searching

Do	Don't
Focus on selling yourself: "My clinical practicum in the ICU at a major health center and my strong organizational skills fit with the entry-level ICU position posted in Nursing Spectrum."	Use many "I"s in the message: "I saw your job posting in Nursing Spectrum, and I have attached my resume."
Use short paragraphs; keep the message short.	Long messages probably will not even be read.
Use highlighting and bullets.	Forget to format for e-mail.
Use an appropriate e-mail address: DKWhitehead431@....	Use a silly or inappropriate e-mail: smartypants@...or partyanimal@...
Use an effective subject: ICU RN position.	Use subjects used by computer viruses or junk e-mailers: Hi, Important, Information.
Send your message to the correct e-mail address.	Assume; if the address is not indicated, call to see what person/address is appropriate.
Send messages individually.	Send a blast message to many recipients; it may be discarded as junk mail.
Treat e-mail with the same care you treat a traditional business application	Slip into informality—remember spelling and grammar checks.
Keep your resume "cyber-safe."	Remove your standard contact information and replace it with your e-mail address
Change the format of your resume: save your word document as an HTML file or an ASCII text file	Assume that everyone is using the same word processing program

Adapted from Job Hunt: The Online Job Search Guide. Retrieved May 13, 2008, from http://www.job-hunt.org/

■ **Where do you see yourself in 5 years?** Most interviewers want to gain insight into your long-term goals as well as some idea whether you are likely to use this position as a brief stop on the path to another job. It is helpful for you to know some of the history regarding the position. For example, how long have others usually remained in that job? Your career planning should be consistent with the organization's needs.

■ **What are your educational goals?** Be honest and specific. Include both professional education, such as RN or bachelor of science in nursing, and continuing education courses. If you want to pursue further education in related areas, such as a foreign language or computers, include this as a goal. Indicate schools to which you have applied or in which you are already enrolled.

■ **Describe your leadership style.** Be prepared to discuss your style in terms of how effectively you work with others, and give examples of how you have implemented your leadership in the past.

■ **What can you contribute to this position? What unique skill set do you offer?** Review your SWOT analysis as well as the job description for the position before the interview. Be specific in relating your contributions to the position. Emphasize your accomplishments. Be specific, and convey that, even as a new graduate, you are unique.

■ **What are your salary requirements?** You may be asked about minimum salary range. Try to find out the prospective employer's salary range before this question comes up. Be honest about your expectations, but make it clear that you are willing to negotiate.

■ **"What if" questions.** Prospective employers are increasingly using competency-based interview questions to determine people's preparation for a job. There is often no single correct answer to these questions. The interviewer may be assessing your clinical decision-making and leadership skills. Again, be concise and specific, focusing your answer in line with the organizational philosophy and goals. If you do not know the answer, tell the interviewer how you would go about finding the answer. You cannot be expected to have all the answers before you begin a job, but you can be expected to know how to obtain answers once you are in the position.

Personal Questions

Personal questions deal with your personality and motivation. Common questions include the following:

- **How would you describe yourself?** This is a standard question. Most people find it helpful to think about an answer in advance. You can repeat some of what you said in your résumé and cover letter, but do not provide an in-depth analysis of your personality.
- **How would your peers describe you?** Ask them. Again, be brief, describing several strengths. Do not discuss your weaknesses unless you are asked about them.
- **What would make you happy with this position?** Be prepared to discuss your needs related to your work environment. Do you enjoy self-direction, flexible hours, and strong leadership support? Now is the time to cite specifics related to your ideal work environment.
- **Describe your ideal work environment.** Give this question some thought before the interview. Be specific but realistic. If the norm in your community is two RNs to a floor with licensed practical nurses and other ancillary support, do not say that you believe a staff consisting only of RNs is needed for good patient care.
- **Describe hobbies, community activities, and recreation.** Again, brevity is important. Many times this question is used to further observe the interviewee's communication and interpersonal skills.

Never pretend to be someone other than who you are. If pretending is necessary to obtain the position, then the position is not right for you.

Additional Points About the Interview

Federal, state, and local laws govern employment-related questions. Questions asked on the job application and in the interview must be related to the position advertised. Questions or statements that may lead to discrimination on the basis of age, gender, race, color, religion, or ethnicity are illegal. If you are asked a question that appears to be illegal, you may wish to take one of several approaches:

- You may answer the question, realizing that it is not a job-related question. Make it clear to the interviewer that you will answer the question even though you know it is not job-related.
- You may refuse to answer. You are within your rights but may be seen as uncooperative or confrontational.
- Examine the intent of the question and relate it to the job.

Just as important as the verbal exchanges of the interview are the nonverbal aspects. These include appearance, handshake, eye contact, posture, and listening skills.

Appearance

Dress in business attire. For women, a skirted suit or tailored jacket dress is appropriate. Men should wear a classic suit, light-colored shirt, and conservative tie. For both men and women, gray or navy blue is rarely wrong. Shoes should be polished, with appropriate heels. Nails and hair for both men and women should reflect cleanliness, good grooming, and willingness to work. The 2-inch red dagger nails worn on prom night will not support an image of the professional nurse. In many institutions, even clear, acrylic nails are not allowed. Paint stains on the hands from a weekend of house maintenance are equally unsuitable for presenting a professional image.

Handshake

Arrive at the interview 10 minutes before your scheduled time (allow yourself extra time to find the place if you have not previously been there). Introduce yourself courteously to the receptionist. Stand when your name is called, smile, and shake hands firmly. If you perspire easily, wipe your palms just before handshake time.

Eye Contact

During the interview, use the interviewer's title and last name as you speak. Never use the interviewer's first name unless specifically requested to do so. Use good listening skills (all those leadership skills you have learned). Smile and nod occasionally, making frequent eye contact. Do not fold your arms across your chest, but keep your hands at your sides or in your lap. Pay attention, and sound sure of yourself.

Posture and Listening Skills

Phrase your questions appropriately, and relate them to yourself as a candidate: "What would be my responsibility?" instead of "What are the responsibilities of the job?" Use appropriate grammar and diction. Words or phrases such as "yeah," "uh-huh," "uh," "you know," or "like" are too casual for an interview.

Do not say "I guess" or "I feel" about anything. These words make you sound indecisive. Remember your action verbs—I analyzed, organized, developed. Do not evaluate your achievements as mediocre or unimpressive.

Asking Questions

At some point in the interview, you will be asked if you have any questions. Knowing what questions you want to ask is just as important as having prepared answers for the interviewer's questions. The interview is as much a time for you to learn the details of the job as it is for your potential employer to find out about you. You will need to obtain specific information about the job, including the type of patients for whom you would care, the people with whom you would work, the salary and benefits, and your potential employer's expectations of you. Be prepared for the interviewer to say, "Is there anything else I can tell you about the job?" Jot down a few questions on an index card before going for the interview. You may want to ask a few questions based on your research, demonstrating knowledge about and interest in the company. In addition, you may want to ask questions similar to the ones listed next. Above all, be honest and sincere (Bhasin, 1998; Bischof, 1993; Johnson, 1999):

- What is this position's key responsibility?
- What kind of person are you looking for?
- What are the challenges of the position?
- Why is this position open?
- To whom would I report directly?
- Why did the previous person leave this position?
- What is the salary for this position?
- What are the opportunities for advancement?
- What kind of opportunities are there for continuing education?
- What are your expectations of me as an employee?
- How, when, and by whom are evaluations done?
- What other opportunities for professional growth are available here?
- How are promotion and advancement handled within the organization?

The following are a few additional tips about asking questions during a job interview:

- *Do not* begin with questions about vacations, benefits, or sick time. This gives the impression that these are the most important part of the job to you, not the work itself.
- *Do* begin with questions about the employer's expectations of you. This gives the impression that you want to know how you can contribute to the organization.
- *Do* be sure you know enough about the position to make a reasonable decision about accepting an offer if one is made.
- *Do* ask questions about the organization as a whole. The information is useful to you and demonstrates that you are able to see the big picture.
- *Do* bring a list of important points to discuss as an aid to you if you are nervous.

During the interview process, there are a few "red flags" to be alert for (Tyler, 1990):

- Much turnover in the position
- A newly created position without a clear purpose
- An organization in transition
- A position that is not feasible for a new graduate
- A "gut feeling" that things are not what they seem

The exchange of information between you and the interviewer will go more smoothly if you review Box 14-2 before the interview.

After the Interview

If the interviewer does not offer the information, ask about the next step in the process. Thank the interviewer, shake hands, and exit. If the receptionist is still there, you may quickly smile and say thank you and good-bye. Do not linger and chat, and do not forget your thank-you letter.

The Second Interview

Being invited for a second interview means that the first interview went well and that you made a favorable impression. Second visits may include a tour of the facility and meetings with a higher-level executive or a supervisor in the department in which the job opening exists and perhaps several colleagues. In preparation for the second interview, review the information about the organization and your own strengths. It does not hurt to have a few résumés and potential references available. Pointers to make your second visit successful

Do's and Don'ts for Interviewing

Do:

Shake the interviewer's hand firmly, and introduce yourself.

Know the interviewer's name in advance, and use it in conversation.

Remain standing until invited to sit.

Use eye contact.

Let the interviewer take the lead in the conversation.

Talk in specific terms, relating everything to the position.

Support responses in terms of personal experience and specific examples.

Make connections for the interviewer. Relate your responses to the needs of the individual organization.

Show interest in the facility.

Ask questions about the position and the facility.

Come across as sincere in your goals and committed to the profession.

Indicate a willingness to start at the bottom.

Take any examinations requested.

Express your appreciation for the time.

Do Not:

Place your purse, briefcase, papers, etc., on the interviewer's desk. Keep them in your lap or on the floor.

Slouch in the chair.

Play with your clothing, jewelry, or hair.

Chew gum or smoke, even if the interviewer does.

Be evasive, interrupt, brag, or mumble.

Gossip about or criticize former agencies, schools, or employees.

Adapted from Bischof, J. (1993). Preparing for job interview questions. Critical Care Nurse, 13(4), 97–100; Krannich, C., & Krannich, R. (1993). Interview for Success. N.Y.: Impact Publications; Mascolini, M., & Supnick, R. (1993). Preparing students for the behavioral job interview. Journal of Business and Technical Communication, 7(4), 482–488; and Zedlitz, R. (2003). How to Get a Job in Health Care. N.Y.: Delmar Learning.

include the following (Knight, 2005; Muha & Orgiefsky, 1994):

- Dress professionally. Do not wear sandals or open-toed shoes. Minimize jewelry and makeup.
- Be professional and pleasant with everyone, including secretaries and housekeeping and maintenance personnel.
- Do not smoke.
- Remember your manners.
- Avoid controversial topics for small talk.
- Obtain answers to questions you might have thought of since your first visit.

In most instances, the personnel director or nurse manager will let you know how long it will be before you are contacted again. It is appropriate to get this information before you leave the second interview. If you do receive an offer during this visit, graciously say "thank you," and ask for a little time to consider the offer (even if this is the offer you have anxiously been awaiting).

If the organization does not contact you by the expected date, do not panic. It is appropriate to call your contact person, state your continued interest, and tactfully express the need to know the status of your application so that you can respond to other deadlines.

Making the Right Choice

You have interviewed well, and now you have to decide among several job offers. Your choice will affect not only your immediate work but also influence your future career opportunities. The nursing shortage of the early 1990s has led to greatly enhanced workplace enrichment programs as a recruitment and retention strategy. Career ladders, shared governance, participatory management, staff nurse presence on major hospital committees, decentralization of operations, and a focus on quality interpersonal relationships are among some of these features. Be sure and inquire about the components of the professional practice environment (Joel, 2003). There are several additional factors to consider.

Job Content

The immediate work you will be doing should be a good match with your skills and interests. Although your work may be personally challenging and satisfying this year, what are the opportunities for growth? How will your desire for continued growth and challenge be satisfied?

Development

You should have learned from your interviews whether your initial training and orientation seem sufficient. Inquire about continuing education to keep you current in your field. Is tuition reimbursement available for further education? Is management training provided, or are supervisory skills learned on the job?

Direction

Good supervision and mentors are especially important in your first position. You may be able to judge prospective supervisors throughout the interview process, but you should also try to get a broader view of the overall philosophy of supervision. You may not be working for the same supervisor in a year, but the overall management philosophy is likely to remain consistent.

Work Climate

The daily work climate must make you feel comfortable. Your preference may be formal or casual, structured or unstructured, complex or simple. It is easy to observe the way people dress, the layout of the unit, and lines of communication. It is more difficult to observe company values, factors that will affect your work comfort and satisfaction over the long term. Try to look beyond the work environment to get an idea of values. What is the unwritten message? Is there an open-door policy sending a message that "everyone is equal and important," or does the nurse manager appear too busy to be concerned with the needs of the employees? Is your supervisor the kind of person for whom you could work easily?

Compensation

In evaluating the compensation package, starting salary should be less important than the organization's philosophy on future compensation. What is the potential for salary growth? How are individual increases? Can you live on the wages being offered?

I Can Not Find a Job (or I Moved)

It is often said that finding the first job is the hardest. Many employers prefer to hire seasoned nurses who do not require a long orientation and mentoring. Some require new graduates to do postgraduate internships. Changes in skill mix with the implementation of various types of care delivery influence the market for the professional nurse. The new graduate may need to be armed with a variety of skills, such as intravenous certification, home assessment, advanced rehabilitation skills, and various respiratory modalities, to even warrant an initial interview. Keep informed about the demands of the market in your area, and be prepared to be flexible in seeking your first position. Even with the continuing nursing shortage, hiring you as a new graduate will depend on you selling yourself.

Even after all this searching and hard work, you still may not have found the position you want. You

may be focusing on work arrangements or benefits rather than on the job description. Your lack of direction may come through in your résumé, cover letter, and personal presentation. As a new graduate, you may also have unrealistic expectations or be trying to cut corners, ignoring the basic rules of marketing yourself discussed in this chapter. Go back to your SWOT analysis. Take another look at your résumé and cover letter. Become more assertive as you start again (Culp, 1999).

The Critical First Year

Why a section on the "first year"? Don't you just get a nursing license and go to work? Aren't nurses always in demand? You have worked hard to succeed in college—won't those lessons help you to succeed in your new position? Some of the behaviors that were rewarded in school are not rewarded on the job. There are no syllabi, study questions, or extra-credit points. Only "A's" are acceptable, and there do not appear to be many completely correct answers. Discovering this has been called "reality shock" (Kramer, 1974), which is discussed elsewhere in this book. Voluminous care plans and meticulous medication cards are out; multiple responsibilities and thinking on your feet are in. What is the new graduate to do?

Your first year will be a transition year. You are no longer a college student, but you are not yet a full-fledged professional. You are "the new kid on the block," and people will respond to you differently and judge you differently than when you were a student. To be successful, you have to respond differently. You may be thinking, "Oh, they always need nurses—it doesn't matter." Yes, it does matter. Many of your career opportunities will be influenced by the early impressions you make. The following section addresses what you can do to help ensure first-year success.

Attitude and Expectations

Adopt the right attitudes, and adjust your expectations. Now is the time to learn the art of being new. You felt like the most important, special person during the recruitment process. Now, in the real world, neither you nor the position may be as glamorous as you once thought. In addition, although you thought you learned much in school, your decisions and daily performance do not always warrant an "A." Above all, people shed the company manners they displayed when you were interviewing, and organizational politics eventually surface. Your leadership skills and commitment to teamwork will get you through this transition period.

Impressions and Relationships

Manage a good impression, and build effective relationships. Remember, you are being watched: by peers, subordinates, and superiors. Because you as yet have no track record, first impressions are magnified. Although every organization is different, most are looking for someone with good judgment, a willingness to learn, a readiness to adapt, and a respect for the expertise of more experienced employees. Most people expect you to "pay your dues" to earn respect from them.

Organizational Savvy

Develop organizational savvy. An important person in this first year is your immediate supervisor. Support this person. Find out what is important to your supervisor and what he or she needs and expects from the team. Become a team player. Present solutions, not problems, as often as you can. You want to be a good leader someday; learn first to be a good follower. Finding a mentor is another important goal of your first year. Mentors are role models and guides who encourage, counsel, teach, and advocate for their mentee. In these relationships, both the mentor and mentee receive support and encouragement (Klein & Dickenson-Hazard, 2000). Mentoring was discussed in Chapter 13.

The spark that ignites a mentoring relationship may come from either the protégé or the mentor. Protégés often view mentors as founts of success, a bastion of life skills they wish to learn and emulate. Mentors often see the future that is hidden in another's personality and abilities (Klein & Dickenson-Hazard, 2000, pp. 20–21).

Skills and Knowledge

Master the skills and knowledge of the position. Technology is constantly changing, and contrary to popular belief, you did not learn everything in school. Be prepared to seek out new knowledge and skills on your own. This may entail extra hours of preparation and study, but no one ever said learning stops after graduation (Holton, 1994; Johnson, 1994).

Advancing Your Career

Many of the ideas presented in this chapter will continue to be helpful as you advance in your nursing career. Continuing to develop your leadership and patient care skills through practice, and further education will be the key to your professional growth. The RN will be expected to develop and provide leadership to other members of the healthcare team while providing competent care to patients. Getting your first job within the nursing shortage may not be so difficult, but advancing in your career will be your own responsibility.

Conclusion

Finding your first position is more than being in the right place at the right time. It is a complex combination of learning about yourself and the organizations you are interested in and presenting your strengths and weaknesses in the most positive manner possible. Keeping the first position and using the position to grow and learn are also a planning process. Recognize that the independence you enjoyed through college may not be the skills you need to keep you in your first position. There is an important lesson to be learned: becoming a team player and being savvy about organizational politics are as important as becoming proficient in nursing skills. Take the first step toward finding a mentor—before you know it, you will become one yourself.

Study Questions

1. Using the SWOT analysis worksheet developed for this chapter, how will you articulate your strengths and weaknesses during an interview?

2. Design a one- to two-page résumé to use in seeking your first position. Are you able to "sell yourself" in one or two pages? If not, what adjustments are you going to make? Develop a cover letter, thank-you letter, acceptance letter, and rejection letter that you can use during the interview process.

3. Using the interview preparation worksheet developed for this chapter, formulate responses to the questions. How comfortable do you feel answering these questions? Share your responses with other classmates to get further ideas.

4. Evaluate the job prospects in the community where you now live. What areas could you explore in seeking your first position?

5. What plans do you have for advancing your career? What plans do you have for finding a mentor?

Case Study to Promote Critical Reasoning

Paul Delane is interviewing for his first nursing position after obtaining his RN license. He has been interviewed by the nurse recruiter and is now being interviewed by the nurse manager on the pediatric floor. After a few minutes of social conversation, the nurse manager begins to ask some specific nursing-oriented questions: How would you respond if a mother of a seriously ill child asks you if her child will die? What attempts do you make to understand different cultural beliefs and their importance in health care when planning nursing care? How does your philosophy of nursing affect your ability to deliver care to children whose mothers are HIV-positive?

Paul is very flustered by these questions and responds with "it depends on the situation," "it depends on the culture," and "I don't ever discriminate."

1. What responses would have been more appropriate in this interview?

2. How could Paul have used these questions to demonstrate his strengths, experiences, and skills?

References

Anderson, J. (1992). Tips on résumé writing. *Imprint*, 39(1), 30–31.

Banis, W. (1994). The art of writing job-search letters. In College Placement Council, Inc. (ed.). *Planning Job Choices*. Philadelphia: College Placement Council, 44–51.

Beatty, R. (1991). *Get the Right Job in 60 Days or Less*. N.Y.: John Wiley & Sons.

Beatty, R. (1989). *The Perfect Cover Letter*. N.Y.: John Wiley & Sons.

Bhasin, R. (1998). Do's and don'ts of job interviews. *Pulp & Paper*, 72(2), 37.

Bischof, J. (1993). Preparing for job interview questions. *Critical Care Nurse*, 13(4), 97–100.

Chestnut, T. (1999). Some tips on taking the fear out of résumé writing. *Phoenix Business Journal*, 19(47), 28.

Costlow, T. (1999). How not to create a good first impression. *Fairfield County Business Journal*, 38(32), 17.

Crowther, K. (1994). How to research companies. In College Placement Council, Inc. (ed.). *Planning Job Choices*. Philadelphia: College Placement Council, 27–32.

Culp, M. (1999). Now's the time to turn the corner on your job search. *San Diego Business Journal*, 20(50), 35.

Ellis, M. (1999). Self-assessment: Discovering yourself and making the best choices for you! *Black Collegian*, 30(1), 30, 3p, 1c.

Eubanks, P. (1991). Experts: Making your résumé an asset. *Hospitals*, 5(20), 74.

Holton, E. (1994). The critical first year on the job. In College Placement Council, Inc. (ed.). *Planning Job Choices*. Philadelphia: College Placement Council, 68–71.

Hunsaker, P. (2001). *Training in Management Skills*. N.J.: Prentice-Hall.

Impollonia, M. (2004), How to impress nursing recruiters to get the job you want. *Imprint*, March.

James, L. (2003). Vitae statistics. *Travel Weekly*, 1695, 70.

Job Hunt: The Online Job Search Guide. Retrieved May 13, 2008, from http://www.job-hunt.org/

Joel, L. (2003). The role of the workplace in your transition from student to nurse. *Imprint*, April.

Johnson, K. (1994). Choose your first job with your whole future in mind. In College Placement Council, Inc. (ed.). *Planning Job Choices*. Philadelphia: College Placement Council, 65–67.

Johnson, K. (1999). Interview success demands research, practice, preparation. *Houston Business Journal*, 30(23), 38.

Klein, E., & Dickenson-Hazard, N. (2000). The spirit of mentoring. *Reflections on Nursing Leadership*, 26(3), 18–22.

Knight, K. (2005). New grad? Be prepared to look great. *Imprint*, January.

Kramer, M. (1974). *Reality Shock: Why Nurses Leave Nursing*. St. Louis: C.V. Mosby.

Krannich, C., & Krannich, R. (1993). *Interview for Success*. N.Y.: Impact Publications.

Marino, K. (2000). *Resumes for the Health Care Professional*. N.Y.: John Wiley & Sons.

Mascolini, M., & Supnick, R. (1993). Preparing students for the behavioral job interview. *Journal of Business and Technical Communication*, 7(4), 482–488.

Muha, D., & Orgiefsky, R. (1994). The 2nd interview: The plant or office visit. In College Placement Council, Inc. (ed.). *Planning Job Choices*. Philadelphia: College Placement Council, 58–60.

Parker, Y. (1989). *The Damn Good Résumé Guide*. Berkeley, Calif.: Ten Speed Press.

Pratt, C. (1994). Successful job-search strategies for the 90's. In College Placement Council, Inc. (ed.). *Planning Job Choices*. Philadelphia: College Placement Council, 15–18.

Rodriguez, K., & Robertson, D. (1992). Selling your talents with a résumé. *American Nurse,* 24(10), 27.

Shingleton, J. (1994). The job market for '94 grads. In College Placement Council, Inc. (ed.). *Planning Job Choices.* Philadelphia: College Placement Council, 19–26.

Tyler, L. (1990). Watch out for "red flags" on a job interview. *Hospitals,* 64(14), 46.

Unknown. (2005). The devil is in the resume details. *Fairfield County Business Journal,* 44(18), 17.

U.S. Health and Human Services. Retrieved May 13, 2008, from http://bhpr.hrsa.gov/healthworkforce/nursingshortage/tech_report/default.htm

Waymon, L., & Baber, A. (1999). Surviving career. *Balance,* 3(2), 10–13.

Zedlitz, R. (2003). *How to Get a Job in Health Care.* N.Y.: Delmar Learning.

⊙ ○ ○ ○ ○ ○ ○ ○ ○ ○

OBJECTIVES

After reading this chapter, the student should be able to:

- Compare and contrast historical and current definitions of nursing.
- Discuss the contribution of nursing leaders to the development of modern nursing: Florence Nightingale, Lillian Wald, Margaret Sanger, Mary Mahoney, Mildred Montag, and Virginia Henderson.
- Discuss the history of men in nursing.
- Differentiate the roles of the American Nurses Association, National League for Nursing, National Organization for Associate Degree Nursing, American Academy of Nursing, and National Institute for Nursing Research.
- Discuss ways for nurses to project a positive image.
- Discuss some of the issues faced by the nursing profession over the past century and today.
- Identify changes that will affect nursing's future
- Describe actions every nurse can take to promote the profession and high quality of care.

Introduction

It is often said that you do not know where you are going until you know where you have been. Over 30 years ago, Beletz (1974) wrote that most people thought of nurses in gender-linked, task-oriented terms: "a female who performs unpleasant technical jobs and functions as an assistant to the physician" (p. 432). Although the image of nurses and nursing has advanced considerably since then, some still think of nurses as helpers who carry out the physician's orders.

In its history, the nursing profession has had many great leaders. There are several who not only demonstrate the strengths of nursing's leaders but also reflect some of the most important issues that the profession has faced over the past 150 years. Each of these leaders initiated change within the social environment of the time, using the strategies of change and conflict resolution discussed earlier in the text.

Nursing Defined

The changes that have occurred in nursing are reflected in the definitions of nursing that have developed over time. In 1859, Florence Nightingale defined the goal of nursing as putting the client "in the best possible condition for nature to act upon him" (Nightingale, 1859, p. 79). In 1966, Virginia Henderson focused her definition on the uniqueness of nursing:

> *"The unique function of the nurse is to assist the individual, sick or well, in the performance of those activities contributing to health or its recovery (or to peaceful death) that he would perform unaided if he had the necessary strength, will or knowledge. And to do this in such a way as to help him gain independence as rapidly as possible" (Henderson, 1966, p. 21).*

Martha Rogers defined nursing practice as "the process by which this body of knowledge, nursing science, is used for the purpose of assisting human beings to achieve maximum health within the potential of each person" (Rogers, 1988, p. 100). Rogers emphasized that nursing is concerned with *all* people, only some of whom are ill.

Florence Nightingale is probably the best known of the historic leaders and is considered the founder of modern nursing. Nightingale brought about change in the care of soldiers, the keeping of hospital records, the status of nurses, and even the profession itself. Her concepts of nursing care became the basis of modern theory development in nursing.

Lillian Wald, founder of the Henry Street Settlement, is a role model for contemporary community health nursing. She developed a model for bringing health care to people.

Margaret Sanger, a political activist like many of the others, is best known for her courageous fight to make birth control information available to everyone who needed or wanted it. Her fight to make Congress aware of the plight of children in the labor force is less well known but led to important changes in the child labor laws. Sanger may have been the first nurse lobbyist.

Mary Eliza Mahoney was the first black graduate nurse in the United States. Her professional attitude helped to change the status of black nurses in this country.

Mildred Montag proposed having two levels of nursing. She developed an associate degree nursing program at Adelphi University.

Virginia Henderson was a 20th century Florence Nightingale. She wrote the nursing fundamentals textbook most commonly used by nurse educators throughout the country for most of the last century.

Many of their characteristics—intelligence, courage, and foresight—are the same ones needed in today's nursing leaders.

Florence Nightingale

Background

Florence Nightingale, an English noblewoman, was born in the city for which she was named—Florence, Italy—on May 12, 1820. Her father was a well-educated, wealthy man who put considerable effort into the education of his two daughters (Donahue, 1985). Florence Nightingale learned French, German, and Italian. Mr. Nightingale personally instructed her in mathematics, classical art, and literature. The family made extended visits to London every year, which provided opportunities for contact with people in the highest social circles. These contacts were very valuable to Nightingale in later years.

Despite her family's ability to shelter her from the meaner side of life, Nightingale always had an interest in the welfare of those less fortunate than herself. She was never quite content with herself, as she was described as a "sensitive, introspective, and somewhat morbid child" (Schuyler, 1992). She was driven to improve herself and the world around her. When she expressed an interest in becoming a nurse, her parents objected strenuously. They wanted her to assume the traditional role of a well-to-do woman of the time: marry, have children, and take her "rightful" place in society.

Becoming a Nurse

In the fall of 1847, Nightingale left England for a tour of Europe with family friends. In Italy, she entered a convent for a retreat. After this retreat, she believed that she had been called by God to help others and became more determined than ever to pursue nursing.

In 1851, Nightingale insisted on going to Kaiserswerth, Germany, to obtain training in nursing. Her family gave her permission on the condition that no one would know where she was. When she returned from Kaiserswerth, she began to work on her plan to influence health care.

Nightingale soon left for France to work with several Catholic nursing sisters. While in France, she received an offer from the committee that regulated the Establishment for Gentlewomen During Illness, a nursing home in London for governesses who became ill. She was appointed superintendent of the home and soon had it well organized, although she did have some difficulties with the committee.

Because of her knowledge of hospitals, Nightingale was often consulted by social reformers and by physicians who also recognized the need for this new type of nurse. She was offered a position as superintendent of nurses at King's College Hospital, but her family objected so strongly that she remained at home until she went to Crimea.

The Need for Reform

Fortunately for Nightingale, it was fashionable to become involved in the reform of medical and social institutions in the middle of the 19th century. After completing the reorganization of the nursing home, she began visiting hospitals and collecting information about nurses' working conditions. She began to realize that, to improve nurses' working conditions, she would first have to improve the nurses.

Up to this time, the guiding principle of nursing had been charity. Nursing services in Europe were provided primarily by the family or by members of religious orders. However, Catholic organizations experienced a decline during the Reformation when the government closed churches and monasteries. Hospitals were no longer run for charitable reasons but as a social necessity. Nursing lost its social standing when the religious orders declined and became a form of domestic service. Nurses were no longer recruited from "respectable" classes but from the lower classes of society, women who needed to earn their keep. Other women who could no longer earn a living by gambling or selling themselves also turned to nursing. Many had criminal backgrounds. They lacked the spirit of self-sacrifice found in the religious orders. They often abused clients and consoled themselves with alcohol and snuff.

The duties of a nurse in those days were to take care of the physical needs of clients and to make sure they were reasonably clean. The conditions in which they had to accomplish these tasks were far from ideal. Hospitals were dirty and unventilated. They were contaminated and spread diseases instead of preventing them. The same bedsheets were used for several clients. The nurses dealt with people suffering from unrelenting pain, hemorrhage, infections, and gangrene (Kalisch & Kalisch, 2004).

To accomplish the needed reforms, Nightingale realized that she had to recruit nurses from higher strata of society, as had been done in the past, and then educate them well. She concluded that this could be accomplished only by organizing a school to prepare reliable, qualified nurses.

The Crimean War

A letter written by war correspondent W.H. Russell comparing the nursing care in the British army unfavorably with that given to the French army created a tremendous stir in England. There was demand for change. In response, the Secretary of War, Sir Sidney Herbert, commissioned Nightingale to go to Crimea (a peninsula in southeastern Ukraine) to investigate conditions there and make improvements.

On October 21, 1854, Nightingale left for Crimea with a group of nurses on the steamer *Vectis* (Griffith & Griffith, 1965). They found a disaster when they arrived. The hospital that had been built to accommodate 1700 soldiers was filled with more than 3000 wounded and critically ill men. There was no plumbing, no sewage disposal facilities.

Mattresses, walls, and floors were soaked with human waste. Rats, lice, and maggots thrived in this filthy environment (Kalisch & Kalisch, 2004).

The nurses went to work. They set up a kitchen, rented a house and converted it into a laundry, and hired soldiers' wives to do the laundry. Money was difficult to obtain, so Nightingale used the *Times* relief fund and her own personal funds to purchase medical supplies, food, and equipment. After the hospital had been cleaned and organized, she began to set up social services for the soldiers.

Nightingale rarely slept. She spent hours giving nursing care, wrote letters to families, prepared requests for more supplies, and reported to London on the conditions she had found and improved. At night, she made rounds accompanied by an 11-year-old boy who held her lamp when she sat by a dying soldier or assisted during emergency surgery. This is how she earned the title "The Lady with the Lamp" from the poet Longfellow (1868).

The physicians and army officers resented the nurses despite their strenuous efforts and enormous accomplishments. They regarded the nurses as intruders who interfered with their work and undermined their authority. There was also some conflict between Nightingale and Dr. John Hall, the chief of the medical staff. At one time, after Dr. Hall had been awarded the Knight Commander of the Order of the Bath, Nightingale sarcastically referred to him as "Dr. Hall, K.C.B., Knight of the Crimean Burial Grounds." When Nightingale contracted Crimean fever, Hall used this as an excuse to send her back to England. However, Nightingale thwarted his resistance and eventually won over the medical staff by creating an operating room and supplying the instruments with her own resources. Although she returned to duty, she never fully recovered from the fever. She returned to England in 1865 a national heroine but remained a semi-invalid for the rest of her life.

A School for Nurses

After her return from Crimea, Nightingale pursued two goals: reform of military health care and establishment of an official training school for nurses. The British public contributed more than $220,000 (a great sum of money at that time) to the Nightingale Fund for the purpose of establishing the school.

Although opposed by most of the physicians in Britain, the Nightingale Training School for Nurses opened in 1860. The school was an independent educational institution financed by the Nightingale Fund. Fifteen probationers were admitted to the first class. Their training lasted a year. Although Nightingale was not an instructor at the school, she was consulted about all of the details of student selection, instruction, and organization. The basic principles on which the Nightingale school was founded are the following:

1. Nurses should be trained technically in schools organized for that purpose.
2. Nurses should come from homes that are of good moral standing.

Her book, *Notes on Nursing: What It Is and What It Is Not*, established the fundamental principles of nursing. The following is an example of her writing:

On What Nursing Ought To Do

   I use the word nursing for want of a better. It has been limited to signify little more than the administration of medicines and the application of poultices. It ought to signify the proper use of air, light, warmth, cleanliness, quiet and the proper selection and administration of diet—all at the least expense of vital power to the patient" (Nightingale, 1859).

This book was one of the first nursing textbooks and is still widely quoted. Many nursing theorists have used Nightingale's thoughts as a basis for constructing their view of nursing.

Nightingale believed that schools of nursing must be independent institutions and that women who were selected to attend the schools should be from the higher levels of society. Many of Nightingale's beliefs about nursing education are still applicable, particularly those involved with the progress of students, the use of diaries kept by students, and the need for integrating theory into clinical practice (Roberts, 1937).

The Nightingale school served as a model for nursing education. Its graduates were sought worldwide. Many of them established schools and became matrons (superintendents) in hospitals in other parts of England, the British Commonwealth, and the United States. However, very few schools were able to remain financially independent of the hospitals and so lost much of their autonomy. This was in contradiction to Nightingale's philosophy that the training schools were educational institutions, not part of any service agency.

Early Health-Care Reform

Nightingale's work marked the beginning of modern military nursing. As a result of her documentation of the conditions in Crimea and the nurses' efforts to improve them, reforms were undertaken.

Nightingale's statistics were so accurate and clearly reported that she was elected a member of the British Statistical Society, the first woman to hold this position. At their conference in 1860, she presented a paper entitled, "Miss Nightingale's Scheme for Uniform Hospital Statistics." Before this paper was written, each hospital had used its own names and classification systems for diseases. Nightingale's opinions on improving health care were solicited constantly. This led to another publication, "Notes on Hospitals."

For more than 40 years, Nightingale played an influential part in most of the important health-care reforms of her time. At the turn of the 20th century, however, her energies had waned, and she spent most of the next 10 years confined to her home on South Street in London. She died in her sleep on August 13, 1910.

Nightingale's Contributions

Nightingale is believed to have been in error in only two areas. First, she did not believe in or appreciate the significance of the germ theory of infection, although her insistence on fresh air, physical hygiene, and environmental cleanliness certainly did a great deal to decrease the transmission of infectious diseases. Second, she did not support a central registry or testing for nurses similar to what was in place for physicians. She was convinced that this would undermine the profession and that a letter of recommendation from the school matron was sufficient to attest to the skill and character of the nurse.

Florence Nightingale was a woman of vision and determination. Her strong belief in herself and her abilities allowed her to pursue and achieve her goals. She was a political activist and a revolutionary in her time. Her accomplishments went beyond the scope of nursing and nursing education, affecting all aspects of health care and social reform.

Lillian Wald

Background

Born in Cincinnati, Ohio, in 1867, Lillian Wald moved to Rochester, New York, where she spent most of her childhood. She received her education at Miss Crittenden's English and French Boarding and Day School for Young Ladies and Little Girls. Her relatives were physicians and had a tremendous influence on her. They encouraged her to choose nursing as a career.

Wald attended the New York Hospital School of Nursing. After graduation, she worked as a nurse in the New York Juvenile Asylum. She felt a need for more medically oriented knowledge, so she entered Women's Medical College in New York.

Turning Point

During this time, Wald and a colleague, Mary Brewster, were asked to go to New York's Lower East Side to give a lecture to immigrant mothers on caring for the sick. Wald and Brewster were shocked by what they discovered there.

While showing a group of mothers how to make a bed, a child came up to Wald and asked for help. The boy took her to a squalid tenement apartment where nine poorly nourished people were living in two rooms. A woman lay on a bed. Although she was seriously ill, it was apparent that no one had attended to her needs for several days (Kalisch & Kalisch, 2004). Miss Crittenden's School had not prepared Wald for this, but she went right to work. She bathed the woman, washed and changed the bedclothes, sent for a physician, and cleaned the room.

This incident was a turning point in her life. Wald left medical school and began a career as an advocate and helper of the poor and sick, joined by Brewster. They soon found that there were thousands of cases similar to the first in just one small neighborhood.

The Visiting Nurses

Wald and Brewster established a settlement house in 1893 in a rented tenement apartment in a poor section of New York's Lower East Side. To be closer to their clients, they gave up their comfortable living quarters and moved into a smaller, upper-floor apartment there.

It did not take long for the women to build up a nursing practice. At first, they had to seek out the sick, but within weeks calls came to them by the hundreds. The people of the neighborhood trusted them and relied on them for help. Gradually, the two developed a reputation among the physicians and hospitals in the area, and requests to see clients came from these sources as well.

Wald and her colleagues brought basic nursing care to the people in their home environment. These nurses were independent practitioners who made their own decisions and followed up on their own assessments of families' needs. Like Nightingale, they were very aware of the effect of the environment on the health of their clients and worked hard to improve their clients' surroundings.

Wald was convinced that many illnesses resulted from causes outside individual control and that treatment needed to be holistic. She said she chose the title *public health nurse* to emphasize the value of the nurse whose work was built on an understanding of the social and economic problems that inevitably accompanied the clients' ills (Bueheler-Wilkerson, 1993).

Because she had the freedom to explore alternatives for care during numerous births, illnesses, and deaths, Wald began to organize an impressive group of offerings, ranging from private relief to services from the medical establishment. She developed cooperative relationships with various organizations, which allowed her access to goods and jobs for her clients. News of her successes spread. Private physicians sought her help and referred their clients to her for care.

The Henry Street Settlement House

Within 2 years, the nurses had outgrown their original quarters. They needed larger facilities and more nurses. With the help of Jacob Schiff, a banker and philanthropist, they moved to a larger building at 265 Henry Street. This became known as the Henry Street Settlement House (Mayer, 1994). Nine graduate nurses moved in soon after.

By 1909, the Henry Street Settlement House had grown into a well-organized social services system with many departments. The staff included 37 nurses, 5 of whom were managers.

Other Accomplishments

Wald is credited with developing school health nursing. Health conditions were so bad in the New York City schools that 15–20 children per school were sent home every day. These ill children were returned to school by their parents in the same condition. As a result, illnesses spread from child to child. Ringworm, scabies, and pediculosis were common.

To prove her point about the value of community health nurses, Wald set up an experiment using one nurse for a month in one school. During that time, the number of children sent home from schools dropped from more than 10,000 to 1100. The New York Board of Health was so impressed that they hired nurses to continue the original nurse's work. Wald's nurses treated illnesses, explained the modes of transmission, and explained the reasons that some children had to be excluded from class and why others did not. The nurses also followed up on the children at home to prevent recurrence of illnesses.

Wald was also responsible for organizing the Children's Bureau, the Nursing Service Division of the Metropolitan Life Insurance Company, and the Town and Country Nursing Service of the American Red Cross. Her dreams of expanding public health nursing, obtaining insurance coverage for home-based preventive care, and developing a national health nursing service have not become a reality. However, in view of today's health-care concerns, she was a visionary who believed that health care belongs in the community and that nurses have a vital role to play in community-based care. She died in 1940 and is remembered as one of the foremost leaders in public health nursing.

Margaret Sanger

Background

Margaret Higgins was born in Corning, New York, on September 14, 1879. After recovering from tuberculosis, which she contracted while caring for her mother, she attended nursing school at the White Plains Hospital School of Nursing. In her autobiography, she described the school as rigid and at times inhuman; perhaps this provides an indication of where her future interests would take her (Sanger, 1938). During her affiliation at the Manhattan Eye and Ear Hospital, she met William Sanger. They married and moved to a suburb of New York, where she stayed at home to raise their three children.

Labor Reformer

Sanger was very concerned about the working conditions faced by people living in poverty. Many workers were paid barely enough to buy food for themselves and their families. At that time, the income for a family with two working parents was about $12–$14 a week. If only the father worked, earnings dropped to $8 a week. When only the mother worked, the family income was lower. A portion of this income was paid back to the company as rent for company housing. Food was often purchased through a company store, and very little was left for other expenses, including health care.

A major strike of industrial workers in Lawrence, Massachusetts, marked the beginning of Sanger's career as an advocate and social reformer. The workers had previously attempted a strike for better conditions, but they conceded because of threatening starvation. If the workers went on strike, then there was no money for food. Strike sympathizers in New York offered to help the workers and to take the children from Lawrence into their homes. Because of her interest in the situation of the underpaid workers and her involvement with New York laborers, Sanger was asked to assist in the evacuation of children from the unsettled and sometimes violent conditions in Lawrence.

Following an outbreak of serious rioting, she was called to Washington to testify before the House Committee on Rules about the condition of the children. She testified that the children were poorly nourished, ill, ragged, and living in conditions worse than those in impoverished city slums.

Two months later, the owners of the mills sat down to talk with the workers and gave in to their demands. Sanger's interventions on behalf of the children had brought the workers' plight to the attention of the general public and to people in Washington.

A New Concern for Sanger

In the spring of 1912, Sanger returned to work as a public health nurse. She was assigned to maternity cases in New York City's Lower East Side. One case became a turning point in her life. Sanger was caring for a 28-year-old mother of three children who had attempted to self-abort. This woman and her husband were already struggling to feed and clothe the children they had and could not afford any more. After 3 weeks, the woman had regained her health. However, during the physician's final visit to her home, he told the young woman that she had been lucky to survive this time but that, if she tried to self-abort again, she would not need his services but those of a funeral director. The young woman pleaded with him for a way to prevent another pregnancy. The doctor replied, "Tell your husband to sleep on the roof" (Sanger, 1938). The young woman then turned to Sanger, who remained silent.

Three months later, Sanger was called to the same home. This time, the woman was in a coma and died within minutes of Sanger's arrival. At that moment, Sanger dedicated herself to learning about and disseminating information about birth control.

Contraception Reform

This task turned out to be far more difficult than Sanger had expected. The Comstock Act of 1873 classified birth control information as obscene. Unrewarding research at the Boston Public Library, the Library of Congress, and the New York Academy of Medicine only increased her frustration. Very little information about birth control was available anywhere in the United States at that time.

But contraception was widely practiced in many European countries, so Sanger went to Europe. She studied methods of birth control in France, and when she returned to the United States, she began to publish a journal called *The Woman Rebel*. This journal carried articles about contraception, family planning, and other matters related to women's rights.

The first birth control clinic in the United States opened at 46 Amboy Street in Brooklyn, New York, in 1916. Sanger operated the clinic with her sister, Ethel Byrne, and another nurse, Fania Mindell. On the first day, more than 150 women asked them for help. Everything went smoothly until a policewoman, masquerading as a client, arrested the three women and recorded the names of all the clients. To bring attention to their plight and to the closing of the clinic, Sanger refused to ride in the police wagon. Instead, she walked the mile to the courthouse.

Several weeks later, Sanger returned to a courthouse overflowing with friends and supporters to face the charges that had been filed against her. The public found it difficult to believe that this attractive mother, flanked by her two sons, was either "demented" or "oversexed," as her adversaries had claimed. She did not deny the charges of disseminating birth control information, but she did challenge the law that made this information illegal. Because she refused to abide by that law, the judge sentenced her to 30 days in a workhouse.

After completing her 30 days, Sanger continued her work for many years. She solicited the support of wealthy women and used their help to gain financial backing to continue her fight. She gave talks and organized meetings. In 1921 she organized the Birth Control Conference in New York (Kalisch & Kalisch, 2004). In 1928 she established the National Committee on Federal Legislation for Birth Control, which eventually became the Planned Parenthood Foundation. Sanger was also an accomplished author, writing *What Every Girl Should Know, What Every Mother Should Know,* and *Motherhood in Bondage.*

Conservative religious and political groups were the most vocal in their opposition to Sanger's work. In the end, however, Sanger won. Planned Parenthood is a thriving organization, and birth control information is available to anyone who seeks it, although some groups oppose its availability on religious or political grounds.

Sanger could fairly be labeled an early example of the liberated woman. She was independent and assertive during a time when it was considered politically incorrect for a woman to behave that way. Her tenacity and her ability to bring the needs of the poor to society's attention represented that part of caring that operates in the political arena to bring about change to improve people's health and save lives.

Mary Eliza Mahoney

Background

Mary Eliza Mahoney was the first African-American registered nurse (RN) in the United States. She was born on May 7, 1845, in Dorchester, Massachusetts. She grew up in Roxbury with her parents and showed an interest in nursing during her adolescence. She worked for 15 years at the New England Hospital for Women and Children (now Dimock Community Health Center). She was a cook, a janitor, a washerwoman, and an unofficial nurse's assistant.

In 1878, at the age of 33, she applied to the hospital's nursing program and was accepted as a student. She spent her training days washing, ironing, and cleaning, expected competencies of that time. Sixteen months later, of the 43 students who began the rigorous course, Mary and 4 white students were the only ones who completed it. After graduation she worked mostly as a private duty nurse. She ended her nursing career as director of an orphanage in Long Island, New York, a position she had held for a decade. She never married.

Contribution to Nursing

Mahoney recognized the need for nurses to work together to advance the status of black nurses within the profession. In 1896 Mahoney became one of the original members of the predominately white Nurses Associated Alumnae of the United States and Canada (later known as the American Nurses Association [ANA]). She cofounded the National Association of Colored Graduate Nurses (NACGN). Mahoney delivered the welcoming speech at the first convention of the NACGN and served as its national chaplain.

Mahoney died on January 4, 1926, and was buried at the Woodlawn Cemetery in Everett, Massachusetts. In 1936, the NACGN created an award in her honor for women who contributed to racial integration in nursing. After the NACGN was dissolved in 1951, the ANA continued to offer this award to black women. In 1976, 50 years after her death, Mary Eliza Mahoney was inducted into the Nursing Hall of Fame.

When she entered nurse's training, Mahoney never envisioned how her simple act of becoming a nurse would change the status of black nurses and help them to attain leadership positions within the profession. Her dedication and effort have been an inspiration to many men and women of color who became dedicated members of the nursing profession.

Mildred Montag

Meeting the Need With Associate Degree Nurses

During World War II, a nursing shortage became evident. To meet the demands for nurses, Congress enacted the Bolton Act of 1943 creating the United States Cadet Nurse Corps. Under the Bolton Act, nurses could be educated in fewer than 3 years but perform the same nursing duties as their counterparts from the traditional 3-year diploma schools (Applegate, 1988). Mildred Montag developed such a program at Adelphi University.

After the war, federal funds were withdrawn, and the numbers of graduates declined. The acute nursing shortage continued. The time for a change in nursing education had come. The postwar era created other job opportunities for women, and hospital-based diploma school was not a popular career choice. The health-care delivery system was disease-oriented.

New technologies had entered the field of health care, requiring nurses to have a stronger background in the sciences and be able to use these technologies at the bedside.

In 1952 a project aimed at developing nursing education programs in junior and community colleges was launched. Montag, now an assistant professor of nursing at Columbia Teacher's College, was appointed the project coordinator. Montag proposed two levels of nursing, creating what she described as the *technical nurse*. This nurse would provide direct, safe nursing care under the supervision of the professional nurse in an acute care setting (Haase, 1990). The curriculum included general education courses to prepare the nurse for social and personal competency as well as skill competency. Today, associate degree programs provide more graduate nurses than any other nursing programs.

Associate degree nursing education has had a profound effect on nursing education. Montag's achievement also increased the shift of nursing education from the hospital to institutions of higher learning.

Virginia Henderson

Background

Virginia Henderson was born November 30, 1897, in Kansas City, Missouri. She attended the U.S. Army School of Nursing during World War I. Her mentor was Annie Goodrich, head of the Army School. Goodrich later became the first dean of the Yale School of Nursing. After the war, Henderson continued her nursing career in public health in New York City and Washington, D.C.

Henderson decided to enter nursing education and took her first faculty position at the Norfolk Virginia Protestant Hospital School of Nursing. In 1929 she returned to New York and enrolled in Columbia Teacher's College to further her nursing education. Here she earned her bachelor's and master's degrees and then joined the faculty of Columbia Teacher's College.

In 1953 she joined the faculty of the Yale School of Nursing in New Haven, Connecticut, as a research associate and spent the last four decades of her life there. She began a 19-year project to review nursing literature and published the four-volume *Nursing Studies Index*, which indexed the English-language nursing literature from 1900 through 1960.

Expanding the Definition of Nursing

Virginia Henderson's most important publication, *Principles and Practice of Nursing*, is considered the 20th century's equivalent to Nightingale's *Notes on Nursing*. Nightingale had emphasized nature as the primary healer but, with the advent of antibiotic therapy and other technological advances, this approach needed expansion (Henderson, 1955).

In her textbook revision in 1955, Henderson first offered her description of nursing: "I say that the nurse does for others what they would do for themselves if they had the strength, the will and the knowledge. But I go on to say that the nurse makes the patient independent of him or her as soon as possible." Henderson wrote three editions of this textbook. Unlike other nursing textbooks, this one emphasized the importance of nursing research. Nurse educators continued using the book throughout the remainder of the century.

Henderson believed that nursing complemented the patient by giving him or her what was needed in "will or strength" to perform the daily activities and carry out the physician's treatment. She believed strongly in "getting inside the skin" of her patients as a way of knowing what he or she needed. As she said, "The nurse is temporarily the consciousness of the unconscious, the love of life for the suicidal, the leg of the amputee, the eyes of the newly blind, a means of locomotion for the infant and the knowledge and confidence of the new mother" (Henderson, 1955).

Her beginnings were in public health, and this influenced her definition of nursing. Because of this background, Henderson was a proponent of publicly financed, universally accessible health-care services. She understood that nurses maintained roots in the communities where they lived, and she believed that nursing belonged in the forefront of health-care reform. She also believed that nurses should take every opportunity to advance the profession by becoming leaders in developing plans for implementing accessible health care. She founded the Interagency Council on Information Resources for Nursing. She was a consultant to the National Library of Medicine and the American Journal of Nursing Company. Henderson received many awards for her work and efforts to increase the status of the nursing profession. The Sigma Theta Tau International Nurses Honor Society named its library in honor of her outstanding contributions to nursing.

Contribution to 20th-Century Nursing

Henderson is thought by many to be the most important nursing figure in the 20th century. Her colleagues refer to her as the 20th century Florence Nightingale (ualberta.ca/~jmorris/nt/henderson.htm, 2000). She represents the essence and the spirit of nursing in the 20th century.

Men in Nursing

Men are not new to nursing. Early Egyptian priests who served the goddess Sekhmet practiced nursing. The first nursing school in the world started in India in about 250 B.C., and only men were considered "pure" enough for admission.

In the Byzantine Empire, nursing was practiced primarily by men and was a separate profession (Kalisch & Kalisch, 2004). During every plague that swept through Europe, men risked their lives to provide nursing care. In 300 A.D. the Parabolani, a group of men, started a hospital to care for victims of the Black Plague. Two hundred years later, St. Benedict founded the Benedictine Nursing Order (Kalisch & Kalisch, 2004). Throughout the Middle Ages, military, religious, and lay orders of men continued to provide nursing care.

The Alexian Brothers, named after St. Alexis, a 5th century nurse, were organized in the 1300s to provide nursing care to those affected by the Black Death. In 1863, the Alexian Brothers opened their first hospital in the United States to educate men as nurses. The Mills School for Nursing and St. Vincent's School for men were organized in New York in 1888. At that time, men did not attend female nursing schools.

Before the Civil War both male and female slaves were employed as "nurses." During the Civil War the Union used mainly female nurse volunteers, although some men also filled this responsibility. The poet Walt Whitman, for example, served as a volunteer nurse in the Union Army. The Confederate Army identified 30 men in each regiment to serve as military nurses. Charged with this responsibility, these men tended to the ill on the battlefields (Clay, 1928).

Modern nursing continued to develop as a predominantly female profession, however, excluding men from schools of nursing and the professional organizations. The Nurses Associated Alumnae of the United States and Canada held its first annual meeting in Baltimore in 1897. Later becoming the

ANA (in 1911), it continued to exclude men until 1930. One of the early acts of the organization was to prevent men from practicing as nurses in the military. The Army Nurse Corps, created in 1901, barred men from serving as nurses (Brown, 1942; Kalisch & Kalisch, 2004).

At the conclusion of the Korean War, the armed services again permitted men to serve as military nurses. Once men entered the military as nurses, their numbers increased in civilian nursing as well. Nursing schools began to admit men, and the numbers of men in nursing gradually increased. Today, although still comparatively few, the number of men pursing nursing careers continues to increase. Men are attaining graduate degrees and specialty certification and continue to enhance nursing by resuming their historical role as caring professionals.

Professional Organizations

ANA

In 1896 delegates from 10 nursing schools' alumnae associations met to organize a national professional association for nurses. The constitution and bylaws were completed in 1907, and the Nurses Associated Alumnae of the United States and Canada was created. The name was changed in 1911 to the American Nurses Association, which in 1982 became a federation of constituent state nurses associations. In 1908, the Canadian Association of Nursing Education created the Canadian National Association of Trained Nurses, which became the Canadian Nurses Association in 1924, with Mary Agnes Snively as its first president (Mansell & Dodd, 2005).

The purposes of the ANA are to:

1. Foster high standards of nursing practice
2. Promote the rights of nurses in the workplace
3. Project a positive and realistic view of nursing
4. Lobby the Congress and regulatory agencies on health-care issues affecting nurses and the public

These purposes, reviewed during each biennial meeting by the House of Delegates, are unrestricted by consideration of age, color, creed, disability, gender, health status, lifestyle, nationality, religion, race, or sexual orientation (ANA, 2007).

The goals of the Canadian Nurses Association are to:

1. Advance the discipline of nursing in the interest of the public

2. Advocate for policy that incorporates the principles of primary health care (access, interdisciplinary, patient and community involvement, health promotion) and respects the Canada Health Act

3. Advance the regulation of RNs in the interest of the public

4. Collaborate with nurses, other providers, stakeholders, and the public to achieve and sustain quality practice environments and positive client outcomes

5. Advance international health

6. Promote awareness of the profession so that the roles and expertise of RNs are understood, respected, and optimized (abbreviated from CAN-AIIC at http://www.CNA-nurses.ca)

The core policy issues identified by the ANA in 2007 were:

- Nursing shortage
- Workplace rights
- Workplace health and safety
- Appropriate staffing
- Patient safety and advocacy

Although more than 2 million people are members of the nursing profession in the United States, only about 10% of the nation's RNs are members of their professional organization. The many different subgroups and numerous specialty nursing organizations contribute to this fragmentation, which makes presenting a united front from which to advocate for nursing difficult. As the ANA works on the goal of preparing nurses during the 21st century, nurses need to work together in their efforts to identify and promote their unique, autonomous role within the health-care system.

Many advantages are available to nurses who join the ANA. Membership offers benefits such as informative publications, group life and health insurance, malpractice insurance, and continuing education courses. As the major voice of nursing in the United States, the ANA lobbies the government to influence laws that affect the practice of nursing and the safety of consumers. The power of the ANA was apparent when nurses lobbied against the American Medical Association's (AMA) proposal to create a new category of health-care worker, the registered care technician, as an answer to the nursing shortage of the 1980s.

The registered care technician category was never established despite the AMA's vigorous support.

The ANA frequently publishes position statements outlining the organization's position on particular topics important to the health and welfare of the public and/or the nurse. Box 15-1 summarizes some of the current position statements available from the ANA, which can be accessed on the ANA Web site (nursingworld.org/) or are available by mail on request. Likewise, the Canadian Nurses Organization publishes position statements on such issues as education, ethics, healthy public policy, leadership, practice, primary health care, protection of the public, and research (Nursing Now, 2005; 2007).

Finally, the ANA offers certification in various specialty areas. Certification is a formal, voluntary process by which the professional demonstrates knowledge of and expertise in a specific area of practice. It is a way to establish the nurse's expertise beyond the basic requirements for licensure and is an important part of peer recognition for nurses. In many areas, certification entitles the nurse to salary increases and position advancement. Some specialty nursing organizations also have certification programs.

National League for Nursing

Another large nursing organization is the National League for Nursing (NLN). Unlike ANA membership, NLN membership is open to other health professionals and interested consumers. Over 1500 nursing schools and health-care agencies and more than 5000 nurses, educators, administrators, consumers, and students are members of the NLN (nln.org/aboutnln/info-history.htm).

The NLN participates in test services, research, and publication. It also lobbies actively for nursing issues and is currently working cooperatively with the ANA and other nursing organizations on health-care reform. To do such things more effectively, the ANA, NLN, American Association of Colleges of Nursing, and American Organization of Nurse Executives have formed a coalition called the TriCouncil for the purpose of dealing with issues that are important to all nurses.

The NLN formed a separate accrediting agency, the National League for Nursing Accrediting Agency (NLNAC). The NLNAC is responsible for the specialized accreditation of nursing education schools and programs, both

box 15-1

Position Statements

American Nurses Association

Bloodborne and Airborne Diseases

Education and Barrier Use for Sexually Transmitted Diseases and HIV Infection

The Health Care Service System and Linkage of Primary Care, Substance Abuse, Mental Health, and HIV/AIDS-Related Services

AIDS/HIV Disease and Socio-Culturally Diverse Populations

Equipment/Safety Procedures to Prevent Transmission of Bloodborne Diseases

Guidelines for Disclosure to a Known Third Party About Possible HIV Infection

HIV Infected Nurse, Ethical Obligations and Disclosure

Tuberculosis and HIV

HIV Disease and Correctional Inmates

Needle Exchange and HIV

Personnel Policies and HIV in the Workplace

Post-Exposure Programs in the Event of Occupational Exposure to HIV/HBV

HIV Exposure from Rape/Sexual Assault

HIV Infection and Nursing Students

Tuberculosis and Public Health Nursing

HIV Infection and U.S. Teenagers

HIV Testing

Travel Restrictions for Persons with HIV/AIDS

HIV Disease and Women

Ethics and Human Rights

Stem Cell Research

Privacy and Confidentiality

Assuring Patient Safety: Registered Nurses' Responsibility in all Roles and Settings to Guard Against Working When Fatigued

Assisted Suicide

Nurses' Participation in Capital Punishment

The Non-Negotiable Nature of the ANA Code for Nurses with Interpretive Statements

Cultural Diversity in Nursing Practice

Discrimination and Racism in Health Care

Nursing Care and Do-Not-Resuscitate Decisions

Ethics and Human Rights

Active Euthanasia

Foregoing Nutrition and Hydration

Mechanisms Through Which SNAs Consider Ethical/Human Rights Issues

Nursing and the Patient Self-Determination Acts

Risk and Responsibility in Providing Nursing Care

Reduction of Patient Restraint and Seclusion in Healthcare Settings

Assuring Patient Safety: The Employers' Role in Promoting

Healthy Nursing Work Hours for Registered Nurses in All Roles and Settings

Pain Management and Control of Distressing Symptoms in Dying Patients

Human Cloning by Means of Blastomere Splitting and Nuclear Transplantation

Social Causes and Health Care

Elimination of Violence in Advertising Directed Toward Children, Adolescents, and Families

Tobacco Use Prevention, Cessation, and Exposure to Second-Hand Smoke

Adult Immunization

Adolescent Immunization

Violence Against Women

Adolescent Health

Environmental Tobacco Smoke

Prevention of Tobacco Use in Youth

Use of Placebos for Pain Management in Patients with Cancer

Home Care for Mother, Infant, and Family Following Birth

Promotion and Disease Prevention

Long-Term Care

Childhood Immunizations

Informal Caregiving

Lead Poisoning and Screening

Nutrition Screening for the Elderly

Reproductive Health

Drug and Alcohol Abuse

Abuse of Prescription Drugs

Polypharmacy and the Older Adult

Opposition to Criminal Prosecution of Women for Use of Drugs While Pregnant

Drug Testing for Health-Care Workers

Nursing Education

Guideline for Commercial Support for Continuing Nursing Education

Nursing Practice

Professional Role Competence

Safety Issues Related to Tubing and Catheter Misconnections

Assuring Safe, High-Quality Health Care in Pre-K Through 12 Educational Settings

Credentialing and Privileging of Advanced Practice Registered Nurses

Providing Patients Safe Access to Therapeutic Marijuana/Cannabis

Privatization and For-Profit Conversion

A National Nursing Database to Support Clinical Nursing Practice

box 15-1

Position Statements—cont'd

Nurse-Midwifery	Polygraph Testing of Health Care Workers
ANA Response to Pew Commission Report	Sexual Harassment
Nursing Research	***Unlicensed Assistive Personnel*** (Note: ANA work on the UAP issue is ongoing)
Education for Participation in Nursing Research	
Consumer Advocacy	Registered Nurses Utilization of Nursing Personnel in All Settings
Referrals to the Most Appropriate Provider	
Mercury in Vaccines	Registered Nurse Education Relating to the Utilization of Unlicensed Assistive Personnel
Elimination of Medication Waste in Long-Term Care Facilities	
Workplace Advocacy	***Joint Statements***
Assuring Patient Safety: The Employers' Role in Promoting Healthy Nursing Work Hours for Registered Nurses in All Roles and Settings	Joint Statement on Delegation American Nurses Association (ANA) and National Council of State Boards of Nursing
Assuring Patient Safety: Registered Nurses' Responsibility in All roles and Settings to Guard Against Working When Fatigued	Authentication in a Computer-Based Patient Record
	On Access to Patient Data
Elimination of Manual Patient Handling to Prevent Work-Related Musculoskeletal Disorders	Computer-Based Patient Record Standards
	Services to Families Following Sudden Infant Death Syndrome
Work Release During a Disaster: Guidelines for Employers	
Registered Nurses' Rights and Responsibilities Related to work Release During a Disaster	Association of Operating Room Nurses Official Statement on RN First Assistants
Opposition to Mandatory Overtime	Maintaining Professional and Legal Standards During a Shortage of Nursing Personnel
Latex Allergy	
The Right to Accept or Reject an Assignment	Role of the Registered Nurse in the Management of Patients Receiving IV Conscious Sedation
Restructuring, Work Redesign, and the Job and Career Security of Registered Nurses	Role of the Registered Nurse in the Management of Analgesia by Catheter Techniques

post-secondary and higher degree (master's degree, baccalaureate degree, associate-degree, diploma, and practical nursing programs).

National Organization for Associate-Degree Nursing

Associate-degree nursing programs prepare the largest number of new graduates for RN licensure. Many of these individuals would never have had the opportunity to become RNs without the access afforded by the community college system. The move to begin a national organization to address associate-degree nursing began in 1986. The organization identified two major goals: to maintain eligibility for licensure for associate-degree graduates and to interact with other nursing organizations. Today, the mission of the National Organization for Associate Degree Nursing (NOADN) includes supporting the associate-degree graduate through:

■ Strong educational programs
■ Dynamic curricula and education of students in a variety of settings

■ Emphasis on lifelong learning
■ Continued interaction with colleges and universities (noadn.org)

American Academy of Nursing

The American Academy of Nursing consists of over 1500 nursing leaders in practice, education, management, and research. Its mission is to advance health policy and practice through the generation, synthesis, and dissemination of nursing knowledge. The mission is accomplished through *Nursing Outlook,* a professional journal; expert panels composed of members of the Academy, a Scholar in Residence program, and supporting appointment of nurses to key policy positions. Membership is through nomination by current Fellows of the Academy (http://www.aannet.org).

National Institute for Nursing Research

The National Institute for Nursing Research (NINR), unlike the other associations described here, is an arm of the federal government, one of the 27 institutes of National Institutes of Health

(NIH). Originally a center at NIH, it became a full-fledged insititute in 1993. NINR supports and conducts basic and clinical research and provides research training in health promotion, disease and disability prevention, quality of life, health disparities, management of symptoms, and end-of-life care encompasing the entire life span (http://www.ninr.nih.gov).

Specialty Organizations

In addition to the national nursing organizations, nurses may join specialty practice organizations focused on practice areas (e.g., critical care, neuroscience, obstetrics) or special interest groups (e.g., male nurses, Hispanic, Philippine, Aboriginal nurses). These organizations provide nurses with information regarding evidence-based practice, trends in the field, and approved standards of specialty practice. Links to nursing organizations may be found at nursingsociety.org/career/nursing_orgs.html or http://www.cna-nurses.ca

Health Care Today

Among the industrialized countries of the world, the United States is the only one that does not provide basic health-care coverage to every citizen (Lieberman, 2003). Forty-seven million Americans have no health insurance (ANA, 2008a), yet the United States has technologically advanced, highly sophisticated health care and spends more per capita (per person) than most countries.

If the United States has the most advanced knowledge and equipment and spends a great deal of money on health care, then why the cause for alarm? What is wrong? Why doesn't everyone have health-care insurance? Why are people so worried about the quality of care? The answer is complex.

For most people, health insurance comes through their place of employment. One problem with this is that many employers are motivated to keep the cost as low as possible or transfer much of the cost to the employee. Another problem is that if one loses one's job, health insurance is also lost.

Managed care was originally designed to reduce the amount spent on health care by emphasizing prevention. Some have said that it has become a way to limit choices and ration care (Mechanic, 2002) rather than prevent illness.

As managed care plans grow and spread across the country, these companies become powerful enough to be able to negotiate reduced rates (discounts) from local hospitals (Trinh & O'Connor, 2002). They can, in effect, say, "We can get an appendectomy for $2300 at hospital A; why should we pay you $2700?" If hospital B does not agree, the hospital may lose all the patients enrolled in that managed care plan. This pressures hospital B to reduce costs and spread staff even thinner than before.

Similar price pressures come from Medicare, Medicaid, and other health insurance companies. To keep costs under control, some states have cut benefits for people receiving Medicaid (state-supported health benefits for low-income people) (Pear, 2002).

With the upsurge in for-profit health plans and the purchase of not-for-profit hospitals by for-profit companies, U.S. health care has become increasingly "corporatized." It was thought that this would yield a highly efficient, responsive system ("the customer is always right"). That has not happened because the "customer" who pays for insurance coverage is actually the employer or the government, not the individual patient. The care provided by the for-profits, in general, appears to be of lesser quality than the old not-for-profit or fee-for-service plans (Mechanic, 2002).

There is a limit to the extent to which cost cutting can increase efficiency without endangering patients. A series of important research studies has shown that increasing the number of RNs providing care in a hospital has a direct effect on improving the outcomes of patient care.

For many years, the United States has been trying to fix its health-care system by applying patches over its worst cracks, but this has apparently not worked very well. Does the system need a major overhaul? Yes. But first, there needs to be a clear vision of what it should be and what it should do (O'Connor, 2002). Whatever way that vision develops, it is certain that nurses will have an important role in a future health-care system. As Aiken and colleagues (2002) wrote, "nurses contribute importantly to surveillance, early detection and timely interventions that save lives" (p. 18).

The ANA, among others, has described the current health-care system in the United States as "sick" and "broken" (ANA, 2008a). As stated before, forty-seven million Americans, including 9 million children, have no health-care insurance. Even worse, two-thirds of the working-age population have a health-care–related financial problem such as unpaid medical bills, being uninsured, or being underinsured. A survey of over 26,000 Americans, half of whom belonged to a union, found that 1 in 3 had decided to do without care because of the cost. Half had stayed in a job just to keep their health-care benefits. More than half reported that their health-care insurance did not cover the care they needed at a price they could afford (Currie, 2008b). More detail about the survey can be found at www.healthcaresurvey.aflcio.org

The quality of the care provided is a second major concern. A 1999 report issued by the Institute of Medicine estimated that 100,000 deaths in hospitals every year were due to errors that could have been prevented (ANA, 2008a). Hospital-acquired drug-resistant infections have become a major problem, having increased a hundredfold over the last 10 years or so. In 1993 there were 3000 hospital discharges that included a diagnosis of drug-resistant microorganism. In 2005 there were 394,000 of these discharges (Currie, 2008a).

Additional concerns include fragmented, impersonal care; failure to consider the whole person when treating a problem; and continuation of disease focus rather than prevention focus. Furthermore, the United States face what Buchan called a "demographic double whammy" of an aging population that will need more health care and, at the same time, an aging workforce (Hewison & Wildman, 2008).

In Canada, a debate over privatization versus public funding of health care continues (Villeneuve & MacDonald, 2006). Health care is still illness- and disease-focused as in the United States. Although there is interest in complementary and alternative treatments, they have not been integrated into general care. Disparities in care of members of minority groups threaten to increase if not addressed more effectively.

Global interconnectedness has brought new concerns about how quickly and easily infectious diseases can cross national borders. HIV, severe acute respiratory syndrome, and the annual waves of influenza that cross the globe are just a few reminders.

Nursing Today

Issues specific to nursing reflect the problems and concerns of the system as a whole. The average bedside RN is in her middle to late 40s (Lillis & O'Brien, 2007). Ninety-percent of nurses are still female, although the number of men is gradually increasing (Dougherty, 2008). Concerns about the supply of RNs and staffing shortages persist in both the United States and Canada.

The related issues of excessive workload, mandatory overtime, scheduling, abuse, workplace violence, and lack of professional autonomy contribute to these concerns (Villeneuve & MacDonald, 2006). On the bright side, there are also some indications of increasing interest in a nursing career as salaries improve and job opportunities expand.

Safe staffing, defined as the appropriate number and mix of nursing staff, is a critical issue for nurses and the people who need their care. A series of research studies has demonstrated the importance of adequate nurse staffing. There is powerful evidence that nurses save lives: there is a 7% increase in the likelihood of a patient dying within 30 days of admission for each additional patient assigned to a nurse (Aiken et al., 2002; Potter & Mueller, 2007). Nurses cannot gain in-depth understanding of their patients, protect their patients, or catch early warning signs of trouble if they are overwhelmed by the number of patients for whom they are responsible. Adequate numbers of nurses affect patient mortality, length of stay, urinary tract infections, fall rates, incidence of hospital-acquired pneumonia, and more. For further information, see www.safestaffingsaveslives.org

Health Care in the Future

Ideally, a new model of health care is needed that offers the following:

- Holistic, person-centered care
- Seamless connections across community, acute-care, and long-term care settings (Pogue, 2007)
- Elimination of health disparities
- Guaranteed accessible, affordable care for everyone (ANA, 2008b)
- Safe care that heals and does not harm the patient
- Equal support for prevention, health promotion, and mental health care
- Healthy environment from green buildings (Trossman, 2007) to the elimination of air, water, soil, and other forms of pollution
- Acknowledgement and addressing of global health concerns: global warming, hunger, poverty, and disease at home and in developing countries

Nursing in the Future

Within the nursing profession, there is much work to do. Cohen (2007) addressed the issue of the image that many nurses present to their public. One is professional appearance and behavior. She quotes Dumont on the question of dress, particularly wearing uniforms covered with cartoon characters: "You're the only thing between the patient and death, and you're covered in cartoons. No wonder you have no authority." The following are some additional suggestions to improve nursing's image:

- Always introduce yourself as a nurse.
- Define professional appearance appropriate to your workplace, and enforce it.
- Define professional behavior, and enforce it.
- Take every opportunity to speak to the public about nursing.
- Document what nurses do and how important they are (Cohen, 2007).

What else can nurses do? It is important that more members of minority groups be brought into nursing so that nursing better reflects the increasing diversity of the population. Collaboration with colleagues in other health professions is also vital to improving health care. Physicians, therapists, social workers, psychologists, aides, assistants, and technicians are concerned about the quality of care provided. Patients and their families are also concerned and personally affected by the quality of care provided. All these groups together would have a stronger voice in health-care reform.

The following are some specific actions you can take to exert leadership in improving health care:

- Learn more about the health-care system and your role in it.
- Join your professional association and specialty associations and support their efforts to improve care.
- Talk with everyone and anyone who will listen.
- Write letters to the editor, speak on local radio and television programs, and participate in online discussions.
- Speak to local, state, and national representatives about these concerns.

In summary, be "visible and vocal" in your support of nursing and improved health care (ANA, 2008a).

Conclusion

As nursing moves forward in the 21st century, the need for courageous and innovative nurse leaders is greater than ever. Society's demand for high-quality health care at an affordable cost is a contemporary force for change.

Nurses began in hospitals, moved to the community, moved back into the hospitals, and are now seeing a move back to the community. Men were the earliest nurses, then left the profession and have now returned, bringing with them new ideas and leadership abilities. Nursing has become as diversified as the populations it serves. You will be the Nightingales, Walds, Sangers, Mahoneys, Montags, and Hendersons of the future; the creativity and dedication of these nurses are part of everyone.

Study Questions

1. Read *Notes on Nursing: What It Is and What It Is Not* by Florence Nightingale. How much of its content is still true today?

2. If Margaret Sanger were alive, how do you think she would view the issue of teaching schoolchildren about AIDS?

3. What do you think Lillian Wald would say about the status of hospitals and health care today?

4. How do you think Florence Nightingale would deal with a physician who is verbally abusive to the nursing staff?

5. If you had been Margaret Sanger, would you have decided to stop teaching women about birth control? Explain your answer.

6. What is your definition of nursing? How does it compare or contrast with Virginia Henderson's definition?

7. Review the mission and purpose of the ANA or another national nursing organization online. Do you believe that nurses should belong to these organizations? Explain your answer.

Case Study to Promote Critical Reasoning

Alina went to nursing school on an Air Force scholarship. She has been directed to lead the planning for establishing a comprehensive primary care and health promotion program clinic on board NASA's newest international space station. The crew is to remain on board the station for 6 months at a time. The crew will consist of military men and women from three countries.

1. What medical and nursing equipment should Alina plan to have in this center?

2. What would the physical environment on board need to have to satisfy Florence Nightingale and Lillian Wald?

3. How do you believe Virginia Henderson would describe the role of the nurse in this environment?

4. Develop a possible nursing research topic for study in this situation.

References

Aiken, L., Clarke, S.P., Sloane, D., Sochalski, J., et al. (2002). Hospital nurse staffing and patient mortality, nurse burnout and job dissatisfaction. *Journal of the American Medical Association, 288*(16), 1987–1993.

American Nurses Association. (2007). Retrieved on October 16, 2007, from http://www.nursinqworld.org/FunctionalMenuCategories/About ANA.aspx

American Nurses Association. (2008a). Health reform: The 2008 elections and beyond. *The American Nurse*, September/October.

American Nurses Association. (2008b). Safe staffing save lives. *The American Nurse*, March/April.

Applegate, M. (1988). Associate degree nursing and health care. In *Perspectives of Nursing 1987–1989*, pp. 207–219.

Beletz, E. (1974). Is nursing's public image up-to-date? *Nursing Outlook, 22*, 432–435.

Brown, D. (1942). Men nurses in the U.S. Navy. *American Journal of Nursing, 42*(5), 499–501.

Bueheler-Wilkerson, K. (1993). Bring care to the people: Lillian Wald's legacy to public health nursing. *American Journal of Public Health, 83*, 1778–1785.

Clay, V. (1928). Home life of a Southern lady. In Hart, Albert B. (ed.). *American History Told by Contemporaries* (vol. 4, p. 244). N.Y.: MacMillan.

Cohen, S. (2007). The image of nursing: How do others see us? How do we see ourselves? *American Nurse Today, 2*(5), 24–26.

Currie, D. (2008a). Drug-resistant could lower costs. *The Nation's Health, 38*(4), 4.

Currie, D. (2008b). One in three forgo care because of cost. *The Nation's Health, 38*(4), 8.

Donahue, H.P. (1985). *Nursing, the Oldest Art*. St. Louis: C.V. Mosby.

Dougherty, C. (2008, May 7). Slowdown's side effect: More nurses. *Wall Street Journal*, pp. D1, D8.

Griffith, G.J., & Griffith, H.J. (1965). *Jensen's history and trends in professional nursing*, 5th ed. St. Louis: C.V. Mosby.

Haase, P. (1990). *The origins and rise of associate degree nursing education*. Durham, N.C.: Duke University Press.

Henderson, V. (1966). *The nature of nursing*. New York: Macmillan.

Henderson, V. (1955). ualberta.ca/-jmorris/nt/henderson.htm Retrieved on May 9, 2000, unc.edu/ehallora/henderson.htm

Hewison, A., & Wildman, S. (2008). Looking back, looking forward: Enduring issues in nursing management. *Journal of Nursing Management, 16*(1), 1–3.

Improving practice environment: Keeping up the momentum. (2007, April): *Nursing Now: Issues and Trends in Canadian Nursing*, Number 22

Kalisch, P.A., & Kalisch, B.J. (2004). *American nursing: A history*. Philadelphia: Lippincott, Williams & Wilkins.

Lieberman, T. (2003). Bruised and broken: The US health system. *AARP Bulletin, 44*(3), 3–5.

Lillis, K., & O'Brien, A. (2007, February 12). Salary survey 2007. *Advance for Nurses*, pp. 11–18.

Longfellow, H.W. (1868). The lady with the lamp. In Williams, M. (1975). *How does a poem mean?* Boston: Houghton Mifflin.

Mansell, D., & Dodd, D. (2005). Professionalism and Canadian nursing. In Bates, C., Bates, D., & Rousseau, N. (eds.) *On all frontiers: Four centuries of Canadian nursing* (pp. 197-211). Ottawa: University of Ottawa Press.

Mayer, S. (1994). Amelia Greenwald: Pioneer in international public health nursing. *Nursing and Health Care, 15*(2), 74–78.

Mechanic, D. (2002). Sociocultural implications of changing organizational technologies in the provision of care. *Social Science and Medicine, 54*, 459–467.

National League for Nursing. Retrieved on May 4, 2006, from http://www.nln.org/aboutnln/info-history.htm

National Organization of Associate Degree Nursing. Retrieved on May 3, 2006, from noadn.org conventionstate.htm

Nightingale, F. (1859). *Notes on nursing: What it is and what it is not*. Reprinted 1992. Philadelphia: J.B. Lippincott.

Nursing leadership in a changing world. (2005, January). *Nursing Now: Issues and Trends in Canadian Nursing*, Number 18.

O'Connor, K. (2002, April 8). Healthcare in need of a fix. *Modern Healthcare,* 27.

Pear, R. (2002, November 20). Report: Health system in crisis. *Sun Sentinel,* 3A.

Pogue, P. (2007). The nurse practitioner role. *Into the Future Nursing Leadership,* 20(2), 34–38.

Potter, P., & Mueller, J.R. (2007). How well do you know your patients? *Nursing Management,* 38(2), 40-41.

Roberts, M. (1937). Florence Nightingale as a nurse educator. *American Journal of Nursing,* 37, 775.

Rogers, M.E. (1988). Nursing science and art: A perspective. *Nursing Science Quarterly,* 1, 99–102.

Sanger, M. (1938). *Margaret Sanger: An autobiography.* New York: W.W. Norton.

Schuyler, C.B. (1992). Florence Nightingale. In *Notes on nursing: What it is and what it is not.* Philadelphia: J.B. Lippincott.

Sigma Theta Tau International Nursing Honor Society. (2006). Retrieved on May 3, 2006, from nursingsociety.org/career/nursing_orgs.html

Trinh, H.Q., & O'Connor, S.J. (2002). Helpful or harmful? The impact of strategic change on the performance of U.S. urban hospitals. *Health Services Research,* 37(1), 145–171.

Trossman, S. (2007). Who says it's not easy being green? Nurses and health care leaders promote healing, environmentally friendly facilities. *The American Nurse,* 39(2), 1, 8.

Villeneuve, M., & MacDonald, J. (2006). *Toward 2020: Visions of nursing.* Ottawa: Canadian Nurses Association.

Codes of Ethics for Nurses

⊙ ○ ○ ○ ○ ○ ○ ○ ○ ○ ○

American Nurses Association Code of Ethics for Nurses

1. The nurse, in all professional relationships, practices with compassion and respect for the inherent dignity, worth, and uniqueness of every individual, unrestricted by considerations of social or economic status, personal attributes, or the nature of health problems.
2. The nurse's primary commitment is to the patient, whether an individual, family, group, or community.
3. The nurse promotes, advocates for, and strives to protect the health, safety, and rights of the patient.
4. The nurse is responsible and accountable for individual nursing practice and determines the appropriate delegation of tasks consistent with the nurse's obligation to provide optimum patient care.
5. The nurse owes the same duties to self as to others, including the responsibility to preserve integrity and safety, to maintain competence, and to continue personal and professional growth.
6. The nurse participates in establishing, maintaining, and improving health care environments and conditions of employment conducive to the provision of quality health care and consistent with the values of the profession through individual and collective action.
7. The nurse participates in the advancement of the profession through contributions to practice, education, administration, and knowledge development.
8. The nurse collaborates with other health professionals and the public in promoting community, national, and international efforts to meet health needs.
9. The profession of nursing, as represented by associations and their members, is responsible for articulating nursing values, for maintaining the integrity of the profession and its practice, and for shaping social policy.

Approved July 2001. Web site: nursingworld. org/ethics/chcode. htm
Reprinted with permission from American Nurses Association, Code of Ethics for Nurses with Interpretive Statements, ©2001 American Nurses Publishing, American Nurses Foundation/American Nurses Association, Washington, DC.

Canadian Nurse Association Code of Ethics for Registered Nurses

The Code of Ethics for Registered Nurses (CNA, 2008) serves as a foundation for nurses' ethical practice. CNA believes that the following seven values, which are described in the code, are central to ethical nursing practice. In the code each of these values is accompanied by a number of responsibility statements, and together they outline the ethical practice that is expected of registered nurses. CNA believes that the quality of the work environment in which nurses practice is also fundamental to their ability to practice ethically.

1. Providing safe, compassionate, competent and ethical care

Nurses provide safe, compassionate, competent and ethical care.

2. Promoting health and well-being

Nurses work with people to enable them to attain their highest possible level of health and well-being.

3. Promoting and respecting informed decision-making

Nurses recognize, respect and promote a person's right to be informed and make decisions.

4. Preserving dignity

Nurses recognize and respect the intrinsic worth of each person.

5. Maintaining privacy and confidentiality

Nurses recognize the importance of privacy and confidentiality and safeguard personal, family and community information obtained in the context of a professional relationship.

6. Promoting justice

Nurses uphold principles of justice by safeguarding human rights, equity and fairness and by promoting the public good.

7. Being accountable

Nurses are accountable for their actions and answerable for their practice. Ethical nursing practice also involves endeavoring to address broad aspects of social justice that are associated with health and well-being. These aspects relate to the need for change in systems and societal structures in order to create greater equity for all. Nurses should endeavor as much as possible, individually and collectively, to advocate for and work toward eliminating social inequities. The code contains thirteen statements entitled "ethical endeavors," which are intended to guide nurses in this area. These statements address the need for awareness and action around such areas as social inequalities, accessibility and comprehensiveness of health care, and major health concerns (e.g., poverty, violence, inadequate shelter) as well as broader global concerns (e.g., war, violations of human rights, world hunger).

Canadian Nursing Association. Web site: www.cna-nurses.ca

Reprinted with permission from the Canadian Nurses Association, 2008.

The International Council of Nurses Code of Ethics for Nurses

Nurses and People

The nurse's primary professional responsibility is to people requiring nursing care.

In providing nursing care, the nurse promotes an environment in which the human rights, values, customs, and spiritual beliefs of the individual, family, and community are respected.

The nurse ensures that the individual receives sufficient information on which to base consent for care and related treatment.

The nurse holds in confidence personal information and uses judgment in sharing this information.

The nurse shares with society the responsibility for initiating and supporting action to meet the health and social needs of the public, in particular those of vulnerable populations.

The nurse also shares responsibility to sustain and protect the natural environment from depletion, pollution, degradation, and destruction.

Nurses and Practice

The nurse carries personal responsibility and accountability for nursing practice, and for maintaining competence by continual learning.

The nurse maintains a standard personal health such that the ability to provide care is not compromised.

The nurse uses judgment regarding individual competence when accepting and delegating responsibility.

The nurse at all times maintains standards of personal conduct which reflect well on the profession and enhance public confidence.

The nurse, in providing care, ensures that use of technology and scientific advances are compatible with safety, dignity, and rights of people.

Nurses and the Profession

The nurse assumes the major role in determining and implementing acceptable standards of clinical nursing practice, management, research, and education.

The nurse is active in developing a core research-based professional knowledge.

The nurse, acting through professional organizations, participates in creating and maintaining equitable social and economic working conditions in nursing.

Nurses and Co-Workers

The nurse sustains a co-operative relationship with co-workers in nursing and other fields.

The nurse takes appropriate action to safeguard individuals when their care is endangered by a co-worker or any other person.

Approved 2000. Web site: cn.ch/ethics.htm

Used with permission International Council of Nurses, Geneva, Switzerland, copyright 2000.

Standards Published by the American Nurses Association*

○ ○ ○ ○ ○ ○ ○ ○ ○ ○

- Faith Community Nursing: Scope and Standards of Practice
- Intellectual and Developmental Disabilities Nursing: Scope and Standards of Practice
- Neonatal Nursing: Scope and Standards of Practice
- Pain Management Nursing: Scope and Standards of Practice
- Plastic Surgery Nursing: Scope and Standards of Practice
- School Nursing: Scope and Standards of Practice
- Scope and Standards for Nurse Administrators
- Scope and Standards of Addictions Nursing Practice
- Scope and Standards of College Health Nursing Practice
- Scope and Standards of Diabetes Nursing Practice
- Scope and Standards of Gerontological Nursing Practice
- Scope and Standards of Home Health Nursing Practice

- Scope and Standards of Hospice and Palliative Nursing Practice
- Scope and Standards of Neuroscience Nursing Practice
- Scope and Standards of Nursing Informatics Practice
- Scope and Standards of Pediatric Nursing Practice
- Scope and Standards of Pediatric Oncology Nursing
- Scope and Standards of Practice for Nursing Professional Development
- Scope and Standards of Psychiatric-Mental Health Nursing Practice
- Scope and Standards of Public Health Nursing Practice
- Scope and Standards of Vascular Nursing Practice
- Standards of Addictions Nursing Practice with Selected Diagnoses and Criteria

*nursingworld.org/books/

Guidelines for the Registered Nurse in Giving, Accepting, or Rejecting a Work Assignment*

⊙ ○ ○ ○ ○ ○ ○ ○ ○ ○ ○

Registered Nurses, as licensed professionals, share the responsibility and accountability along with their employer to ensure that safe, quality nursing care is provided. The scope of professional nurses' accountability involves legal, ethical, and professional guidelines for assuring safe, quality patient care. Legal responsibility for the provisions, delegation and supervision of patient care is specified in the Nurse Practice Act 464.001, and the Administrative Rules Chapter 59S. The American Nurses Association (ANA) Code for Nurses with Interpretive Statements (1985) guides ethical conduct and decision making of professional nurses. The ANA Standards and Scope of Practice (1997) provides a systematic application of nursing process for patient care management across patient care settings. In addition, the ANA Restructuring Survival Kit (1996) suggests common strategies to assist the professional nurse facing assignment and delegation issues during reassignment and reorganization, temporary or permanent. Lastly, the employer requirements for safe, competent staffing are outlined in facility policies and guidelines.

Within ethical and legal parameters the nurse exercises informed judgment and uses individual competence and qualifications as criteria in seeking consultation, accepting responsibilities and delegating nursing activities to others. The nurse's decision regarding accepting or making work assignments is based on the legal, ethical and professional obligation to assume responsibility for nursing judgment and action.

The document offers strategies for problem solving as the staff nurse, nurse manager, chief nurse executive and administrator practice within the complex environment of the health care system.

Nursing Care Delivery

Only a Registered Nurse (RN) will assess, plan and evaluate a patient's or client's nursing care needs. No nurse shall be required or directed to delegate nursing activities to other personnel in a manner inconsistent with the Nurse Practice Act, the standards of the Joint Commission on Accreditation of Health Organizations, the ANA Standards of Practice or Hospital Policy. Consistent with the preceding sentence, the individual RN has the autonomy to delegate (or not delegate) those aspects of nursing care the nurse determines appropriate based on the patient assessment.

When a nurse is floated to a unit or area where the nurse receives an assignment that is considered unsafe to perform independently, the RN has the right and obligation to request and receive a modified assignment, which reflects the RN's level of competence.

The Florida Nurses Association (FNA), the Florida Organization of Nurse Executives (FONE), and the FNA Labor Employee Relations Commission (LERC) recognize that changes in the health care delivery system have occurred and will continue to occur, while emphasizing the common goal to provide safe quality patient care. The parties also recognize that RNs have a right and responsibility to participate in decisions affecting delivery of nursing care and related terms and conditions of employment. All parties have a mutual interest in developing systems, which will provide quality care on a cost efficient basis without jeopardizing patient outcomes. Thus, commitment to measuring the impact of staffing and assignments to patient outcomes is a shared commitment of all professional nurses irrespective of organizational structure.

Assignment Despite Objection (ADO)/Documentation of Practice Situation (DOPS)

Staff nurses today face often untenable assignments that need to be documented as such. Critical, clinical judgment should be utilized when evaluating the appropriateness of an assignment. Refusal to accept an assignment without appropriate discussion within the chain of command can be defined as insubordinate behavior. Each Registered Nurse should become familiar with organizational policies, procedures and documentation regarding refusal to accept an unsafe assignment. ANA has recently adopted a position statement and model ADO form available for use by SNA members. (Please contact Florida Nurses Association for further information.)

Staffng

In the event a Registered Nurse determines in his/her professional opinion that he/she has been given an assignment that does not allow for appropriate patient care, he/she shall notify the Supervisor or designee who shall review the concerns of the nurse. If the nurse's concerns cannot be resolved by telephone, the Supervisor or designee, except in instances of compelling business reasons that preclude him/her from doing so, will then come to the unit within four (4) hours of being contacted by the nurse to assess the staffing. Such assessment shall be documented with a copy given to the nurse. Nothing herein shall prohibit a Registered Nurse from completing and submitting a protest of assignment form.

Nurse Practice Act, 1994, Administrative Rules Chapt. 59S, 14.001 Definitions (4/29/96)

"Assignments" - are the normal daily functions of the UAPs based on institutional or agency job duties which do not involve delegation of nursing functions or nursing judgment.

"Competency" - is the demonstrated ability to carry out specified tasks or activities with reasonable skill and safety that adheres to the prevailing standard of practice in the nursing community.

"Delegation" - is the transference to a competent individual the authority to perform a selected nursing task or activity in a selected situation by a nurse qualified by licensure and experience to perform the task or activity.

"Supervision" - is the provision of guidance by a qualified nurse and periodic inspection by the nurse for the accomplishment of a nursing task or activity, provided the nurse is qualified and legally entitled to perform such task or activity. The supervisor may be the delegator or a person of equal or greater licensure to the delegator.

Scenario

■ Suppose you are asked to care for an unfamiliar patient population or to go to a unit for which you feel unqualified—what do you do?
■ Suppose you are approached by your supervisor and asked to work an additional shift. Your immediate response is that you don't want to work another shift—what do you do?

Such situations are familiar and emphasize the rights and responsibilities of the RN to make informed decisions. Yet all members of the health care team, from staff nurses to administrator, share a joint responsibility to ensure that quality patient care is provided. At times, though, difference in interpretation of legal or ethical principles may lead to conflict.

Guidelines for decision making are offered to assist RNs problem-solve work assignment issues. Applications of these guidelines are presented in the form of scenarios, examples of unsafe assignments experienced by RNs.

Guidelines for Decision Making

The complexity of the delivery of nursing care is such that only professional nurses with appropriate education and experience can provide nursing care. Upon employment with a health care facility, the nurse contracts or enters into an agreement with that facility to provide nursing services in a collaborative practice environment.

It is the Registered Nurse's Responsibility to:

■ provide competent nursing care to the patient
■ exercise informed judgment and use individual competence and qualifications as criteria in seeking consultation, accepting responsibilities and delegating nursing activities to others
■ clarify assignments, assess personal capabilities, jointly identify options for patient care assignments when he/she does not feel personally competent or adequately prepared to carry out a specific function
■ refuse an assignment that he/she does not feel prepared to assume after appropriate consultation with supervisor

It is Nursing Management's Responsibility to:

- ensure competent nursing care is provided to the patient
- evaluate the nurse's ability to provide specialized patient care
- organize resources to ensure that patients receive appropriate nursing care
- collaborate with the staff nurse to clarify assignments, assess personal capabilities, jointly identify options for patient care assignments when the nurse does not feel personally competent or adequately prepared to carry out a specific function
- take appropriate disciplinary action according to facility policies
- communicate in written policies to the staff the process to make assignment and reassignment decisions
- provide education to staff and supervisory personnel in the decision making process regarding patient care assignments and reassignments, including patient placement and allocation of resources
- plan and budget for staffing patterns based upon patient's requirements and priorities for care
- provide a clearly defined written mechanism for immediate internal review of proposed assignments, which includes the participation of the staff involved, to help avoid conflict

Issues Central to Potential Dilemmas Are:

- the right of the patient to receive safe professional nursing care at an acceptable level of quality
- the responsibility for an appropriate utilization and distribution of nursing care services when nursing becomes a scare resource
- the responsibility for providing a practice environment that assures adequate nursing resources for the facility, while meeting the current socioeconomic and political realities of shrinking health care dollars

Legal Issues

Behaviors and activities relevant to giving, accepting, or rejecting a work assignment that could lead to disciplinary action include:

- practicing or offering to practice beyond the scope permitted by law, or accepting and performing professional responsibilities

which the licensee knows or has reason to know that he or she is not competent to perform
- performing, without adequate supervision, professional services which the licensee is authorized to perform only under the supervision of a licensed professional, except in an emergency situation where a person's life or health is in danger
- abandoning or neglecting a patient or client who is in need of nursing care without making reasonable arrangements for the continuation of such care
- failure to exercise supervision over persons who are authorized to practice only under the supervision of the licensed professional

Of the above, the issue of abandonment or neglect has thus far proven the most legally devastating. Abandonment or neglect has been legally defined to include such actions as insufficient observation (frequency of contact), failure to assure competent intervention when the patient's condition changes (qualified physician not in attendance), and withdrawal of services without provision for qualified coverage. Since nurses at all levels most frequently act as agents of the employing facility, the facility shares the risk of liability with the nurse.

Application of Guidelines for Decision Making

Two clinical scenarios are presented for the RN to demonstrate appropriate decision making when faced with an unsafe assignment. Sometimes an example or two can help the RN objectively examine legal, ethical and professional issues prior to making a final decision. Additional resources are listed following the scenarios.

Scenario—A Question of Competence

An example of a potential dilemma is when an evening supervisor pulls a psychiatric nurse to the coronary care unit because of a lack of nursing staff. The CCU census has risen and there is not additional qualified staff available.

Suppose you are asked to care for an unfamiliar patient population or to go to a unit for which you feel unqualified—what do you do?

1. CLARIFY what it is you are being asked to do.
   - How many patients will you be expected to care for?

- Does the care of these patients require you to have specialty knowledge and skills in order to deliver safe nursing care?
- Will there be qualified and experienced RNs on the unit?
- What procedures and/or medications will you be expected to administer?
- What kind of orientation do you need to function safely in the unfamiliar setting?

2. ASSESS yourself. Do you have the knowledge and skill to meet the expectations that have been outlined for you? Have you had experience with similar patient populations? Have you been oriented to this unit or a similar unit? Would the perceived discrepancies between your abilities and the expectations lead to an unsafe patient care situation?

3. IDENTIFY OPTIONS and implications of your decision.
   a) If you perceive that you can provide safe patient care, you should accept the assignment. You would now be ethically and legally responsible for the nursing care of these patients.
   b) If you perceive there is a discrepancy between abilities and the expectations of the assignment, further dialogue with the nurse supervisor is needed before you reach a decision. At this point it may be appropriate to consult the next level of management, such as the house supervisor or the chief nurse executive.

In further dialogue, continue to assess whether you are qualified to accept either a portion or the whole of the requested assignment. Also point out options which might be mutually beneficial. For example, obviously it would be unsafe for you to administer chemotherapy without prior training. However, if someone else administered the chemotherapy, perhaps you could provide the remainder of the required nursing care for that patient. If you feel unqualified for the assignment in its entirety, the dilemma becomes more complex.

At this point the RN must be aware of the legal rights of the facility. Even though the RN may have legitimate concern for patient safety and one's own legal accountability in providing safe care, the facility has legal precedent to initiate disciplinary action, including termination, if you refuse to accept an assignment. Therefore, it is important to continue to explore options in a positive manner, recognizing that both the RN

and the facility have a responsibility for safe patient care.

4. POINT OF DECISION/IMPLICATIONS: If none of the options are acceptable, you are at your final decision point.
   a) Accept the assignment, documenting carefully your concern for patient safety and the process you used to inform the facility (manager) of your concerns. Keep a personal copy of this documentation and send a copy to the manager(s) involved. Once you have reached this decision it is unwise to discuss the situation or your feelings with other staff or patients. Now you are legally accountable for these patients. From this point, withdrawal from the agreed upon assignment may constitute abandonment.
   b) Refuse the assignment, being prepared for disciplinary action. Document your concern for patient safety and the process you used to inform the facility (manager) of your concerns. Keep a personal copy of this documentation and send a copy to the nurse executive. Courtesy suggests that you also send a copy to the manager(s) involved.
   c) Document the steps taken in making your decision. It may be necessary for you to use the facility's grievance procedure.

Scenario—A Question of an Additional Shift

An example of another potential dilemma is when a nurse who recognizes his/her fatigue and its potential for patient harm is required to work an additional shift.

Suppose you are approached by your supervisor and asked to work an additional shift. Your immediate response is that you don't want to work another shift—what do you do?

1. CLARIFY what it is you are expected to do.
   - For example, would the additional shift be with the same patients you are currently caring for, or would it involve a new patient assignment?
   - Is your reluctance to work another shift because of a new patient assignment you do not feel competent to accept? (If the answer is yes, then refer to the previous example, "A Question of Competence.")
   - Is your reluctance due to work fatigue, or do you have other plans?

- Is this a chronic request due to poor scheduling, inadequate staffing, or chronic absenteeism?
- Are you being asked to work because there is no relief nurse coming for your present patient assignment? Because your unit will be short of professional staff on the next shift? Because another unit will be short of professional staff on the next shift?
- How long are you being asked to work—the entire shift or a portion of the shift?

2. ASSESS yourself.
- Are you really tired, or do you just not feel like working? Is your fatigue level such that your care may be unsafe? Remember, you are legally responsible for the care of your current patient assignment if relief is not available.

3 IDENTIFY OPTIONS and implications of your decision.
a) If you perceive that you can provide safe patient care and are willing to work the additional shift, accept the assignment.
b) If you perceive that you can provide safe patient care but are unwilling to stay due to other plans or the chronic nature of the request, inform the manager of your reasons for not wishing to accept the assignment.
c) If you perceive that your fatigue will interfere with your ability to safely care for patients, indicate this fact to the manager.

If you do not accept the assignment and the manager continues to attempt to persuade you it may be appropriate to consult the next level of management, such as the house supervisor or the nurse executive.

In further dialogue, continue to weigh your reasons for refusal versus the facility's need for an RN. If you have a strong alternate commitment, such as no child care, or if you seriously feel your fatigue will interfere with safe patient care, restate your reasons for refusal.

At this point, it is important for you to be aware of the legal rights of the facility. Even though you may have legitimate concern for patient safety and your own legal accountability in providing safe care, or legitimate concern for the safety of your children or other commitments, the facility has legal precedent to initiate disciplinary action,

including termination, if you refuse to accept an assignment. Therefore, it is important to continue to explore options in a positive manner, recognizing both you and the facility have a responsibility for safe patient care.

4. POINT OF DECISION/IMPLICATIONS
a) Accept the assignment, documenting your professional concern for patient safety and the process you used to inform the facility (manager) of your concerns. Keep a personal copy of this documentation and send a copy to the nurse executive. Courtesy suggests that you also send a copy to the manager(s) involved. Once you have reached this decision it is unwise to discuss the situation of your feelings with other staff and/or patients.
b) Accept the assignment, documenting your professional concerns for the chronic nature of the request and possible long-term consequences in reducing the quality of care. Documentation should follow the procedures outlined in (a).
c) Accept the assignment, documenting your personal concerns regarding working conditions in which management decides the legitimacy of employee personal commitments. This documentation should go to your manager. You may wish to request a meeting with your manager to discuss the incident and your concerns regarding future requests.
d) Refuse the assignment, being prepared for disciplinary action. If your reasons for refusal were patient safety or an imperative personal commitment, document this carefully, including the process you used to inform the facility (nurse manager) of your concerns. Keep a personal copy of this documentation and send a copy to the chief nurse executive. Courtesy suggests that you also send a copy to the manager(s) involved.
e) Document the rationale for your decision. It may be necessary to use the facility's grievance procedure.

Summary

Two scenarios of how an RN may apply the guidelines for decision making in the actual work situation have been presented. Staffing dilemmas will always be present and mandate that active communication between staff nurses and all levels of nursing management be maintained to assure patient safety. The likelihood of a satisfactory solution will increase if there is prior consideration of the choices available. This consideration of available alternatives should include recognition that professional nurses are intelligent adults who should be involved in the decision making process. Professional nurses are accountable for nursing judgments and actions regardless of the personal consequences. Providing safe nursing care to the patient is the ultimate objective of the professional nurse and the health care facility.

The Florida Nurses Association Labor and Employment Relations Commission acknowledges:

- the Florida Organization of Nurse Executives for input and collaboration in this document and the development of the previous 1989 edition of this document.
- the **Florida Nurses Association Labor and Employment Relations Commission** for final preparation of the revised 1999 edition of this document.

Resources

To maintain current and accurate information on accountability of registered nurses for giving, accepting, or rejecting a work assignment, the following resources are suggested:

- **Health Care Facility:** Nurses are encouraged to seek consultation with their nurse manager/ executives to discuss the facility's missions and goals as well as policies and procedures.

- The **Florida Nurses Association,** the largest statewide organization for registered nurses, represents nursing in the governmental, policy making arena and maintains current information and publications relative to the nurse's practice environment. Contact FNA or check out our website http://www.floridanurse.org for the benefits and services of membership, as well as priorities and activities of the Association.
- The **American Nurses Association** serves as the national clearing-house of information and offers publications on contemporary issues, including standards of practice, nursing ethics, as well as legal and regulatory issues. Contact ANA for a complimentary copy of the Publications Catalogue.
- *ANA Survival Kit* (1996) available through the American Nurses Association.
- *ANA Basic Guide to Safe Delegation* available through the American Nurses Association.
- *ANA Code of Ethics for Nurses* (1998) available through the American Nurses Association.
- *ANA Standards and Scope of Practice* (1997) available through the American Nurses Association.
- Nurse Practice Act (Florida Statutes 464, January 1994) and Administrative Rules (59S).
- Board of Nursing. A complimentary copy of the Nurse Practice Act is available to each registered nurse upon request.

*Reproduced with permission of Florida Nurses Association, 1999, Orlando, Florida.

Index

○○○○○○○○○○

A

Abandonment
  legal issues in patient, 263
Abilities
  as delegation criterion, 121, 123
Acceptance letters
  job search, 225–226, 229f
Accident
  patient safety and, 147
Accountability
  in codes of ethics, 257–258
  principle of, 47
  in standards of practice, 28
Acknowledgment of others
  in effective communication,
    75, 75t
Acting
  health-care reform and, 151–152
  in values clarification, 42, 42b
Active listening
  in communication, 74, 74b
  in evaluative feedback, 84
Active resistance
  to change, 107, 107t
Addictions
  workplace, 185–186
Administrative law, 23, 24
Advance directives
  in ethical dilemmas, 50
  legal issues in, 32–33
Advancement
  career, 236
Adverse event
  patient safety and, 147
African-American registered nurses
  Mahoney as first, 246
Age
  distributive justice and, 45–46
Agencies
  quality and safety support from,
    148b, 148–150
Agency for Healthcare Research and
    Quality
  quality indicators of, 149
  Web site of, 148b
Aggressiveness
  assertiveness versus, 75
Aging
  of population and nursing workforce,
    145–146
Agreements
  collective bargaining, 98–99, 99b

Alarm
  in stress response, 198
Alcohol use
  as licensure violation, 36
  workplace, 185–186
Algorithms
  in quality improvement, 137
Allergy
  latex, 181–183, 182t
Alternative medicine
  health-care resources and, 144
Ambulatory care center
  organizational structure of, 63f
American Academy of Nursing, 251
American Hospital Association
  on nursing shortage, 145
  Patient's Bill of Rights of, 27
  unlicensed assistive personnel survey
    of, 119
American Nurses Association
  Code of Ethics for Nurses of, 47,
    188, 257
  on delegation, 116–117
    criteria for, 121
    definition of, 120–121
  on disabled nurses' rights, 189
  on disaster and terrorism readiness,
    189–190
  Do Not Resuscitate orders and, 32
  ergonomic guidelines of, 185
  on health-care crisis, 252–253
  health-care reform agenda of, 151–152
  history of, 248
  on mandatory overtime, 187
  overview of, 248–249
  position statements of, 249,
    250b–251b
  publications of, 259
  quality of care and, 139, 148b, 149
  on reporting questionable practices,
    188–189, 189b
  safety and, 149, 174–175
  on sexual harassment, 181
  on staffing ratios, 188
  standards of practice of, 27, 139, 259
  unlicensed assistive personnel and, 188
Americans With Disabilities Act
  disabled nurses' rights and, 189
  as statutory law, 22
Anxiety
  as barrier to effective communication,
    75–76
  in work-related stress, 198

Appearance
  in job interview, 232
  professional image and, 254
Appropriateness
  in delegation, 124
Artifact level
  in organizational culture, 59
Assault
  overview of, 26
  workplace, 177
Assertiveness
  aggressiveness versus, 75
Assessment
  in delegation, 118
  in ethical dilemmas, 49–50, 50b
  in SBAR communication model,
    80, 81t
  in work assignment guidelines,
    262–265
Assignment
  delegation of tasks and, 118–119,
    120f, 126
  despite objection, 262
  Nurse Practice Act definition of,
    262
  refusal of, 163
Assignment sheets
  in time management, 162
Assistants
  power sources of, 65
Assisted suicide
  as ethical issue, 52
Associate degree nursing education
  history of, 246–247
Assumptions
  in organizational culture, 59
Attitudes
  in effective leadership, 9
  in new job, 235–236
Authoritarian leadership style, 6, 6t
Authority
  as power source, 64
Autocratic leadership style, 6, 6t
Automation
  in time management, 166
Autonomy
  in codes of ethics, 257–258
  in empowerment, 65
  principle of, 44
Avoidance
  in response to conflict, 93b
Awareness
  in stress management, 207, 207b